Acceptance and Commitment Therapy for Insomnia

Renatha El Rafihi-Ferreira
Editor

Acceptance and Commitment Therapy for Insomnia

A Session-By-Session Guide

Springer

Editor
Renatha El Rafihi-Ferreira
Department of Clinical Psychology
Universidade de São Paulo
São Paulo, São Paulo, Brazil

ISBN 978-3-031-50709-0 ISBN 978-3-031-50710-6 (eBook)
https://doi.org/10.1007/978-3-031-50710-6

This Springer imprint is published by the registered company Springer Nature Switzerland AG
The registered company address is: Gewerbestrasse 11, 6330 Cham, Switzerland

Paper in this product is recyclable.

Foreword

Healthy sleep is an essential pillar of good mental and physical health. Chronic lack of sleep or disturbed sleep is associated with multiple adverse health outcomes including increased risks for depression, hypertension, and premature cognitive impairments. Sleep problems also produce major consequences on occupational health and increase both absenteeism and presenteeism at work, as well as increased risks of accidents on the road and at work.

In this 24/7 society with constant pressure to perform and produce, it is no surprise that insomnia is the most prevalent of all sleep disorders, affecting at least 10% of adults on a chronic basis and another 20–30% occasionally. These prevalence rates increased by at least twofold during the COVID-19 pandemic. Persistent insomnia affects all segments of the population, including children, teenagers, adults, and elderly people. It is especially prevalent among people with mental health problems, particularly among those with mood and anxiety disorders, in patients with medical problems such as chronic pain, and in individuals with atypical work schedules such as shift workers. Given its high prevalence and impact, there is a definite need for effective insomnia therapies.

The most widely used and readily accessible treatment for insomnia is medication. Many people do not even seek professional help for this problem, but instead go to their drug stores and buy all sorts of highly advertised over-the-counter products of unknown risks and benefits. When a patient sees a healthcare professional for insomnia, usually a family doctor, a sleeping pill is often the only recommendation made to the patient, either because of lack of time or lack of knowledge about other effective therapies for insomnia.

Cognitive behavioral therapy is now recognized by several professional and sleep organizations around the world as the first-line therapy for insomnia. When a patient has the great fortune to find a therapist with CBT-I expertise, this is like winning a lottery. Indeed, there is now solid evidence that CBT-I is not only effective for improving sleep, but it also produces clinically meaningful daytime benefits, and may even prevent depression in at-risk individuals. Of course, not all patients with chronic insomnia respond or remit with standard CBT-I, and there is a need for alternative, evidence-based, therapies.

Acceptance and Commitment Therapy for Insomnia: A Session-by-Session Guide, by Renatha El Rafihi-Ferreira and colleagues, provides a welcome addition to the insomnia treatment literature. ACT is part of the third-wave cognitive behavioral therapies which has proven effective for several psychological problems. In this book, Professor El Rafihi-Ferreira and her colleagues have very nicely crafted ACT for patients with insomnia disorder. The book is well organized with a step-by-step treatment protocol complemented by "real-world" case studies illustrating the effective use of ACT in clinical practice. It provides a clear description of the theoretical framework of ACT, along with its key concept of psychological flexibility and underlying processes of acceptance, cognitive "defusion", and mindfulness, to name a few. The book is also packed with clinically useful information about the assessment and differential diagnosis of insomnia and a description of the more standard behavioral and cognitive procedures for treating insomnia.

This treatment manual provides a novel approach that is likely to be a useful guide for any clinicians working with patients who suffer from chronic insomnia, either as the primary problem or comorbid with other mental or medical problems. ACT can be used as a stand-alone treatment or it can be combined with the more standard behavioral (stimulus control, sleep restriction, relaxation) and cognitive procedures (cognitive restructuring). *Acceptance and Commitment Therapy for Insomnia* is definitely a value-added, hands-on resource for any behavioral sleep medicine specialist and psychotherapist working with insomnia patients.

Charles M. Morin
Professor of Psychology and Canada Research
Chair in Behavioral Sleep Medicine
Université Laval,
Quebec City, QC, Canada

Preface

This book was written to prepare clinical psychologists for the growing demand for effective insomnia treatment options. Within this context, the book addresses the theoretical model of Acceptance and Commitment Therapy (ACT) for the treatment of insomnia.

Insomnia is associated with numerous harms, a fact that reinforces the need for evidence-based treatments, especially those that do not require the use of medications. Cognitive Behavioral Therapy for Insomnia (CBT-I) is the treatment of choice; however, there are patients who have difficulties in adhering to some therapeutic components (stimulus control and sleep restriction), while others are refractory to this modality. Another important aspect is the plurality of individuals and that not all of them identify with the same therapeutic approach; hence, more options other than CBT-I are needed.

Recently, the application of ACT to treat insomnia has shown effective results and may provide another approach to deal with the cognitive components involved in sleep difficulties. ACT represents a change in the insomnia paradigm that could improve the effectiveness of treatment because it does not focus exclusively on sleep problems and symptom control, but also on the patient as a whole in an attempt to enhance quality of life and psychological flexibility, reducing the severity of insomnia. ACT can be applied in conjunction with behavioral therapy components that are associated with better insomnia treatment outcomes, such as stimulus control and sleep restriction. This modality can also be applied as monotherapy in patients who are resistant to behavioral components such as stimulus control and bedtime restriction.

The primary goal of ACT is the development of psychological flexibility, which can be achieved through the processes of acceptance, cognitive defusion, being present, self as context, values, and committed action. This book on ACT is divided into five parts, each consisting of three to five chapters.

The first part "Sleep and Insomnia" is dedicated to the understanding of normal sleep, changes in sleep patterns throughout life, sleep architecture, sleep functions, consequences of sleep deprivation, and the definition and classification of the different subtypes of insomnia, all of them part of psychoeducation. This part also discusses comorbidities of insomnia, differential diagnoses, and hypnotic dependence and withdrawal. The part is divided into five chapters: (1) Chapter 2: Sleep and Its Functions; (2) Chapter 3: Effects of Sleep Deprivation; (3) Chapter 4: Insomnia; (4) Chapter 5: Insomnia: Its Comorbidities and Differential Diagnosis, and (5) Chapter 6: Hypnotic Dependence and Withdrawal.

The second part "Assessment of Insomnia" covers the assessment process of insomnia. In this part, the initial interview, the use of retrospective measures for patient assessment and the use of prospective measures for follow-up of the therapeutic process are discussed. The part is divided into three chapters: (1) Chapter 7: Initial Interview in the Therapeutic Setting; (2) Chapter 8: Evaluation and Retrospective Measurements, and (3) Chapter 9: The Role of Actigraphy and Sleep Diaries in Assessing Sleep in Adults with Insomnia.

The third part "Behavioral Treatment for Insomnia" deals with behavioral treatment options for insomnia and is divided into three chapters: (1) Chapter 10: Sleep Hygiene; (2) Chapter 11: Stimulus Control Therapy for Insomnia, and (3) Chapter 12: Sleep Restriction.

The fourth part "ACT for Insomnia" explains the theoretical model of ACT and the concept of psychological flexibility and its six processes (acceptance, cognitive defusion, mindfulness, self as context, values, and committed action) and provides a brief review of the evidence on ACT-based therapy for insomnia. A model of a flexible ACT protocol for insomnia (ACT-I) using resources such as metaphors, mindfulness exercises, and poetry is presented. The therapeutic processes of this ACT protocol for insomnia are also discussed. The chapters that make up this part are: (1) Chapter 13: Acceptance and Commitment Therapy; (2) Chapter 14: Evidence of Acceptance and Commitment Therapy-Based Therapies for Insomnia; (3) Chapter 15: A Session-by-Session Guide for Acceptance and Commitment Therapy for Insomnia, and (4) Chapter 16: ACT Therapeutic Processes in the ACT-I Protocol.

The fifth and last part of this book "Application of ACT-I and ACT-BBI-I" is dedicated to examples of clinical cases in which the ACT protocol for insomnia was applied in different modalities: group format, individual format, and use of behavioral components for insomnia management. This part is divided into three chapters: (1) Chapter 17: Case Example: Application of ACT-I in a Group Intervention; (2) Chapter 18: Case Example: Application of ACT-I in an Individual Intervention, and (3) Chapter 19: Case Example: Application of ACT-BBI-I in an Individual Intervention.

São Paulo, Brazil Renatha El Rafihi-Ferreira

Contents

About the Authors

Daniel Guilherme Suzuki Borges Daniel G. Suzuki Borges is attending physician at Sleep Group at Hospital of Clinics – University of Sao Paulo. Residency: Psychiatry University of Sao Paulo – USP (2015), Sleep Medicine: University of Sao Paulo – USP (2016). MD University of Sao Paulo – USP (2011). Certifications: Board Certification: Psychiatry, Brazilian Medical Association (2016), Sleep Medicine, Brazilian Medical Association (2017).

Bárbara Araújo Conway Psychologist with expertise in Sleep Psychology. Master's student in the Graduate Program in Psychiatry at the Faculty of Medicine of the University of São Paulo (FMUSP), with a scholarship from the State of São Paulo Research Foundation (FAPESP). Volunteer psychologist at the Sleep Outpatient Clinic of the Institute of Psychiatry (ASONO) and the Sleep Outpatient Clinic of the Division of Neurological Clinic, both at Hospital das Clínicas da FMUSP (HCFMUSP).

Silvia Gonçalves Conway Clinical psychologist by Universidade de São Paulo (USP). Specialist in non-pharmacological intervention for Post-Traumatic Stress Disorder and sleep disturbs. Certified in Sleep Psychology by Associação Brasileira do Sono (ABS) and Sociedade Brasileira de Psicologia. Master in Science by Universidade Federal de São Paulo (UNIFESP). Member of the Sleep Department and coordinator of Sleep Psychology course at Instituto de Psiquiatria da USP. Founding partner of AkasA – Formação & Conhecimento. Meditation practitioner and student since 2002. Pathwork® facilitator. USP – University of São Paulo. Associação Brasileira do Sono – Brazilian Sleep Association. Sociedade Brasileira de Psicologia – Brazilian Psychological Society. Universidade Federal de São Paulo – Federal University of São Paulo. Instituto de Psiquiatria da USP – Psychiatry Institute of Clinical Hospital from University of São Paulo.

Israel Soares Pompeu de Sousa Brasil Title of specialist in Neurology and Sleep Medicine by the Brazilian Academy of Neurology/Brazilian Medical Association (ABN/AMB). Attending physician of the Neurology Residency Program at Instituto de Assistência Médica do Servidor Público Estadual de São Paulo (IAMSPE), São Paulo-São Paulo, Brasil. Collaborating physician from the sleep clinic at Instituto de Psiquiatria do Hospital das Clínicas da Faculdade de Medicina da Universidade de São Paulo (IPq-HCFMUSP).

Marwin do Carmo Ph.D. student in Psychology at the University of California, Davis. MSc. in Psychiatry at University of São Paulo (USP) – São Paulo, Brazil. Bachelor in Psychology at Universidade do Estado do Rio de Janeiro (UERJ) – Rio de Janeiro, Brazil. mmcarmo@ucdavis.edu.

Renatha El Rafihi-Ferreira Professor at the Department of Clinical Psychology at the Institute of Psychology at the University of São Paulo. Advisor at the Graduate Program in Clinical Psychology at the University of São Paulo. Support from the FAPESP Young Researcher Program (2018/19506-5) to conduct research on behavioral therapy for insomnia. Psychologist. Master in Behavior Analysis from the State University of Londrina (UEL). PhD and Post-Doctorate in Clinical Psychology from the University of São Paulo (USP). Certified in Sleep Psychology by the Brazilian Association of Sleep and the Brazilian Society of Psychology. rerafihi@usp.br.

Rosa Hasan MD, Neurologist and specialist in Sleep Medicine. Director of the Sleep Laboratory and Sleep Outpatient Clinic at the Psychiatry Institute of the Hospital das Clínicas of the Medical School of the University of São Paulo.

Roberta Kovac PhD in Clinical Psychology (USP) and Master in Experimental Psychology: Behavior Analysis (PUC-SP). Academic Director, professor and advisor at Instituto Par Educação (former Centro Paradigma de Ciências do Behavior). Coordinator of the research laboratory RFTAC (Theory of Relational Frames applied to the clinic) also at Instituto Par. Member of the Brazilian Association of Behavioral Sciences (ABPMC) and the Association for Contextual Behavioral Sciences (ACBS). Past President of the ACBS Chapter – Brazil. He works mainly in the clinical area, in contextual behavioral therapies and in teaching, training therapists and researchers. Author of several articles and book chapters related to Behavior Analysis and Contextual Behavioral Sciences.

Ila Marques Porto Linares Graduation in Psychology (UFSCar), Master in Neurology (USP), PhD in Mental Health (USP), Pos Doctoral in progress (USP), Specialization in Clinical Behavioural Analysis (Núcleo Paradigma), Certified in Sleep Psychology by the Brazilian Sleep Association and the Brazilian Society of Psychology. Volunteer psychologist at the sleep outpatient clinic at Instituto da Criança, Hospital das Clínicas, Faculty of Medicine, University of São Paulo (HC-FMUSP).

Léo Paulos-Guarnieri PhD student in Psychiatry at the Faculty of Medicine of the University of São Paulo (USP) – São Paulo, Brazil, with research support from the São Paulo State Research Support Foundation (FAPESP) [grant #2023/06859-5]. Bachelor in Psychology at the Pontifical Catholic University of São Paulo (PUC-SP) – São Paulo, Brazil.

Maria Laura Nogueira Pires Psychologist, Master in Psychobiology and PhD in Sciences from the Departament of Psychobiology at Universidade Federal de São Paulo-Unifesp. FAPESP funding post-doctoral fellowship at the Sleep and Mood Disorders Laboratory at Oregon Health & Science University (OHSU, USA). Board certified in sleep psychology by the Brazilian Sleep Association-ABS and Brazilian Society of Psychology-SBP. Former professor of psychology at public university (Universidade Estadual Paulista-Unesp), now work in private sector with sleep psychology and actigraphy (LP Actigrafia & Sono). laurapires@actigrafia.org

Michaele Terena Saban-Bernauer Master in Experimental Psychology and specialist in Behavior Analysis, professor and coordinator of the ACT course at Hospital das Clínicas, Faculty of Medicine, University of São Paulo. Author of the book "Introduction to Acceptance and Commitment Therapy", and co-author of the book "Third Generation Behavioral Therapies", "The Treatment of Chemical Dependence and Cognitive Behavioral Therapies", among others of the ACT Brazilian literature. Founding President of the Brazilian Association for Contextual Behavioral Science – ACBS Brasil, and was part of the founding board of the ACBS Foundation.

Ksdy Maiara Moura Sousa Psychologist, specialists in Neuropsychology from the Neurological Institute of São Paulo. Master and PhD in Sciences with an emphasis on Medicine and Sleep Biology by the Department of Psychobiology at the Universidade Federal de São Paulo. Pedagogical coordinator of the neuropsychology course at Nepsi MG, Sleep Psychologist certified by the Associação Brasileira do Sono, researcher at the Universidade Federal de São Paulo.

Andrea Cecilia Toscanini Graduated in Biomedicine and Medicine, area of expertise "Sleep Medicine". PhD concluded in 2005 Medical School of University of São Paulo (FMUSP), researcher since then in basic and clinical area. At the moment, works as a physician at the sleep clinic at the Institute of Psychiatry at the Hospital das Clínicas at FMUSP. andrea.toscanini@uol.com.br

Chapter 1
Introduction

Renatha El Rafihi-Ferreira

1.1 Why to Use Acceptance and Commitment Therapy for Insomnia?

Chronic insomnia is associated with clinical and psychiatric health problems and is a burden on the healthcare system (Hargens et al., 2013; Hertenstein et al., 2019; Laugsand et al., 2011). CBT-I is recognized as the treatment of choice for insomnia, with several studies supporting its effectiveness (Riemann & Espie, 2018; Van Straten et al., 2018). CBT-I is a directive and structured treatment that consists of behavioral and cognitive techniques (Morin et al., 2006). The behavioral strategies, which include sleep hygiene, stimulus control, sleep restriction, and relaxation, focus on behaviors and habits that contribute to good sleep quality. The cognitive therapeutic strategy is cognitive restructuring, which involves refuting and restructuring dysfunctional beliefs about sleep (Harvey et al., 2014).

Although studies have reported positive results, CBT-I does not lead to remission of insomnia disorder in 20–25% of patients with insomnia without comorbidities (Morin et al., 2006) and in approximately 60% of patients with psychiatric or medical comorbidities (Wu et al., 2015). Furthermore, adherence to stimulus control and sleep restriction techniques is difficult for many individuals (Harvey & Tang, 2003).

Considering that some individuals do not respond to traditional CBT-I approaches and that adherence remains difficult for many individuals, a modified treatment may be useful to enhance the effects of existing insomnia treatments and to improve outcomes in a larger number of individuals. In addition, the effect sizes of CBT for insomnia are less representative than for other psychological complaints (Harvey & Tang, 2003). The combination of these factors justifies the need for new therapeutic modalities for insomnia.

R. El Rafihi-Ferreira (✉)
Department of Clinical Psychology, University of São Paulo, São Paulo, Brazil
e-mail: rerafihi@usp.br

R. El Rafihi-Ferreira (ed.), *Acceptance and Commitment Therapy for Insomnia*,
https://doi.org/10.1007/978-3-031-50710-6_1

The need for new therapeutic modalities is supported by the following factors: (a) pre-sleep cognition is associated with insomnia and arousal; (b) thought suppression strategies increase the levels of pre-sleep cognitive activity and arousal, and (c) CBT-I primarily uses thought control strategies for the management of pre-sleep cognitive activity. It is, therefore, plausible to argue that the reduced effect sizes associated with CBT-I may be in part due to the use of thought control strategies. Thus, interventions that do not focus on control, such as those using acceptance and mindfulness, may be able to effectively address pre-sleep cognition and related arousal (Espie et al., 2006).

Within this context, over the last decades, third-wave behavioral therapies have proposed a different approach to private events (thoughts and feelings). Unlike cognitive therapy, which involves refuting beliefs and thought content, contextual therapies focus on context and are more concerned with the function of a behavior rather than modifying its content. Third-wave therapies include ACT, functional analytic psychotherapy (FAP), dialectical behavior therapy (DBT), and mindfulness-based therapies. Taylor et al. (2015) evaluated the effect of third-wave therapies for insomnia and concluded that these therapies demonstrate efficacy and effectiveness in treating insomnia, particularly mindfulness-based therapies. In the book *Mindfulness-Based Therapy for Insomnia* Ong (2016) introduces mental health practitioners to an evidence-based treatment: mindfulness-based therapy for insomnia (MBTI). Although third-wave therapies show some similarities, their theoretical basis is different. This book focuses on ACT.

1.2 Acceptance and Commitment Therapy for Insomnia

ACT is a behavioral therapy based on functional contextualism, a philosophy that seeks to predict behavior accurately and thoroughly, and on the relational frame theory (RFT), an accurate and empirically sound post-Skinnerian assumption of language and cognition (Barbosa & Murta, 2014). The central goal of ACT is the development/enhancement of behavioral and psychological flexibility, that is, the ability to contact the present moment more fully as a conscious human being and, based on what the situation offers, to change or persist in behavior in order to serve valued ends (Hayes et al., 2003). This therapeutic modality involves the clarification of personal values and value-based action planning. As such, ACT links processes of acceptance and mindfulness to processes of commitment and behavior change (Hayes & Strosahl, 2004). Psychological flexibility is established through six core ACT processes: acceptance, cognitive defusion, being present, self as context, values, and committed action (Luoma et al., 2007).

The six ACT processes are overlapping and interrelated, and their aim is to develop psychological flexibility. The core principles of ACT can be applied to different problems and can be useful for treating insomnia, as many people with insomnia have difficulty controlling their sleep problems since they struggle to fall asleep (Dalrymple et al., 2010).

Regarding control strategies for insomnia, Espie et al. (2006) point out that the process of falling asleep is relatively automatic and can be inhibited by focused attention and repeated attempts to fall asleep. The intense effort of trying to fall asleep, as well as trying to control the insomnia, actually exacerbates and further worsens sleep difficulties. According to Hayes et al. (2006), many strategies that focus directly on solving the problems end up becoming the problem, that is, by trying to control the symptoms, they become even more central, salient, and influential.

According to Lundh (2005), the process of acceptance proposed by ACT can reduce the effort to fall asleep, increasing acceptance of physiological and mental arousal, in addition to the commitment proposed by this modality that includes the planning of value-based actions. Espie et al. (2006) highlight that insomniacs often place an exacerbated value on sleep problems and eventually leave aside other aspects of their lives.

Considering this paradigm, a treatment that goes beyond the sleep complaint may be an effective strategy (Hertenstein et al., 2014) since the focus shifts from symptom control to acceptance of the feelings and thoughts associated with it through value-based actions. ACT is thus an appropriate intervention for the treatment of insomnia since it does not focus on a single symptom but on improving overall quality of life (Hayes et al., 2012).

Within the context of insomnia, the clinician simultaneously addresses the processes of acceptance, defusion, being present, and self as context through the use of metaphors for mindfulness and meditation, in which the patient is invited to observe his/her relationship with sleep (e.g., the fear of not being able to sleep, daytime tiredness, thoughts like "my day will be ruined if I don't sleep tonight," "what will happen if I can't sleep") without judgment in order to promote a posture of impartial observer in relation to these experiences without changing their content. In parallel, the patients' values are explored in different domains (professional, personal, and family, among others) and compared with their current choices in order to plan actions based on values and not on avoidance of experiences. For example, by questioning their values, patients may discover that they are devoting little time to the personal domain in order to avoid experiences of frustration and thereby increase their workflow, which may compromise their quality of sleep and quality of life. In an attempt to avoid pain, the individual often makes choices based on avoidance rather than values. ACT applied to insomnia does not focus exclusively on the sleep complaint but rather on the patient as a whole person and on the different domains that encompass his/her experiences.

Studies using the ACT conceptual model for insomnia have reported favorable results. A recent systematic review (Paulos-Guarnieri et al., 2022) on the level of evidence and characteristics of interventions using ACT for insomnia indicated beneficial effects on sleep and insomnia symptoms. ACT can be applied as monotherapy (ACT-I) or in combination with the behavioral components of stimulus control and sleep restriction (ACT-BBI-I). According to the authors of the review, ACT-BBI-I can improve adherence to stimulus control and sleep restriction techniques (Paulos-Guarnieri et al., 2022). In a randomized controlled trial, El Rafihi-Ferreira et al. (2021) reported that ACT-BBI-I was as effective as CBT-I in treating patients with chronic insomnia. In addition, the use of ACT-BBI-I increased sleep efficiency and reduced sleep onset latency, nocturnal awakenings, and insomnia symptoms. This modality also improved anxiety and psychological flexibility and reduced sleep-related dysfunctional beliefs.

Studies investigating ACT as monotherapy for the treatment of insomnia are still incipient. Recently, El Rafihi-Ferreira et al. (2022) compared the efficacy of ACT as monotherapy and CBT-I for the treatment of insomnia. The results showed that both treatment modalities significantly reduced the severity of insomnia. The proportion of treatment responders was higher in the CBT-I group than in the ACT-I group (64.7% versus 50.0%, respectively). Six months later, additional improvements were observed in the ACT-I group, while there was a reduction in the treatment response in the CBT-I group (58.8% versus 55.6%, respectively). The results suggest a better short-term response for CBT-I, while the response to ACT-I is slower but more sustained, with better long-term results. Since this was the first study comparing CBT-I versus ACT as monotherapy for insomnia, the results have important clinical implications. Because many individuals have difficulty adhering to stimulus control and sleep restriction, ACT-I may be a viable option for people resistant to CBT-I.

Preliminary data from an ongoing randomized clinical trial (El Rafihi-Ferreira et al.) have demonstrated favorable outcomes of ACT for insomnia, with a significant reduction in insomnia severity and a parallel decrease in the scores assessing depression, beliefs about sleep, and non-acceptance of sleep problems.

ACT represents a shift in the insomnia paradigm that can improve therapeutic effectiveness because it does not focus exclusively on sleep problems and symptom control, but also on the patient as a whole in an attempt to enhance quality of life and psychological flexibility, reducing the severity of insomnia. ACT for insomnia has beneficial effects on sleep and insomnia symptoms and can be applied in different formats and with different intervention components. The use of ACT for insomnia can be divided into two categories: ACT-I (i.e., ACT as monotherapy for insomnia) and ACT-BBI-I (i.e., ACT plus behavioral components of stimulus control and sleep restriction).

Although the empirical support for ACT-based interventions in treating insomnia is not the same as that for established treatments (i.e., CBT-I), the former can serve as an alternative treatment for insomnia and contribute to the building of a process-based approach.

References

Barbosa, L. M., & Murta, S. G. (2014). Terapia de aceitação e compromisso: história, fundamentos, modelo e evidências. *Revista Brasileira de Terapia Comportamental e Cognitiva, 16*(3), 34–49. https://www.rbtc.org.br/detalhe_artigo.asp?id=209

Dalrymple, K. L., Fiorentino, L., Politi, M. C., & Posner, D. (2010). Incorporating principles from acceptance and commitment therapy into cognitive-behavioral therapy for Insomnia: A case example. *Journal of Contemporary Psychotherapy, 40*, 209–217. https://contextualscience.org/files/Dalrymple%20et%20al%20ACT%20for%20insomnia.pdf

El Rafihi-Ferreira, R., Morin, C. M., Toscanini, A. C., Lotufo Neto, F., Brasil, I. S., Gallinaro, J. G., Borges, D. S., Conway, S. G., & Hasan, R. (2021). Acceptance and commitment therapy-based behavioral intervention for insomnia: A pilot randomized controlled trial. *Brazilian Journal of Psychiatry, 43*(5), 1–6. https://doi.org/10.1590/1516-4446-2020-0947

El Rafihi-Ferreira, R., Morin, C. M., Hasan, R., Brasil, I. S., Ribeiro Júnior, J. H. Z., & Toscanini, A. C. (2022). A pilot randomized controlled trial (RCT) of acceptance and commitment therapy versus cognitive behavioral therapy for chronic insomnia. *Behavioral Sleep Medicine, 2022*, 193. https://doi.org/10.1080/15402002.2022.2071272

El Rafihi-Ferreira, R. et al. (on-going). Acceptance and Commitment Therapy for Insomnia (ACTI). ClinicalTrials.gov Identifier: NCT04866914.

Espie, C. A., Broomfield, N. M., MacMahon, K., Macphee, L. M., & Taylor, L. M. (2006). The attention-intention-effort pathway in the development of psychophysiologic insomnia: A theoretical review. *Sleep Medicine Reviews, 10*(4), 215–245. https://doi.org/10.1016/j.smrv.2006.03.002

Hargens, T. A., Kaleth, A. S., Edwards, E. S., & Butner, K. L. (2013). Association between sleep disorders, obesity, and exercise: A review. *Nature and Science of Sleep, 5*, 27–35. https://doi.org/10.2147/NSS.S34838

Harvey, A. G., & Tang, N. K. Y. (2003). Cognitive behaviour therapy for primary insomnia: Can we rest yet? *Sleep Medicine Reviews, 7*(3), 237–262. https://doi.org/10.1053/smrv.2002.0266

Harvey, A. G., Bélanger, L., Talbot, L., Eidelman, P., Beaulieu-Bonneau, S., Fortier-Brochu, É., Ivers, H., Lamy, M., Hein, K., Soehner, A. M., Mérette, C., & Morin, C. M. (2014). Comparative efficacy of behavior therapy, cognitive therapy, and cognitive behavior therapy for chronic insomnia: A randomized controlled trial. *Journal of Consulting and Clinical Psychology, 82*(4), 670–683. https://doi.org/10.1037/a0036606

Hayes, S. C., & Strosahl, K. D. (Eds.). (2004). *A practical guide to acceptance and commitment therapy*. Springer.

Hayes, S. C., Strosahl, K. D., & Wilson, K. G. (2003). *Acceptance and commitment therapy: An experimental approach to behavior change*. The Guilford Press.

Hayes, S. C., Luoma, J. B., Bond, F. W., Masuda, A., & Lillis, J. (2006). Acceptance and commitment therapy: Model, processes and outcomes. *Behavior Research and Therapy, 44*(1), 1–25. https://doi.org/10.1016/j.brat.2005.06.006

Hayes, S. C., Strosahl, K. D., & Wilson, K. G. (2012). *Acceptance and commitment therapy: The process and practice of mindful change* (2nd ed.). Guilford.

Hertenstein, E., Thiel, N., Luking, M., Kulz, A. K., Scharamm, E., Baglioni, C., Spiegelhalder, K., Riemann, D., & Nissen, C. (2014). Quality of life improvements after acceptance and commitment therapy in nonresponders to cognitive behavioral therapy for primary insomnia. *Psychotherapy and Psychosomatics, 83*(6), 371–373.

Hertenstein, E., Feige, B., Gmeiner, T., Kienzler, C., Spiegelhalder, K., Johann, A., Jansson-Fröjmark, M., Palagini, L., Rücker, G., Riemann, D., & Baglioni, C. (2019). Insomnia as a predictor of mental disorders: A systematic review and meta-analysis. *Sleep Medicine Reviews, 43*, 96–105. https://doi.org/10.1016/j.smrv.2018.10.006

Laugsand, L. E., Vatten, L. J., Platou, C., & Janszky, I. (2011). Insomnia and the risk of acute myocardial infarction: A population study. *Circulation, 124*(19), 2073–2081. https://doi.org/10.1161/CIRCULATIONAHA.111.025858

Lundh, L. G. (2005). The role of acceptance and mindfulness in the treatment of insomnia. *Journal of Cognitive Psychotherapy: An International Quarterly, 19*(1), 29–39. https://contextualscience.org/system/files/Lundh,2005.pdf

Luoma, J. B., Hayes, S. C., & Walser, R. D. (2007). *Learning ACT: An acceptance and commitment therapy skills-training manual for therapists*. New Harbinger Publications.

Morin, C. M., Bootzin, R. R., Buysse, D. J., Edinger, J. D., Espie, C. A., & Lichstein, K. L. (2006). Psychological and behavioral treatment of insomnia: Update of the recent evidence (1998-2004). *Sleep, 29*(11), 1398–1414. https://doi.org/10.1093/sleep/29.11.1398

Ong, J. C. (2016). *Mindfulness-based therapy for insomnia* (1st ed.). American Psychological Association.

Paulos-Guarnieri, L., Linares, I. P. M., & El Rafihi-Ferreira, R. (2022). Evidence and characteristics of Acceptance and Commitment Therapy (ACT)-based interventions for insomnia: A systematic review of randomized and non-randomized trials. *Journal of Contextual Behavioral Science, 23*(1), 1–14. https://doi.org/10.1016/j.jcbs.2021.11.001

Riemann, D., & Espie, C. (2018). Evidence-based psychological therapies for insomnia. *The Lancet, 392*(10149), 735. https://doi.org/10.1016/S0140-6736(18)31819-1

Taylor, H. L., Hailes, H. P., & Ong, J. (2015). Third-wave therapies for insomnia. *Current Sleep Medicine Reports, 1*, 166–176. https://doi.org/10.1007/s40675-015-0020-1

Van Straten, A., van der Zweerde, T., Kleiboer, A., Cuijpers, P., Morin, C. M., & Lancee, J. (2018). Cognitive and behavioral therapies in the treatment of insomnia: A meta-analysis. In A. van Straten (Ed.), *Sleep medicine reviews* (Vol. 38, pp. 3–16). W.B. Saunders Ltd.. https://doi.org/10.1016/j.smrv.2017.02.001

Wu, J. Q., Appleman, E. R., Salazar, R. D., & Ong, J. C. (2015). Cognitive behavioral therapy for Insomnia comorbid with psychiatric and medical conditions: A meta-analysis. *JAMA Internal Medicine, 175*(9), 1461–1472. https://doi.org/10.1001/jamainternmed.2015.3006

Part I
Sleep and Insomnia

Chapter 2
Sleep and Its Functions

Andrea Cecilia Toscanini and Rosa Hasan

The classic definition of sleep is generally based on physiological characteristics observed in mammals, including decrease in muscle activity, reduced response to external stimuli, closed eyes, lower respiratory rates, typical body position and characteristic brain wave architecture evaluated by polysomnography (Zielinski et al., 2016) (see Table 2.1).

REM and NREM Sleep

Normal human sleep comprises two states: REM (Rapid Eye Movement) and NREM (Non-Rapid Eye Movement) that cyclically alternate during a period of sleep (Fig. 2.1), with the larger proportion of REM sleep occurring in the second half of this period.

Sleep alterations are common as an individual ages, considering that sleep is a dynamic state (Ohayon et al., 2004). Therefore, newborns have approximately 50% REM sleep that reduces to 20–25% at 2 years old, maintaining this percentage throughout adulthood, and possibly reducing again after age 60 (Lenehan et al., 2023). Conversely, the opposite occurs with NREM sleep slow waves which are not present at birth but appear during the first 2 years of life. These slow waves reduce

---

Sleep is the intermediate state between wakefulness and death;
wakefulness being regarded as the active state
of all the animal and intellectual functions,
and death as that of their total suspension (Macnish, R. (1830). *The Philosophy of Sleep*. W. R. McPhun.).

A. C. Toscanini (✉)
Institute of Psychiatry, School of Medicine, University of São Paulo, Sao Paulo, Brazil
e-mail: a.toscanini@hc.fm.usp.br; andrea.toscanini@uol.com.br

R. Hasan
Institute of Psychiatry, School of Medicine, Hospital das Clínicas, FMUSP, Sao Paulo, Brazil
e-mail: r.hasan@hc.fm.usp.br

R. El Rafihi-Ferreira (ed.), *Acceptance and Commitment Therapy for Insomnia*,
https://doi.org/10.1007/978-3-031-50710-6_2

Table 2.1 Physiological characteristics of wakefulness, NREM and REM

Wakefulness	NREM	REM
Fine motor activity	Decrease in motor activity	Muscle atony
Open eyes	Closed eyes	Closed eyes (movement)
Response to environmental stimuli	Reduced response to environmental stimuli	Reduced response to environmental stimuli
Varied body positon	Typical body position	Typical body position
Varied respiratory rates	Regular respiratory rate	Varied respiratory rates

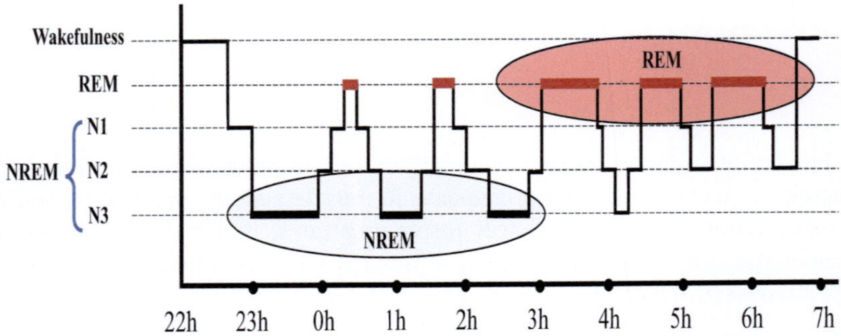

Fig. 2.1 Schematic progression of sleep stages across a single night

by around 40% during adolescence compared to previous years and continue to reduce until old age, curiously, more so in men than in women.

Besides age and sex, other factors alter sleep in a predictable way, such as premorbid sleep history, circadian rhythm, chronotype, temperature, environmental conditions, medications, and other substances potentially being used, clinical or psychiatric disorders, and other sleep disorders.

Sleep–Wakefulness Cycle Regulation

The two-process sleep–wakefulness cycle regulation, proposed tree decades ago, postulate that are two different mechanisms: homeostatic and circadian acting in opposition and synchronization throughout the 24-hour cycle (Borbély et al., 2016) (Fig. 2.2).

The "S" process is expressed as sleep drive that exponentially increases during wakefulness and abruptly decreases during sleep. During the increase in the "S" process, there is an accumulation of sleep-promoting substances in the central nervous system, such as adenosine, which would be eliminated during sleep. The "C" or circadian process, on the other hand, involves 24-hour biological rhythms, self-sustaining and synchronized with environmental cues (zeitgerbers) such as the light-dark cycle, meals, physical activity, and social commitments. This process is controlled by the circadian timing system located in the suprachiasmatic nucleus (Achermann and Borbély, 2017).

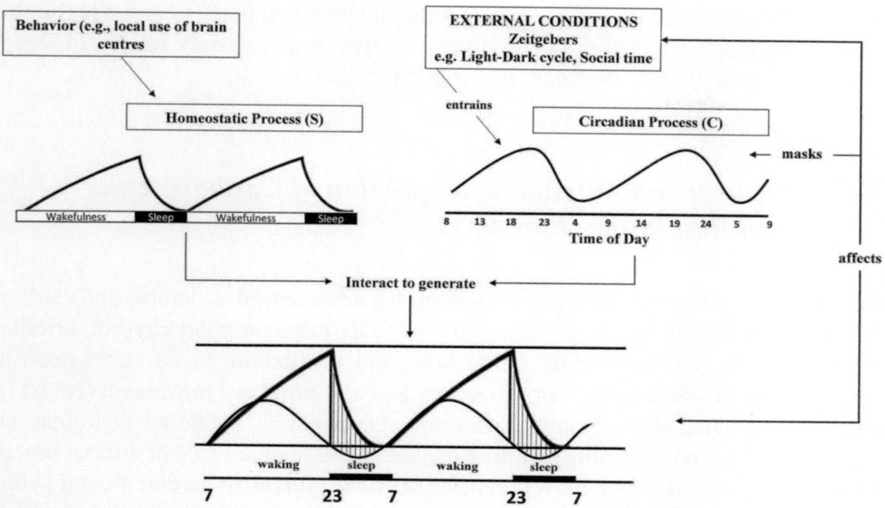

Fig. 2.2 The two-process sleep–wakefulness cycle regulation model. (Modified from Borbély (1982) and from Daan et al. (1984))

Legend for Fig. 2.2: Sleep propensity, reflected by the homeostatic process S, builds up during wakefulness and declines during sleep. The two thresholds (T1 and T2) delimiting S are modulated by a circadian process (C). A circadian pacemaker entrained by external Zeitgebers generates or synchronizes various physiological circadian oscillations. The masking effect in this context is considered as the overruling by external factors of the expression of the endogenous rhythm. Behavior or more specifically the local use of brain centers as induced, for example, by a learning task might have an impact on the local sleep homeostatic drive (e.g., Huber et al., 2004). External circumstances also affect the final output of these two processes to define our specific sleep–wake behavior (Schmidt et al., 2007).

2.1 Sleep Functions

Humans spend roughly one-third of their lives sleeping, and other animals sleep even more (Cirelli and Tononi, 2008). Despite how much time is spent in this offline state, why we sleep remains a mystery. There are various candidate answers related to the immune system, hormonal systems, thermoregulatory systems, and basic metabolic processes, as sleep is essential for all these bodily functions. Although the entire body benefits from sleep (Knutson et al., 2007), the most immediate, detrimental, and unavoidable consequences of sleep loss impact the brain and the various cognitive functions it supports (Zamore and Veasey, 2022). This insight has led some researchers to conclude that "sleep is of the brain, by the brain, and for the brain."

Far from the arduous task of dealing with all sleep functions, here we highlight some important ones in the social context we live in and closely related to sleep disorders that are highly prevalent in our population.

2.1.1 Central and Autonomic Regulation of Cardiovascular and Respiratory Functions

Because of the close neurohumoral coupling between central structures and cardiorespiratory function, a special coordination exists between heart rhythm, arterial blood pressure, coronary artery blood flow, and ventilation. Sleep states exert a major impact on cardiorespiratory function, and non-rapid eye movement (NREM) sleep is associated with relative autonomic stability and functional coordination between respiration, pumping action of the heart, and maintenance of arterial blood pressure. During rapid eye movement (REM) sleep, surges in cardiac-bound sympathetic and parasympathetic nerve activity provoke accelerations and pauses in heart rhythm, respectively (Harper et al., 2012).

In general, the autonomic stability of NREM sleep, with hypotension, bradycardia, and reduced cardiac output and systemic vascular resistance, provides a relatively salutary neurohumoral background during which the heart has an opportunity for metabolic restoration. REM sleep can disrupt cardiorespiratory homeostasis, due to its characteristics explained above. Furthermore, accessory and upper airway muscles diminish activity (REM atonia) while neurons serving the principal diaphragmatic respiratory muscles are spared the generalized inhibition. Cardiac efferent vagus nerve tone generally is suppressed during REM sleep, and the highly irregular breathing patterns can lead to lower oxygen levels (Mancia, 1993).

An important consideration in preserving circulatory homeostasis during sleep is coordination of control over two systems: the respiratory system, essential for oxygen exchange, and the cardiovascular system, for blood transport. The coordination of two motor systems, one for somatic musculature and the other for autonomic regulation is a unique task during sleep.

2.1.1.1 Immune System Regulation and Maintenance

Over the last 15 years, research following a system approach of neuroimmunology has accumulated surprisingly strong evidence that sleep enhances immune defense, in agreement with the popular wisdom that "sleep helps healing."

Life is organized in rhythms. A multi-oscillatory system with cellular clocks in many, if not all cells of the organism which are synchronized by a hypothalamic pacemaker, the suprachiasmatic nuclei, regulates the circadian (~24 h) rhythm of body functions and behavior. The sleep–wake cycle can be regarded as the most prominent manifestation of the circadian rhythm.

The nocturnal sleep period in humans is characterized by a profound downregulation of the two stress systems, the hypothalamus–pituitary–adrenal (HPA) axis and the sympathetic nervous system (SNS), with a concomitant drop in blood levels of cortisol, epinephrine, and norepinephrine. In contrast, mediators serving cell growth, differentiation, and restoration like the pituitary growth hormone (GH) and prolactin and the pineal hormone: melatonin. This hormone shows a steep increase in their blood levels during the night, when humans sleep (Haus, 2007; Reis et al., 2011). In parallel, increases of leptin that is released by adipocytes are assumed to prevent sleep-disturbing feelings of hunger during this time (Baccelli et al., 1969).

Despite their very different cellular sources, GH, prolactin, melatonin, and leptin exert remarkably synergistic actions on the immune system. They are pro-inflammatory signals that support immune cell activation, proliferation, differentiation, and the production of pro-inflammatory cytokines like interleukin (IL)-1, IL-12, tumor necrosis factor (TNF)-α, and of Th1 cytokines like interferon (IFN)-γ (Hattori, 2009; Kelley et al., 2007; Radogna et al., 2010). In contrast, cortisol and catecholamines generally suppress these immune functions in an anti-inflammatory manner (Elenkov et al., 2008), although some specific aspects of immunity may be supported by these signals.

On this background, numerous experiments have shown a consistent and intriguing pattern of endocrine and immune rhythms reflecting an "inflammatory peak" during nocturnal sleep whereas wakefulness is associated with prevalent anti-inflammatory activity (Lange et al., 2010; Scheff et al., 2010). In addition to the effects of hormones and danger signals, immune rhythms are regulated by intrinsic cellular clocks.

What triggers pro-inflammatory cytokine production throughout the body with the beginning of the rest period? Neuroendocrine rhythms with the prevalent release of pro-inflammatory hormones and a suppression of anti-inflammatory hormones during the early SWS-rich portion in combination with endogenous and exogenous danger signals throughout the active wake period and the intrinsic clock gene activity synergistically impact immune and nonimmune cells to boost immune activation during the rest period. This pro-inflammatory function of sleep can be beneficial.

Thus, sleep after vaccination can enhance the subsequent adaptive immune response like an adjuvant. How does sleep affect immunity during a genuinely ongoing immune response? There are a few studies that investigated the effects of sleep on the response to vaccinations used as an experimental model of infection. Intriguingly, these studies consistently demonstrate that sleep enhances the adaptive immune response against the invading antigen. Compared with subjects who stayed awake during the night after a single vaccination against hepatitis A in the morning before, subjects who regularly slept on this first night after vaccination, 4 weeks later, displayed a twofold increase in antigen-specific antibody titres (Lange, 2003).

The proportion of pro-inflammatory and Th1 cytokine (IL-2, IFN-γ, TNF-α) producing T cells was also profoundly reinforced by sleep. Importantly, these immuno-enhancing effects of sleep were still present at a one-year follow-up, indicating that sleep in enhancing the initial formation of an adaptive immune response also supports the long-term maintenance of the antigenic memory, a function hallmarking the immune system.

Collectively, these findings provide strong evidence for the notion that processes of immune activation and proliferation involving pro-inflammatory signals, antigen-presenting cells (APC), naïve and central memory T cells in lymph nodes are timed to the resting period. The reason for this timing is not clear. However, inflammation, if present during waking, causes malaise, fatigue, immobility, pain, and other aspects of sickness behavior that are incompatible with the demands of mental and physical activity required during the day.

Hence, confining major immunological response to sleep time seems reasonable (Petrovsky, 2001). In addition, immune activation, especially protein synthesis and cell proliferation, needs energy, and the endocrine changes during sleep allow for the allocation of energy-rich fuels like glucose from insulin-dependent tissues (e.g., muscle) to the immune system (Straub et al., 2010). Finally, inflammation leads to oxidative stress and cell injury that are efficiently counteracted by melatonin scavenging free radicals and by hematopoietic stem cells providing cellular supply. These may be just some reasons favoring the sleep period as suitable time for initiating adaptive immune responses and associated pro-inflammatory activity.

2.2 Thermoregulation and Energy Conservation

Core body temperature (CBT) comprises the temperature of the brain and the abdominal cavity, and is regulated between thermoeffector thresholds, which are subject to circadian oscillations (Kräuchi, 2007). Circadian rhythms in mammals are generated by the self-sustaining central pacemaker located in the suprachiasmatic nuclei (SCN) of the hypothalamus and are usually coupled to the 24-hour solar day mainly synchronized by light (Moore and Danchenko, 2002).

The regulation of CBT results from the concerted action of the homeostatic and circadian processes. In humans, the daily decline of CBT in the evening results from a regulated decline in the thermoregulatory thresholds of heat production and heat loss; the inverse happens in the morning.

Under resting conditions, about 70% of heat production depends on the metabolic activity of inner organs, whereas body heat loss is initiated by heat redistribution from the core to the shell through blood flow to the distal skin regions (Kräuchi, 2007). Thermoregulatory distal skin blood flow is regulated by the autonomic nervous system by constriction or dilation of arteriovenous anastomoses.

Nocturnal secretion of melatonin, which is under control of the SCN, plays a crucial role in the endogenous downregulation of CBT in the evening. Administration of melatonin in the afternoon, when endogenous melatonin levels are low, provokes exactly the same thermophysiological effects, as observed naturally in the evening (Kräuchi et al., 2006). Whether melatonin induces distal vasodilation in humans by acting directly on blood vessel receptors, indirectly through modulation of sympathetic nerve activity, or both, remains to be determined. In addition, both subjective ratings of sleepiness and the level of activity in the electroencephalogram (EEG) theta and alpha rhythms as an objective outcome of the sleep–wake state are increased (Kräuchi et al., 2006).

Moreover, it is noteworthy that rise in melatonin secretion in the evening belongs to a well-orchestrated circadian physiological regulation controlled by the SCN, which in turn downregulates CBT, increases sleepiness, and promotes sleep. The most evident explanation for whether and why the sleep regulatory and thermoregulatory systems are interrelated is that "sleep is for energy conservation" (Berger, 1984). All species sleep or rest when their energy expenditure is low. Rest or quiet wakefulness is a prerequisite for sleep in all species.

2.3 Memory Processing

Humans can learn, store, and remember various types of information in different ways and for variable periods of time, from conscious acquisition strategies to incidental detection of environmental events.

Long-term memories in humans may further belong to multiple systems, primarily delineated between declarative and nondeclarative memories. Declarative memory further comprises semantic and episodic memory components. Semantic memory is the receptacle for our general knowledge about the world, regardless of the spatiotemporal context of knowledge acquisition. Conversely, episodic memory refers to the system that stores events and information along with their contextual location in time and space. On the other hand, distinctive features of nondeclarative memories are that they are not easily accessible to verbal description and can be acquired and reexpressed implicitly. It means that our behavioral performance can be affected by the new memory even if we are not necessarily consciously aware that new information has been encoded or is retrieved.

Importantly, memory abilities aggregated under the nondeclarative label also include skills, habits, priming, and conditioning.

Scientific evidence suggests two main models:

(a) Sleep and associated processes of brain plasticity (Maquet et al., 2003) are major players in time-dependent processes of memory consolidation, acting as key constituents in the chain of transformations that help integrate information for the long term. According to the *dual-process hypothesis*, REM and NREM sleep act differently on memory traces depending on the memory system or process to which they belong.
(b) Memory processing during sleep takes place in a sequential manner whereby particular transitions from one sleep state to another each handle particular aspects of memory consolidation (Stickgold et al., 2000).

Both approaches assume that it is sleep on the first post-training night that is important for memory consolidation. On the other hand, during wakefulness, processes of memory consolidation have also been observed, and for this reason it is inappropriate to claim that *only* sleep may achieve the necessary conditions to consolidate novel memories in the nervous system (Peigneux, 2006; Brown and Robertson, 2007; Robertson et al., 2004).

In addition to the sleep functions mentioned here, the importance of sleep is present in endocrine physiology (affecting activity of the hypothalamic-pituitary axes, carbohydrate metabolism, appetite regulation, and the hormone control of blood pressure and body-fluid balance), in motor and sensory processing, and in as many as other systems as those that may appear in our organism. It should be remembered that the most studied and didatic way to learn about the functions of sleep is simply to verify the effects of its deprivation.

References

Achermann, P., & Borbély, A. A. (2017). Sleep homeostasis and models of sleep regulation. In M. Kryger, T. Roth, & W. C. Dement (Eds.), *Principles and practice of sleep medicine* (6th ed., pp. 377–387). Elsevier.

Baccelli, G., Guazzi, M., Mancia, G., et al. (1969). Neural and non-neural mechanisms influencing circulation during sleep. *Nature, 223*, 184–185. PMID: 5791726.

Berger, R. J. (1984). Slow wave sleep, shallow torpor and hibernation: Homologous states of diminished metabolism and body temperature. *Biological Psychology, 19*, 305–326. PMID: 6395910.

Borbély, A. A., Daan, S., Wirz-Justice, A., & Deboer, T. (2016). The two-process model of sleep regulation: A reappraisal. *Journal of Sleep Research, 25*, 131–143.

Borbély A. A. (1982). A two process model of sleep regulation. *Hum Neurobiol,1*, 195–204.

Brown, R., & Robertson, E. (2007). Off-line processing: Reciprocal interactions between declarative and procedural memories. *The Journal of Neuroscience, 27*, 10468–10475. PMID: 17898218.

Cirelli, C., & Tononi, G. (2008). Is sleep essential? *PLoS Biology, 6*, e216.

Daan S, Beersma D. G. M., & Borbély A. A. (1984). Timing of human sleep: recovery process gated by a circadian pacemaker. *Am J Physiol, 246*, R161–178.

Elenkov, I. J., Kvetnansky, R., Hashiramoto, A., Bakalov, V. K., Link, A. A., Zachman, K., Crane, M., Jezova, D., Rovensky, J., Dimitrov, M. A., Gold, P. W., et al. (2008). Low- versus high-baseline epinephrine output shapes opposite innate cytokine profiles: Presence of Lewis- and Fischer-like neurohormonal immune phenotypes in humans? *Journal of Immunology, 181*, 1737–1745.

Harper, R. M., Kumar, R., Macey, P. M., et al. (2012). Functional neuroanatomy, and sleep-disordered breathing: Implications for autonomic regulation. *The Anatomical Record (Hoboken), 295*, 1385–1395.

Hattori, N. (2009). Expression, regulation and biological actions of growth hormone (GH) and ghrelin in the immune system. *Growth Hormone & IGF Research, 19*, 187–197.

Haus, E. (2007). Chronobiology in the endocrine system. *Advanced Drug Delivery Reviews, 59*, 985–1014.

Huber, R., Hill, S. L., Holladay, C., Biesiadecki, M., Tononi, G., & Cirelli, C. (2004). Sleep homeostasis in Drosophila melanogaster. *Sleep, 27*(4), 628–39. https://doi.org/10.1093/sleep/27.4.628. PMID: 15282997.

Kelley, K. W., Weigent, D. A., & Kooijman, R. (2007). Protein hormones and immunity. *Brain, Behavior, and Immunity, 21*, 384–392.

Knutson, K. L., Spiegel, K., Penev, P., & Van Cauter, E. (2007). The metabolic consequences of sleep deprivation. *Sleep Medicine Reviews, 11*, 163–178.

Kräuchi, K. (2007). The thermophysiological cascade leading to sleep initiation in relation to phase of entrainment. *Sleep Medicine Reviews, 11*, 439–451.

Kräuchi, K., Cajochen, C., Pache, M., et al. (2006). Thermoregulatory effects of melatonin in relation to sleepiness. *Chronobiology International, 23*, 475–484.

Lange, T., Perras, B., Fehm, H. L., & Born, J. (2003). Sleep enhances the human antibody response to hepatitis A vaccination. *Psychosomatic Medicine, 65*, 831–835.

Lange, T., Dimitrov, S., & Born, J. (2010). Effects of sleep and circadian rhythm on the human immune system. *Annals of the New York Academy of Sciences, 1193*, 48–59.

Lenehan, S. M., Fogarty, L., O'Connor, C., Mathieson, S., & Boylan, G. B. (2023). The architecture of early childhood sleep over the first two years. *Maternal and Child Health Journal, 27*(2), 226–250. https://doi.org/10.1007/s10995-022-03545-9. Epub 2022 Dec 31. PMID: 36586054; PMCID: PMC9925493.

Mancia, G. (1993). Autonomic modulation of the cardiovascular system during sleep. *The New England Journal of Medicine, 328*, 347–349. PMID: 8419822.

Maquet, P., Smith, C., & Stickgold, R. (2003). *Sleep and brain plasticity*. Oxford University Press.

Moore, R. Y., & Danchenko, R. L. (2002). Paraventricular-subparaventricular hypothalamic lesions selectively affect circadian function. *Chronobiology International, 19*, 345–360. PMID: 12025929.

Ohayon, M., Carskadon, M. A., Guilleminault, C., et al. (2004). Meta-analysis of quantitative sleep parameters from childhood to old age in healthy individuals: Developing normative sleep values across the human lifespan. *Sleep, 27*, 1255–1273.

Peigneux, P., Orban, P., Balteau, E., et al. (2006). Offline persistence of memory-related cerebral activity during active wakefulness. *PLoS Biology, 4*, e100. PMID: 16602824.

Petrovsky, N. (2001). Towards a unified model of neuroendocrine–immune interaction. *Immunology and Cell Biology, 79*, 350–357.

Radogna, F., Diederich, M., & Ghibelli, L. (2010). Melatonin: A pleiotropic molecule regulating inflammation. *Biochemical Pharmacology, 80*, 1844–1852.

Reis, E. S., Lange, T., Kohl, G., Herrmann, A., Tschulakow, A. V., Naujoks, J., Born, J., & Kohl, J. (2011). Sleep and circadian rhythm regulate circulating complement factors and immunoregulatory properties of C5a. *Brain, Behavior, and Immunity, 25*(7), 1416–1426.

Robertson, E. M., Pascual-Leone, A., & Press, D. Z. (2004). Awareness modifies the skill-learning benefits of sleep. *Current Biology, 14*, 208–212. PMID: 14761652.

Scheff, J. D., Calvano, S. E., Lowry, S. F., & Androulakis, I. P. (2010). Modeling the influence of circadian rhythms on the acute inflammatory response. *Journal of Theoretical Biology, 264*, 1068–1076.

Schmidt, C., Collette, F., Cajochen, C., & Peigneux, P. (2007). A time to think: Circadian rhythms in human cognition. *Cognitive Neuropsychology, 24*(7), 755–789. https://doi.org/10.1080/02643290701754158. PMID: 18066734.

Stickgold, R., Whidbee, D., Schirmer, B., et al. (2000). Visual discrimination task improvement: A multi-step process occurring during sleep. *Journal of Cognitive Neuroscience, 12*, 246–254. PMID: 10771409.

Straub, R. H., Cutolo, M., Buttgereit, F., & Pongratz, G. (2010). Energy regulation and neuroendocrine–immune control in chronic inflammatory diseases. *Journal of Internal Medicine, 267*, 543–560.

Zamore, Z., & Veasey, S. C. (2022). Neural consequences of chronic sleep disruption. *Trends in Neurosciences, 45*, 678–691.

Zielinski, M. R., McKenna, J. T., & MCCarley RW. (2016). Functions and mechanisms of sleep. *AIMS Neuroscience, 3*(1), 67–104.

Chapter 3
Effects of Sleep Deprivation

Andrea Cecilia Toscanini and Rosa Hasan

Sleep is a vital biological function, so its existence is conditioned to a series of mechanisms inherent to life itself, its evolution and maintenance. The need to quantify the necessary sleep time to keep our body functioning properly is the subject of numerous studies and represents more than simply "hours of sleep" for adequate physical and mental functioning, there is an important political and economic impact directly and indirectly caused by sleep deprivation (Hafner et al., 2017).

The American Academy of Sleep Medicine (AASM) and the National Sleep Foundation (NSF) recommend that school-age children should receive at least 10 hours of sleep daily while the minimum requirement for adults is 7–8 hours. The reality, however, is that large proportions of the population are sleeping far less than these recommended minimums. Population-based studies indicate that nearly 30% of American adults report sleeping an average of six or fewer hours per night, while 69% of high school students report having an average of less than 8 hours of sleep on school nights (CDC, 2009).

Previous research has shown that sleeping patterns are related to quality of life (QoL) and that key aspects are the time when individuals sleep, sleep duration, and sleep quality. People who obtain sufficient high-quality sleep at proper times were found to have better general health and overall quality of life. By contrast, individuals who sleep too much or sleep poorly exhibit diminished quality of life (Kudrnáčová & Kudrnáč, 2023).

In recent decades, studies have shown an important association between sleep duration and mortality risk, finding the lowest risk among those individuals who

A. C. Toscanini (✉)
Institute of Psychiatry, Faculty of Medicine, University of São Paulo, Sao Paulo, Brazil
e-mail: a.toscanini@hc.fm.usp.br

R. Hasan
Institute of Psychiatry, Hospital das Clínicas, FMUSP, Sao Paulo, Brazil
e-mail: r.hasan@hc.fm.usp.br

R. El Rafihi-Ferreira (ed.), *Acceptance and Commitment Therapy for Insomnia*,
https://doi.org/10.1007/978-3-031-50710-6_3

sleep between 7 and 9 hours/night (Vgontzas et al., 2010). In the United States, sleep deprivation is directly associated with 5 of the 15 leading causes of death (Kochanek et al., 2014).

Sleep deprivation is a global and growing problem in modern society, largely attributed to the 24/7 social pattern in which we live, where there are long working hours and "virtually" 24 hours of wakefulness. Currently, the main cause of excessive daytime sleepiness is chronic sleep deprivation. Studies around the world indicate rates of 2.5–26% of the population with excessive daytime sleepiness (Hayley et al., 2014; Bixler et al., 2005).

Insufficient sleep was reported by 23%, 12%, and 9% in representative surveys from Japan, Sweden, and Finland, respectively. In 2008, the Centers for Disease Control (CDC) examined data from over 400,000 subjects throughout the USA and found that 11.1% reported that they had had insufficient rest or sleep every day during the preceding 30 days (Ford et al., 2015).

Sleep deprivation may be a result of behavior which may range from a person's decision to restrict sleep time, even unconsciously, in pursuit of other activities or consumption of stimulants such as coffee and tea close to bedtime. The disruption of sleep cycles is commonly seen among shift workers and frequent business travelers. The growing levels of stress and unrealistic targets and time pressures at workplaces have an adverse impact on sleep. Sleep deprivation is also becoming very common among school-age children and adolescents as their schedules and demands are preventing them from having sufficient sleep, although it is recommended these groups should try to sleep more than adults (Chattu et al., 2018).

According to the International Classification of Sleep Disorders (ICSD), "Insufficient sleep syndrome occurs when an individual persistently fails to obtain the amount of sleep required to maintain normal levels of alertness and wakefulness. The individual is chronically sleep deprived because of failure to achieve necessary sleep time due to reduced time in bed."

3.1 Consequences of Insufficient Sleep Syndrome (ISS)

In general, the most prevalent consequences of insufficient sleep (low performance, cognitive changes, and drowsiness) are largely unrecognized and not valued, many of them being confused with overworking, mood swings, tiredness, or even aging. When it comes to children, this may present as low school performance, irritability, and impairment of social activities (Kohyama et al., 2018).

ISS can lead to serious consequences for all the systems present in our organism, affecting the physiological homeostasis in each one of them. However, cognitive impairment, obesity, hypertension, and insulin resistance are the most pronounced, a decrease in immune function and an increase in inflammatory markers are also observed, in addition to the dysregulation of several hormones, including sexual and thyroid axes (Table 3.1) (Aldabal & Bahammam, 2011).

Table 3.1 Summary of the major adverse effects of insufficient sleep

Complications	Effects
Daytime sleepiness	Inadvertently fall asleep during sedentary activities, such as meetings, reading, watching television or movies, or while driving and increased risk for motor vehicle accidents
Emotional disturbances	Results in a more negative mood, with reduced optimism and sociability Complaints of pain were also observed Worsens mood states in healthy adolescents, with females having heightened vulnerability
Effects on functions of the brain	Cognitive impairment, prefrontal cortex dysfunction, Novelty detection, a mechanism that involves the frontal lobes, gets negatively affected Memory disorders
Effects on the structure of the brain	Reduction of cells in the dentate gyrus of the hippocampus Structural changes in the cortical neurons Degeneration of locus ceruleus neurons
Effects on body weight	Weight gain during insufficient sleep reverses when normal sleep is resumed Decrease of appetite-suppressing hormone leptin while levels of ghrelin, a hunger
Glucose metabolism	Glucose tolerance test shows a pre-diabetic state in otherwise normal persons Changes in insulin sensitivity and body weight Increased insulin resistance in diabetes
Cardiovascular system	Hypertension, arrhythmia, oxidative stress, endothelial dysfunction, inflammation, and metabolic disorder in coronary heart disease patients Coronary heart disease
Reproductive system	Impairment of sperm health
Genes linked with immune and inflammatory processes	Fraternal twins have shown that resiliency and vulnerability to sleep loss are highly heritable Variant in the ABCC9 gene that explains approximately 5% of the variation in sleep duration Genetic polymorphisms related to orexin signaling are important for predicting an individual's vulnerability to overeating and gaining weight when sleep deprived
Circardian rhythms	Reduction in circardian transcripts in whole blood
Immune system, inflammation, and infection	Decrease antibody production following influenza vaccination Dampened the normal circadian T-cell function and regulation Associated with a 1.39 relative risk of developing pneumonia Alterations in interleukin 6 and tumor necrosis factor alpha Leading to cardiovascular disease, insulin resistance, and osteoporosis

Table 3.1 shows a summary of the major adverse effects of insufficient sleep (Chattu et al., 2018).

Depending upon chronicity and extent of sleep loss, individuals with this condition may show irritability, concentration and attention deficits, reduced vigilance, distractibility, reduced motivation, anergia, dysphoria, fatigue, restlessness, lack of coordination, and malaise. Secondary symptoms may become the focus of the patient, serving to obscure the primary cause of the difficulties. Psychologically and somatically normal individuals who chronically obtain less sleep than they physiologically require typically experience daytime sleepiness. Situational factors such as demands of the family and work schedule may make it very difficult to obtain adequate sleep (Sateia, 2014).

In humans, sleep is responsible for orchestrating our metabolism during a third of our lives. For this reason, it would be impossible to cite "all" the consequences of its deprivation, but it is certainly possible to group some of them. Thus, in a didactic and modest way, there are three groups of alterations frequently found in sleep-deprived patients:

1. Mental health impairment: cognition and mood.
2. Metabolic alterations.
3. Immune function and inflammatory response modifications.

3.1.1 Mental Health Impairment: Cognition and Mood

Sleep deprivation (SD) is one of the reasons for the etiopathogenesis of various neurological disorders, and it impairs long-term potentiation and brain-derived neurotrophic factors and is linked to dementia and cognitive decline (Bishir et al., 2020). SD also causes accumulation or misfolding of proteins and its role in neurodegenerative diseases like Alzheimer's Disease (Wang & Holtzman, 2020), Parkinson's Disease (Dong et al., 2019), and cerebral stroke (Novati et al., 2011) is well documented. SD is associated with an imbalance in the immune axis leading to increased release of cytokines, autoimmune diseases (multiple sclerosis) (Kaminska et al., 2011), and glioma (Lee et al., 2004). In summary, it is apparent that SD plays a role in adversely modulating several key proteins and cellular/molecular cascades in various neurological disorders (Table 3.2). Based on the data gathered from literature and clinical studies on SD, it is apparent that the impact is enormous and profound and needs urgent attention.

In the field of psychiatry, it is believed that most psychiatric disorders can be aggravated, if not precipitated, by sleep deprivation, and we have to remember that in addition to traditional sleep deprivation (the imposition of a routine that provides fewer hours of sleep), there are unwanted conditions that also reduce total sleep time, such as insomnia, and lead to the same consequences as sleep deprivation itself.

Anxiety disorders are commonly seen in primary care settings where patient complaints of sleep problems are often prominent.[1] Sleep disturbances are included among the diagnostic features of generalized anxiety disorder (GAD), separation

[1] Sleep difficulties and sleep deprivation can lead to worsening of anxiety symptoms, including panic attacks, in patients with panic disorder.

Table 3.2 Sleep deprivation and neurological disorders associated

	References
Alzheimer's disease (AD)	Wang and Holtzman, *Neuropsychopharmacology* 2020 Ramanathan et al., *Frontiers in aging neuroscience* 2015 Lucey et al., *Neurology* 2018
Parkinson's disease (PD)	Currie et al., *Neurology* 1997 Dong et al., *Frontiers in neuroscience* 2019
Multiple sclerosis (MS)	Rudick and Goelz, *Experimental cell research* 2011 Papantoniou et al., *Occup and environmental medicine* 2019 Chalah and Ayache, *J of inflammation research* 2018
Stroke	Baumann et al., *Sleep* 2006 Gao et al., *Sleep* 2010
Huntingtons's disease (HD)	Essa et al., *Neurotoxicity research* 2019 Herzog-Krzywoszanska and L. Krzywoszanska, *Frontiers in psychiatry* 2019.
Learning and cognition impairment	McDermott et all, *The J of neurosciences* 2003 Hagewoud et al., *J sleep research* 2010
Epilepsy	M. Steriade, *Trends in neurosciences* 2005 Lanigar and Bandyopaghyay, *Missouri medicine* 2017 Staniszewska et al., *Neuropsychitric disease* 2017
Glioma	Hardeland and Pandi-Perumal, *Nutrition and metabolism* 2005 Jung and Ahmad, *Cancer research* 2006 Bieganska et al., J *of molecular neuroscience* 2012
Autism spectrum disorders (ASD)	Buckley et al., *Archieves of pediatrics* 2010 National Sleep Foundation, 2019
Neuropathic pain	Kundermann et al., *Pain research and management* 2004 Onen et al., *Brain research* 2001 Murk et al., *Neuropsychobiology* 2002

anxiety disorder, and post-traumatic stress disorder (PTSD). Polisomnography studies of anxiety disorders indicate that there are abnormalities in initiating and maintaining sleep and in sleep stage distribution. Sleep difficulties and sleep deprivation can lead to worsening of anxiety symptoms, including panic attacks, in patients with panic disorder (Roy-Byrne et al., 1986).

Mood disorders are the second-most common category of psychiatric disorders after anxiety disorders (Kessler et al., 2005). Subjective sleep complaints are some of the most consistent symptoms associated with major depression. Disruption of typical sleep patterns (insomnia or hypersomnia) is a diagnostic criterion for depressive episodes in the Diagnostic and Statistical Manual of Mental Disorders (DSM5) (Kessler et al., 2005). Sleep has been studied more extensively in patients with depression than in those with any other psychiatric disorder, and in addition to the subjective reports, objective, robust, and relatively specific changes in sleep architecture have been identified as correlates with the underlying neurobiology of depression. On the other hand, sleep deprivation, alone or in combination with pharmacological treatment, and as part of a chronotherapy package, is potentially used for people with major depressive episodes; however, the evidence base is still conflicting (Mitter et al., 2022).

A range of sleep and circadian disturbances are prominent features of bipolar disorder. Sleep disturbance persists during the interepisode period; up to 70% of adults with bipolar disorder report clinically significant sleep disturbance between episodes (Harvey et al., 2005). There is also evidence that sleep disturbance can precede the onset of the disorder by several years. Sleep disturbances during mood episodes and interepisode periods of bipolar disorder may include insomnia, hypersomnia, reduced sleep need, delayed sleep phase, and irregular sleep patterns. More specifically, insomnia is highly prevalent in bipolar disorder. As many as 100% of people with bipolar disorder report experiencing insomnia while depressed (Nofzinger et al., 1991), and 55% report having insomnia during the interepisode period. Reduced need for sleep is often exhibited during mania and mixed episodes and is characterized by a decrease in total sleep time. Furthermore, people with bipolar disorder are more likely to report circadian dysfunction, such as a delayed sleep phase preference, compared with healthy individuals. All these conditions converge in a decrease in total sleep time, and literature does not clarify the cause-consequence relationship clearly.

Up to 70% of children with ADHD have been reported to have mild to severe "sleep problems" (Sung et al., 2008). In terms of adult ADHD, there are no epidemiologic studies that investigate subjective sleep complaints, but sleep disturbances are also considered to be common in adults with ADHD (Philipsen et al., 2006). The most recent meta-analysis on sleep disturbances in ADHD, which focused on children and adolescents (Cortese et al., 2009), found significantly more sleep problems in children with ADHD than in healthy controls without ADHD based on subjectively rated sleep items, including bedtime resistance, sleep-onset difficulties, night awakenings, difficulties with morning awakenings, sleep-disordered breathing, and daytime sleepiness and, compared with controls, children with ADHD had less total sleep time based on actigraphy.

3.1.2 Metabolic Alterations

Metabolism is defined as the whole range of biochemical processes that occur within a living organism. It constitutes the two processes of anabolism (build up) and catabolism (break down). It is believed that during normal sleep, the metabolic rate reduces by around 15% and reaches a minimum in the morning in a standard circadian pattern (Goldberg, 1988). Although impact of sleep on glucose regulation has been known and studied for some time, metabolic dysregulation with sleep loss has only recently been understood. Studies done by Hampton et al. revealed that when subjects were made to simulate shift work, it resulted in alterations in postprandial glucose and lipid metabolism (Hampton et al., 1996).

The mechanism of sleep deprivation causing metabolic dysregulation may be multifactorial. Changes in hormonal secretion profile as discussed above may have profound effect on glucose regulation (Scheen et al., 1996). Sympathetic stimulation has been shown to occur with sleep deprivation (Vgontzas et al., 2004) and might contribute to the metabolic dysregulation. The third possible mechanism is inflammation. Experimental sleep deprivation has been found to alter immune response and increase proinflammatory markers such as IL-6, TNF-α, and PCR (Meier-Ewert et al., 2004).

Epidemiological data increasingly suggests that short sleep duration or chronic partial sleep deprivation may increase the risk of type II diabetes. A Swedish study with more than 2000 people followed for over 10 years revealed that short duration of sleep (<5 hours) and difficulty in initiating and maintaining sleep were associated with higher incidence of diabetes in men (but not in women) even after adjusting for confounding factors (Mallon et al., 2005). In another study by Yaggi and colleagues, a large cohort of men without diabetes at baseline was followed for more than 15 years in a longitudinal study. Subjects who self-reported less than 6 hours of sleep were twice as likely to develop diabetes (Yaggi et al., 2006). Although epidemiological studies do not establish causality, these studies are consistent with the physiological data discussed earlier.

More than two dozen epidemiological studies from around the globe looking at sleep deprivation and BMI in humans have shown association between decreased obesity and an increase in sleep duration. These studies, however, do not establish a causal relationship. Few studies revealed a U-shaped curve with lowest mean BMI associated with 7.7 hours/night (Taheri et al., 2004; Cournot et al., 2004). Apart from cross-sectional studies, there have been around nine prospective/longitudinal studies in adults and children, eight of which have shown similar findings of sleep deprivation and a higher prevalence of obesity (Patel et al., 2006; Lumeng et al., 2007). Epidemiological data is suggestive of weight gain with sleep deprivation though a few studies have also noted weight gain with prolonged sleep. Based on data on sleep duration and weight, sleep hygiene counseling could form an important tool in management of obesity (Sharma and Kavuru, 2010).

Mechanistically, sleep and circadian rhythm exert considerable influences on hormones involved in appetite regulation and energy metabolism. As such, data from experimental sleep deprivation in humans demonstrate that insufficient sleep induces a positive energy balance with resultant weight gain, due to increased energy intake that far exceeds the additional energy expenditure of nocturnal wakefulness, and adversely impacts glucose metabolism (Duan et al., 2023).

3.1.3 Immune Function and Inflammatory Response

The role that sleep plays in the maintenance and function of the immune system has not been completely elucidated. Some studies have shown that sleep deprivation can have important effects on immune function, levels of cytokines, and inflammation markers, also decreasing the function of NK cells, T lymphocytes, and monocytes. This is consistent with evidence accumulated in recent years, which show that sleep increases defense immunity by several mechanisms, among others, the increase in

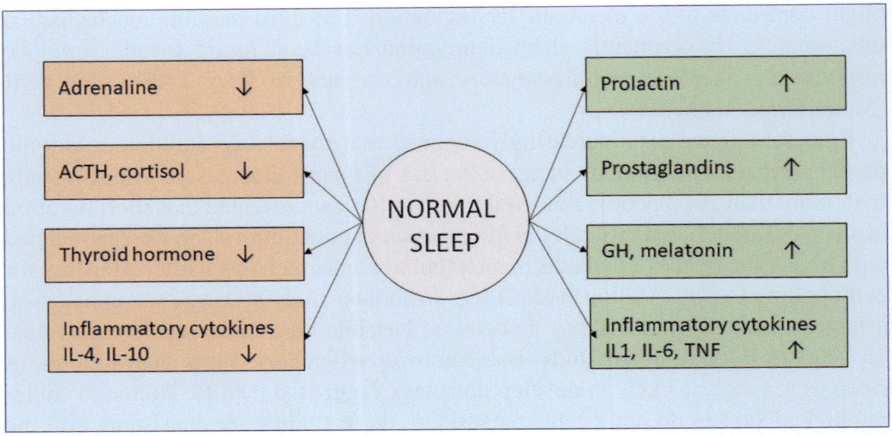

Fig. 3.1 Main cytokines and hormones presented and regulated during normal sleep. In orange boxes those that increase during sleep, and in green boxes those that decrease. (Adapted from Rico-Rosillo and Vega-Robledo, 2018)

immunological memory and the proinflammatory, and activating functions that develop during this time (Fig. 3.1) (Rico-Rosillo and Vega-Robledo, 2018).

Repeated partial sleep deprivation for several days produces an increase in the production of C-reactive protein (PCR) (Grandner et al., 2013), IL-6 (Ferrie et al., 2013), TNF (Chennaoui et al., 2011), and IL-1β (Frey et al., 2007), which persists even after a full night's sleep recovery. These molecules activate NF-κB, the key transcriptional control pathway in the inflammatory signaling cascade. Sleep disturbance, possibly through effects on inflammation, may contribute to the development of chronic inflammatory diseases (Kinucan et al., 2013). Studies carried out on people who sleep less than 5 hours show that they have a greater risk of presenting cardiovascular events (Sabanayagam et al., 2011), with a linear relationship between the duration of sleep and the possible risks (Chien et al., 2010). They suggest that the duration of optimal sleep is between 7 and 8 hours.

In addition to the alterations exposed here, there are certainly other physical and mental conditions modulated by sleep deprivation. However, besides the impact on health, it is necessary to remember the economic and social impact that sleep deprivation entails, considering that it is the most prevalent sleep disorder in the world.

References

Aldabal, L., & Bahammam, A. S. (2011). Metabolic, endocrine, and immune consequences of sleep deprivation. *Open Respiratory Medicine Journal, 5*, 31–43.

Baumann, C. R., Kilic, E., Petit, B., et al. (2006). Sleep EEG changes after middle cerebral artery infarcts in mice: Different effects of striatal and cortical lesions. *Sleep, 29*(10), 1339–1344.

Biegańska, K., Sokołowska, P., Jöhren, O., & Zawilska, J. B. (2012). Orexin A suppresses the growth of rat C6 glioma cells via a caspase-dependent mechanism. *Journal of Molecular Neuroscience, 48*(3), 706–712.

Bishir, M., Bhat, A., Essa, M. M., Ekpo, O., Ihunwo, A. O., Veeraraghavan, V. P., Mohan, S. K., Mahalakshmi, A. M., Ray, B., Tuladhar, S., Chang, S., Chidambaram, S. B., Sakharkar, M. K., Guillemin, G. J., Qoronfleh, M. W., & Ojcius, D. M. (2020). Sleep deprivation and neurological disorders. *BioMed Research International, 2020*, 5764017. https://doi.org/10.1155/2020/5764017. PMID: 33381558; PMCID: PMC7755475.

Bixler, E. O., Vgontzas, A. N., Lin, H. M., Calhoun, S. L., Vela-Bueno, A., & Kales, A. (2005). Excessive daytime sleepiness in a general population sample: The role of sleep apnea, age, obesity, diabetes, and depression. *The Journal of Clinical Endocrinology and Metabolism, 90*(8), 4510–4515.

Buckley, A. W., Rodriguez, A. J., Jennison, K., et al. (2010). Rapid eye movement sleep percentage in children with autism compared with children with developmental delay and typical development. *Archives of Pediatrics & Adolescent Medicine, 164*(11), 1032–1037.

Centers for Disease Control and Prevention (CDC). (2009). Perceived insufficient rest or sleep among adults - United States, 2008. *MMWR. Morbidity and Mortality Weekly Report, 58*(42), 1175–1179.

Chalah, M. A., & Ayache, S. S. (2018). Is there a link between inflammation and fatigue in multiple sclerosis? *Journal of Inflammation Research, 11*, 253–264.

Chattu, V. K., Sakhamuri, S. M., Kumar, R., Spence, D. W., BaHammam, A. S., & Pandi-Perumal, S. R. (2018). Insufficient Sleep Syndrome: Is it time to classify it as a major noncommunicable disease? *Sleep Science, 11*(2), 56–64. https://doi.org/10.5935/1984-0063.20180013. PMID: 30083291; PMCID: PMC6056073.

Chennaoui, M., Sauvet, F., Drogou, C., Van-Beers, P., Langrume, C., Guillard, M., et al. (2011). Effect of one night of sleep loss on changes in tumor necrosis factor alpha (TNF-alpha) levels in healthy men. *Cytokine, 56*(2), 318–324. https://doi.org/10.1016/j.cyto.2011.06.002

Chien, K. L., Chen, P. C., Hsu, H. C., Su, T. C., Sung, F. C., Chen, M. F., et al. (2010). Habitual sleep duration and insomnia and the risk of cardiovascular events and all-cause death: Report from a community-based cohort. *Sleep, 33*(2), 177–184.

Cortese, S., Faraone, S. V., Konofal, E., & Lecendreux, M. (2009). Sleep in children with attention-deficit/hyperactivity disorder: Meta-analysis of subjective and objective studies. *Journal of the American Academy of Child and Adolescent Psychiatry, 48*, 894–908.

Cournot, M., Ruidavets, J. B., Marquie, J. C., Esquirol, Y., Baracat, B., & Ferrieres, J. (2004). Environmental factors associated ` with body mass index in a population of southern France. *European Journal of Cardiovascular Prevention and Rehabilitation, 11*(4), 291–297.

Currie, L. J., Bennett, J. P., Harrison, M. B., Trugman, J. M., & Wooten, G. F. (1997). Clinical correlates of sleep benefit in Parkinson's disease. *Neurology, 48*(4), 1115–1117.

Dong, H., Wang, J., Yang, Y. F., Shen, Y., Qu, W. M., & Huang, Z. L. (2019). Dorsal striatum dopamine levels fluctuate across the sleep–wake cycle and respond to salient stimuli in mice. *Frontiers in Neuroscience, 13, 242*.

Duan, D., Kim, L. J., Jun, J. C., & Polotsky, V. Y. (2023). Connecting insufficient sleep and insomnia with metabolic dysfunction. *Annals of the New York Academy of Sciences, 1519*(1), 94–117. https://doi.org/10.1111/nyas.14926. Epub 2022 Nov 13. PMID: 36373239; PMCID: PMC9839511.

Essa, M. M., Moghadas, M., Ba-Omar, T., et al. (2019). Protective effects of antioxidants in Huntington's disease: An extensive review. *Neurotoxicity Research, 35*(3), 739–774.

Ferrie, J. E., Kivimaki, M., Akbaraly, T. N., Singh-Manoux, A., Miller, M. A., Gimeno, D., et al. (2013). Associations between change in sleep duration and infl ammation: Fi ndings on C-reactive protein and interleukin 6 in the Whitehall II study. *American Journal of Epidemiology, 178*(6), 956–961. https://doi.org/10.1093/aje/kwt072

Ford, E. S., Cunningham, T. J., Giles, W. H., & Croft, J. B. (2015). Trends in insomnia and excessive daytime sleepiness among U.S. adults from 2002 to 2012. *Sleep Medicine, 16*(3), 372–378.

Frey, D. J., Fleshner, M., & Wright, K. P. (2007). The effect of 40 hours of total sleep deprivation on infl ammatory markers in healthy young adults. *Brain, Behavior, and Immunity, 21*(8), 1050–1057. https://doi.org/10.1016/j.bbi.2007.04.003

Gao, B., Cam, E., Jaeger, H., Zunzunegui, C., Sarnthein, J., & Bassetti, C. L. (2010). Sleep disruption aggravates focal cerebral ischemia in the rat. *Sleep, 33*(7), 879–887.

Goldberg, G. R., Prentice, A. M., Davies, H. L., & Murgatroyd, P. R. (1988). Overnight and basal metabolic rates in men and women. *European Journal of Clinical Nutrition, 42*(2), 137–144.

Grandner, M. A., Buxton, O. M., Jackson, N., Sands-Lincoln, M., Pandey, A., & Jean-Louis, G. (2013). Extreme sleep durations and increased C-reactive protein: Effects of sex and ethnoracial group. *Sleep, 36*(5), 769–779. https://doi.org/10.5665/sleep.2646

Hafner, M., Stepanek, M., Taylor, J., Troxel, W. M., & van Stolk, C. (2017). Why sleep matters: The economic costs of insufficient sleep: A cross-country comparative analysis. *Rand Health Quarterly, 6*(4), 11.

Hagewoud, R., Havekes, R., Novati, A., Keijser, J. N., Van der Zee, E. A., & Meerlo, P. (2010). Sleep deprivation impairs spatial working memory and reduces hippocampal AMPA receptor phosphorylation. *Journal of Sleep Research, 19*(2), 280–288.

Hakki Onen, S., Alloui, A., Jourdan, D., Eschalier, A., & Dubray, C. (2001). Effects of rapid eye movement (REM) sleep deprivation on pain sensitivity in the rat. *Brain Research, 900*(2), 261–267.

Hampton, S. M., Morgan, L. M., Lawrence, N., et al. (1996). Postprandial hormone and metabolic responses in simulated shift work. *Journal of Endocrinology, 151*(2), 259–267.

Hardeland, R., & Pandi-Perumal, S. R. (2005). Melatonin, a potent agent in antioxidative defense: Actions as a natural food constituent, gastrointestinal factor, drug and prodrug. *Nutrition & Metabolism, 2*(1), 22.

Harvey, A. G., Schmidt, D. A., Scarna, A., et al. (2005). Sleep-related functioning in euthymic patients with bipolar disorder, patients with insomnia, and subjects without sleep problems. *The American Journal of Psychiatry, 162*, 50–57.

Hayley, A. C., Williams, L. J., Kennedy, G. A., Berk, M., Brennan, S. L., & Pasco, J. A. (2014). Prevalence of excessive daytime sleepiness in a sample of the Australian adult population. *Sleep Medicine, 15*(3), 348–354.

Herzog-Krzywoszanska, R., & Krzywoszanski, L. (2019). Sleep disorders in Huntington's disease. *Frontiers in Psychiatry, 10*, 221.

Jung, B., & Ahmad, N. (2006). Melatonin in cancer management: Progress and promise: Figure 1. *Cancer Research, 66*(20), 9789–9793.

Kaminska, M., Kimoff, R. J., Schwartzman, K., & Trojan, D. A. (2011). Sleep disorders and fatigue in multiple sclerosis: Evidence for association and interaction. *Journal of the Neurological Sciences, 302*(1–2), 7–13.

Kessler, R. C., Berglund, P., Demler, O., et al. (2005). Lifetime prevalence and age-of-onset distributions of DSM-IV disorders in the National Comorbidity Survey Replication. *Archives of General Psychiatry, 62*(6), 593–602.

Kinucan, J. A., Rubín, D. T., & Ali, T. (2013). Sleep and inflammatory bowel disease: Exploring the relationship between sleep disturbances and infl ammation. *Gastroenterology and Hepatology (New York), 9*(11), 718–727.

Kochanek, K. D., Murphy, S. L., Xu, J., & Arias, E. (2014). Mortality in the United States, 2013. *NCHS Data Brief*, (178), 1–8.

Kohyama, J., Anzai, Y., Ono, M., Kishino, A., Tamanuki, K., Takada, K., Inoue, K., Horiuchi, M., & Hatai, Y. (2018). Insufficient sleep syndrome: An unrecognized but important clinical entity. *Pediatrics International, 60*(4), 372–375. https://doi.org/10.1111/ped.13519. Epub 2018 Feb 28. PMID: 29337407.

Kudrnáčová, M., & Kudrnáč, A. (2023). Better sleep, better life? Testing the role of sleep on quality of life. *PLoS One, 18*(3), e0282085. https://doi.org/10.1371/journal.pone.0282085. PMID: 36920893; PMCID: PMC10016705.

Kundermann, B., Krieg, J. C., Schreiber, W., & Lautenbacher, S. (2004). The effect of sleep deprivation on pain. *Pain Research and Management, 9*(1), 32.

Lanigar, S., & Bandyopadhyay, S. (2017). Sleep and epilepsy: A complex interplay. *Missouri Medicine, 114*(6), 453–457.

Lee, K., Cho, M., Miaskowski, C., & Dodd, M. (2004). Impaired sleep and rhythms in persons with cancer. *Sleep Medicine Reviews, 8*(3), 199–212.

Lucey, B. P., Hicks, T. J., McLeland, J. S., et al. (2018). Effect of sleep on overnight cerebrospinal fluid amyloid β kinetics. *Annals of Neurology, 83*(1), 197–204.

Lumeng, J. C., Somashekar, D., Appugliese, D., Kaciroti, N., Corwyn, R. F., & Bradley, R. H. (2007). Shorter sleep duration is associated with increased risk for being overweight at ages 9 to 12 years. *Pediatrics, 120*(5), 1020–1029.

Mallon, L., Broman, J. E., & Hetta, J. (2005). High incidence of diabetes in men with sleep complaints or short sleep duration: A 12-year follow-up study of a middle-aged population. *Diabetes Care, 28*(11), 2762–2767.

McDermott, C. M., LaHoste, G. J., Chen, C., Musto, A., Bazan, N. G., & Magee, J. C. (2003). Sleep deprivation causes behavioral, synaptic, and membrane excitability alterations in hippocampal neurons. *The Journal of Neuroscience, 23*(29), 9687–9695.

Meier-Ewert, H. K., Ridker, P. M., Rifai, N., et al. (2004). Effect of sleep loss on C-reactive protein, an inflammatory marker of cardiovascular risk. *Journal of the American College of Cardiology, 43*(4), 678–683.

Mitter, P., De Crescenzo, F., Loo Yong Kee, K., Xia, J., Roberts, S., Chi, W., Kurtulmus, A., Kyle, S. D., Geddes, J. R., & Cipriani, A. (2022). Sleep deprivation as a treatment for major depressive episodes: A systematic review and meta-analysis. *Sleep Medicine Reviews, 64*, 101647. https://doi.org/10.1016/j.smrv.2022.101647. Epub 2022 May 26. PMID: 35700677.

Murck, H., Struttmann, T., Czisch, M., Wetter, T., Steiger, A., & Auer, D. P. (2002). Increase in amino acids in the pons after sleep deprivation: A pilot study using proton magnetic resonance spectroscopy. *Neuropsychobiology, 45*(3), 120–123.

National Sleep Foundation. (2019, October). *Why do we need sleep?* https://www.sleepfoundation.org/articles/why-do-we-need-sleep

Nofzinger, E. A., Thase, M. E., Reynolds, C. F., 3rd, et al. (1991). Hypersomnia in bipolar depression: A comparison with narcolepsy using the multiple sleep latency test. *The American Journal of Psychiatry, 148*, 1177–1181.

Novati, A., Hulshof, H. J., Koolhaas, J. M., Lucassen, P. J., & Meerlo, P. (2011). Chronic sleep restriction causes a decrease in hippocampal volume in adolescent rats, which is not explained by changes in glucocorticoid levels or neurogenesis. *Neuroscience, 190*, 145–155.

Papantoniou, K., Massa, J., Devore, E., et al. (2019). Rotating night shift work and risk of multiple sclerosis in the Nurses' Health Studies. *Occupational and Environmental Medicine, 76*(10), 733–738.

Patel, S. R., Malhotra, A., White, D. P., Gottlieb, D. J., & Hu, F. B. (2006). Association between reduced sleep and weight gain in women. *American Journal of Epidemiology, 164*(10), 947–954.

Philipsen, A., Hornyak, M., & Riemann, D. (2006). Sleep and sleep disorders in adults with attention deficit/hyperactivity disorder. *Sleep Medicine Reviews, 10*, 399–405.

Ramanathan, A., Nelson, A. R., Sagare, A. P., & Zlokovic, B. V. (2015). Impaired vascular-mediated clearance of brain amyloid beta in Alzheimer's disease: The role, regulation and restoration of LRP1. *Frontiers in Aging Neuroscience, 7*, 136.

Rico-Rosillo, M. G., & Vega-Robledo, G. B. (2018). Sueño y sistema immune [Sleep and immune system]. *Revista Alergia México, 65*(2), 160–170. https://doi.org/10.29262/ram.v65i2.359. Spanish. PMID: 29983013.

Roy-Byrne, P. P., Uhde, T. W., & Post, R. M. (1986). Effects of one night's sleep deprivation on mood and behavior in panic disorder. Patients with panic disorder compared with depressed patients and normal controls. *Archives of General Psychiatry, 43*(9), 895–899.

Rudick, R. A., & Goelz, S. E. (2011). Beta-interferon for multiple sclerosis. *Experimental Cell Research, 317*(9), 1301–1311.

Sabanayagam, C., Shankar, A., Buchwald, D., & Goins, R. T. (2011). Insomnia symptoms and cardiovascular disease among older American Indians: The Native Elder Care Study. *Journal of Environmental and Public Health, 2011*, 964617. https://doi.org/10.1155/2011/964617

Sateia, M. J. (2014). International classification of sleep disorders-third edition: Highlights and modifications. *Chest, 146*(5), 1387–1394. https://doi.org/10.1378/chest.14-0970. PMID: 25367475.

Scheen, A. J., Byrne, M. M., Plat, L., Leproult, R., & Van Cauter, E. (1996). Relationships between sleep quality and glucose regulation in normal humans. *American Journal of Physiology, 271*(2), E261–E270.

Sharma, S., & Kavuru, M. (2010). Sleep and metabolism: An overview. *International Journal of Endocrinology, 2010*, 270832. https://doi.org/10.1155/2010/270832. Epub 2010 Aug 2. PMID: 20811596; PMCID: PMC2929498.

Staniszewska, A., Mąka, A., Religioni, U., & Olejniczak, D. (2017). Sleep disturbances among patients with epilepsy. *Neuropsychiatric Disease and Treatment, 13*, 1797–1803.

Steriade, M. (2005). Sleep, epilepsy and thalamic reticular inhibitory neurons. *Trends in Neurosciences, 28*(6), 317–324.

Sung, V., Hiscock, H., Sciberras, E., & Efron, D. (2008). Sleep problems in children with attention-deficit/hyperactivity disorder: Prevalence and the effect on the child and family. *Archives of Pediatrics & Adolescent Medicine, 162*, 336–342.

Taheri, S., Lin, L., Austin, D., Young, T., & Mignot, E. (2004). Short sleep duration is associated with reduced leptin, elevated ghrelin, and increased body mass index. *PLoS Medicine, 1*(3), e62.

Vgontzas, A. N., Zoumakis, E., Bixler, E. O., et al. (2004). Adverse effects of modest sleep restriction on sleepiness, performance, and inflammatory cytokines. *Journal of Clinical Endocrinology and Metabolism, 89*(5), 2119–2126.

Vgontzas, A. N., Liao, D., Pejovic, S., Calhoun, S., Karataraki, M., Basta, M., et al. (2010). Insomnia with short sleep duration and mortality: The Penn State cohort. *Sleep, 33*(9), 1159–1164.

Wang, C., & Holtzman, D. M. (2020). Bidirectional relationship between sleep and Alzheimer's disease: Role of amyloid, tau, and other factors. *Neuropsychopharmacology, 45*(1), 104–120.

Yaggi, H. K., Araujo, A. B., & McKinlay, J. B. (2006). Sleep duration as a risk factor for the development of type 2 diabetes. *Diabetes Care, 29*(3), 657–661.

Chapter 4
Insomnia

Israel Soares Pompeu de Sousa Brasil and Renatha El Rafihi-Ferreira

4.1 Insomnia: A Multiple Condition

Insomnia is the most common sleep disorder in the general population (Schutte-Rodin et al., 2008). But what are we talking about exactly: The complaint? The symptom? Or the disorder? Do these phenomena refer to the same patient profile or do their characteristics lead to differences in terms of evolution and prognosis? Hence, one of the main challenges involving insomnia today is how to delineate universal concepts for such a multifaceted condition.

Nosologically, insomnia has been included in more and more categories over time. It can be evaluated as a symptom (when it is part of the presentation of other diseases, for example, major depression), as a disorder (when it becomes a syndromic condition with its own course and prognosis), or even denominating diseases such as fatal familial insomnia (Poon et al., 2021). Despite so many features, it is as a disorder that insomnia demonstrates all its strength; the investigation of insomnia disorder facilitates the understanding of its pathophysiology and repercussions on the patient's life and it is, therefore, the chosen condition in studies on insomnia. Within this context, insomnia disorder is defined as a persistent difficulty with sleep initiation, duration, consolidation, or quality that occurs despite favorable circumstances and opportunities to fall asleep, resulting in daytime impairments (American Academy of Sleep Medicine, 2014). Its chronic and recurrent nature is one of the characteristics that reinforce the concept of a disorder within the insomnia spectrum.

I. S. P. de Sousa Brasil (✉)
Institute of Medical Assistance to State Civil Servants of São Paulo (IAMSPE), São Paulo, Brazil

R. El Rafihi-Ferreira
Department of Clinical Psychology, University of São Paulo, São Paulo, Brazil
e-mail: rerafihi@usp.br

R. El Rafihi-Ferreira (ed.), *Acceptance and Commitment Therapy for Insomnia*,
https://doi.org/10.1007/978-3-031-50710-6_4

Previous versions of the International Classification of Sleep Disorders (ICSD) distinguished between primary (and its subtypes: psychophysiological, idiopathic, associated with inadequate sleep hygiene, and paradoxical) and secondary insomnia (when associated with a comorbidity). The current version of the ICSD no longer differentiates the different types of insomnia and combines all of them in a single entity—the aforementioned insomnia disorder. In addition to reflecting observations made in clinical practice, that is, patients hardly fit into a single category, this apparent simplification also reinforces the importance of the syndromic diagnosis of insomnia as an entity that requires specific assessment and treatment. Nevertheless, remembering these subdivisions can be useful in the etiological investigation of insomnia (Hasan & Brasil, 2019).

Assessing the course of a patient's complaint of sleep difficulty can be the key to determining not only the classification of insomnia as a symptom or disorder but also the clinical and environmental factors that explain its occurrence. It is not rare that the conversion of a symptom into insomnia disorder occurs along a continuum that involves the outbreak of a precipitating factor and the progressive development of poor habits and dysfunctional beliefs about sleep that will perpetuate the disruption promoted by that factor, as proposed by Spielman's theoretical model (Spielman et al., 1987). At this point, the focus of attention of insomnia is no longer the alteration that caused the sleep difficulty (e.g., pain, anguish, or dyspnea) but sleep itself, which is intrinsically unstructured in the patient's view (Espie et al., 2006). This degeneration process may not necessarily last 3 months, the interval suggested by the diagnostic criteria for insomnia disorder (see below), but much less; the patient may already require a more robust therapeutic approach within a few weeks, as recommended for cases of the disorder (Perlis et al., 2022).

The above considerations highlight the complexity of insomnia whose manifestation is specific for each patient. The full understanding of this condition requires the specialist to consider temporal, emotional, cognitive, and environmental factors of the insomnia patient, which form the basis of a more assertive and effective treatment.

4.2 Epidemiological Characteristics

Both clinical practice and research confirm that insomnia is the most common sleep disorder in the population. However, a more precise epidemiological notion of this problem is still difficult to obtain because of the already-mentioned nosological variability of the condition (Poon et al., 2021). More detailed studies indicate a global prevalence of 30% to 35% of insomnia symptoms and of 3.9% to 22.1% of insomnia disorder (American Academy of Sleep Medicine, 2014). The annual incidence can reach 7–15% (Morphy et al., 2007). Unlike initiating sleep and early morning awakening, the difficulty staying asleep seems to be the most common complaint among individuals with insomnia, as demonstrated by an European group (Ohayon & Reynolds, 2009).

Complaints of insomnia are more common among women and older adults, especially when accompanied by other medical and psychiatric comorbidities or by substance/medication use. Female predominance is reflected by a female/male ratio of 1.4 for insomnia symptoms and of 2.0 for insomnia disorder (Singareddy et al., 2012); hormonal and psychosocial factors are usually related to this female predominance (Johnson et al., 2006). The higher prevalence in older age groups can be explained by the greater sleep fragmentation found in this population and by the higher frequency of comorbidities and medication use (Ohayon et al., 2004).

The environmental dimension of insomnia is illustrated by the higher prevalence of cases in lower socioeconomic strata, among retired and unemployed individuals, and among widowers and divorced/separated individuals. This scenario also reflects the impact of the association with psychiatric disorders such as anxiety and depression. Mental health is so intrinsically linked to sleep that it is not surprising that depressive and anxiety disorders are the most common comorbidities in patients with insomnia; these disorders maintain a bidirectional relationship of cause and consequence, influencing both the development and the prognosis of each condition (Hertenstein et al., 2018).

4.3 Diagnostic Criteria

Defining a clinical entity based on diagnostic criteria must consider fundamental features of the disease that differentiate it from other diseases and, at the same time, are sensitive so that the condition does not pass unrecognized. This definition is especially difficult in the case of insomnia, given its aforementioned nosological multiplicity. It is no coincidence that such criteria have changed over the years and should continue to change as new perspectives emerge.

The Diagnostic and Statistical Manual of Mental Disorders (DSM), now in its fifth edition, was the first manual that combined all insomnia variants in a single diagnosis, that is, insomnia disorder (American Psychiatric Association, 2013). It can be further divided into different types according to specifications associated with comorbidities (psychiatric condition, clinical comorbidity, other sleep disorder) and course (episodic: 1 to 3 months; persistent: more than 3 months; recurrent: 2 or more episodes per year). The criteria of the DSM-V are given in Box 4.1.

Box 4.1: Criteria of the DSM-V

A. Dissatisfaction with sleep quantity or quality, associated with one (or more) of the following symptoms:

   1. Difficulty initiating sleep.
   2. Difficulty maintaining sleep, characterized by frequent awakenings or problems returning to sleep after awakenings.
   3. Early morning awakening with difficulty returning to sleep.

B. The sleep disturbance causes clinically significant impairment in social, occupational, educational, academic, and behavioral functioning or any other important area.
C. The sleep difficulty occurs at least three nights per week.
D. The sleep difficulty is present for at least 3 months.
E. The sleep difficulty occurs despite adequate opportunity for sleep.
F. Insomnia is not better explained by or does not occur exclusively during the course of another sleep disorder (narcolepsy, breathing-related sleep disorder, circadian rhythm disorder, parasomnia).
G. Insomnia is not attributable to the physiological effects of a substance (e.g., a drug of abuse and a medication).
H. A mental disorder or medical condition does not adequately explain the predominant complaint of insomnia.

The third edition of the ICSD (ICSD-3), published in 2014 and revised in 2023 (ICSD-3R), followed the pattern established by the DSM-V and also proposed a single diagnosis of chronic insomnia disorder (American Academy of Sleep Medicine, 2014). This manual also mentions other varieties based on time course (short-term; other insomnia disorder). It is worth mentioning that criteria for behavioral insomnia of childhood have also been incorporated into the classification of insomnia disorder. The complaint of "non-restorative sleep" was eliminated as a diagnostic criterion from both the DSM-V and the ICSD-3R because of its subjective nature, the lack of specificity (much more frequent attribution to other diseases such as sleep apnea and fibromyalgia), and the lack of association with more objective markers. The criteria of the ICSD-3R are given in Box 4.2.

Box 4.2: Criteria of the ICSD-3

Criteria A–F must be present:

A. The patient reports, or caregivers observe, one or more of the following characteristics:

1. Difficulty initiating sleep.
2. Difficulty maintaining sleep.
3. Waking up earlier than desired.
4. Resistance to going to bed on appropriate schedule.
5. Difficulty falling asleep without parent or caregiver intervention.

B. The patient reports, or caregivers observe, one or more of the following difficulties related to nighttime sleep:

1. Fatigue/malaise.
2. Attention, concentration, or memory impairment.
3. Impaired social, family, occupation, or academic performance.
4. Mood disturbance/irritability.
5. Daytime sleepiness.
6. Behavioral problems (e.g., hyperactivity, impulsivity, aggression).
7. Reduced motivation/energy/initiative.
8. Proneness for errors/accidents.
9. Concerns about or dissatisfaction with sleep.

C. The reported sleep/wake complaints cannot be explained by inadequate opportunity (i.e., enough time is allotted for sleep) or inadequate circumstances (i.e., the environment is safe, dark, quiet, and comfortable) for sleep.

D. The sleep disturbance and associated daytime symptoms occur at least three times per week.

E. The sleep disturbance and associated daytime symptoms have been present for at least 3 months.

F. The sleep disturbance and associated daytime symptoms are not solely due to another current sleep disorder, medical disorder, mental disorder, or medication/substance use.

The latest version of the International Classification of Diseases (ICD-11), which came into effect in 2022, also follows the precepts determined by the aforementioned manuals, with codes for three modalities: chronic insomnia disorder, short-term insomnia disorder, and insomnia disorders, unspecified (World Health Organization, 2018). This classification also allows characterization based on their severity, with codes for mild, moderate, and severe insomnia. Although the ICD-11 determines the threshold of 3 months for characterizing chronic insomnia, it does not specify a minimum frequency of symptoms per week (as occurs in the other manuals).

4.4 Etiological Factors of Insomnia

Insomnia is often explained from different pathophysiological perspectives, reflecting its multifaceted nature. When understood as a sleep continuity disorder linked to psychological, cognitive, and functional repercussions, insomnia may be considered to involve different mechanisms in different contexts.

From an anatomophysiological point of view, it is still difficult to specify how insomnia emerges. The hypervigilant state, a phenomenon considered to be the underlying clinical condition of patients with insomnia, has been illustrated by several studies, which indicate possible mechanisms for this pattern: hyperactivation of the hypothalamic-pituitary-adrenal axis and the sympathetic nervous system, dysfunction of homeostatic sleep regulatory mechanisms, and circadian alterations associated with the sleep-wake cycle, among others (Coelho & Rizzo, 2019). Recently, polymorphisms in genes related to stress reactivity and neuronal excitability that could be linked to insomnia disorder have been described (Ban et al., 2011; Jansen et al., 2019). Nevertheless, none of these findings fully explains the entire cascade involved in the genesis of insomnia, nor do they help to effectively understand the development of the disease in each patient.

Theoretical models have been developed in recent decades in an attempt to explain key points in the course of insomnia that could contribute to the investigation and treatment of patients. These models are much more useful and didactic than previous ones in the clinical approach to insomnia. The behavioral model proposed by Spielman and collaborators (1987) is the oldest, most articulated, and most cited regarding the etiology of chronic insomnia. Also known as the 3P model, it postulates that predisposing, precipitating, and perpetuating factors are involved in the genesis of insomnia (Conway et al., 2019).

Predisposing factors refer to factors that increase vulnerability to developing insomnia, such as old age, female gender, an irregular sleep–wake cycle, a hyperalert condition, a personal and/or family history of insomnia, and the presence of psychiatric comorbidities (anxiety and/or depression) (Rafihi-Ferreira & Soares, 2012; Spielman et al., 1987). Insomnia is commonly precipitated by stressful events, for example, the diagnosis of an illness, unemployment, divorce, interpersonal conflicts, difficulties at work, and financial losses. These factors contribute to the development of short-term insomnia (Conway et al., 2019; Spielman et al., 1987). The factors that perpetuate insomnia are related to behaviors that prolong the duration of this condition. Spending excessive time in bed and taking daytime naps can lead to an irregular sleep–wake cycle. Furthermore, if the bed or the room becomes a place for carrying out daily activities like studying, working, eating, watching TV, or using cell phones, tablets and notebooks, the reflex conditioning involving bed-relaxation-sleep will be broken. In addition to inadequate behaviors for good quality sleep, patients may have erroneous and dysfunctional beliefs regarding sleep ("if I don't sleep 8 hours per night, I will have countless damages to my health"; "if I don't sleep well tonight, I won't be able to study tomorrow"; "my insomnia is the result of some chemical dysfunction"). These beliefs function as mediators of insomnia, contributing to its perpetuation (Graci, 2005; Paltiel & Greenwald, 2008).

In general, a set of factors is associated with the development of insomnia. The constant interaction between biological, behavioral, and environmental factors of the individual must be considered to understand the etiology of insomnia (Rafihi-Ferreira & Soares, 2012). Within this context, predisposing, precipitating, and perpetuating factors can interfere with the homeostatic process and increase arousal and alertness, resulting in insomnia (Berger, 2009).

4.5 Clinical Presentation

Clinical manifestations can be as varied as the factors that modulate the presentation of insomnia, so that each patient becomes the bearer of his own characteristics and course. This variability encourages the discussion about the delimitation of new phenotypes of the disease (see below). Nevertheless, it is possible to identify elements that are commonly found in cases of insomnia and that would help with the recognition of the condition. For didactic purposes, the clinical presentation of insomnia can be divided into daytime and nighttime symptoms, as shown in Table 4.1.

It can be noted that insomnia disorder is a 24-h condition, affecting the individual in physical, psychological, and functional domains, although nocturnal phenomena are the defining factors of the disease. The difficulty in initiating and maintaining sleep is the trigger for a series of symptoms that simultaneously cause and perpetuate the condition. The patient develops irritability and anguish in the face of the obstacle, which can give rise to the feeling of impotence and hopelessness. Ruminating thoughts is a phenomenon that permeates this whole scenario and is a major barrier to the process of falling asleep. The hyperarousal state probably even modulates the perception of time, which helps explain the fact that many individuals with insomnia underestimate their sleep time, reaching extremes as in cases of poor sleep perception (or paradoxical insomnia). This negative context usually occurs in

Table 4.1 Clinical characteristics of insomnia

Daytime symptoms	Nighttime symptoms
Fatigue	Ruminating thoughts
Irritability	Somatic symptoms
Anxiety	Irritability
Somatic symptoms	Anxiety
Excessive concern about sleep	Hyperalertness
Depressive mood	
Malaise	
Cognitive symptoms	
Excessive sleepiness	

the supposed sleep environment—the bed, which involuntarily transforms it into a scenario of conflict and agony, with persistence of symptoms.

The individual with insomnia shows during the day many of the consequences of a bad night's sleep, although there is a wide variation in these symptoms among patients. Fatigue, tiredness, malaise, and irritability can be cited. Anxious, depressive, and cognitive symptoms (e.g., difficulty concentrating and forgetfulness) are common and usually have a great functional impact, affecting the individual in the family, occupational, and academic spheres, among others. The risk of errors and accidents is increased and there is great loss of quality of life (Ohayon & Reynolds, 2009). It must be noted that a proportion of this population does not experience excessive sleepiness, reflecting the hyperarousal state that is so typical of this condition. Individuals with insomnia who are drowsy may not rarely exhibit reduced objective total sleep time; in addition, they may have other sleep disorders, a fact reinforcing the importance of paying attention to this symptom since it indicates a more severe condition and poor prognosis (Vgontzas & Fernandez-Mendoza, 2013).

4.6 Phenotypes of Insomnia

Diseases characterized by a broad spectrum of symptoms are usually divided or categorized for better identification and even for more specific treatments. This requirement perfectly applies to insomnia but its categorization is still incipient, a fact that can probably be explained by the phenomenological complexity of the disease.

A priori phenotypic classification of a disease based on its clinical presentation and/or associated etiological factors is common. This applies to insomnia, for which subdivisions based on its possible causes are available but were abandoned by the latest editions of clinical manuals, as reported earlier, while classification based on clinical presentation, which is more practical and simpler, has been maintained (see Table 4.2).

It must be noted that the classification based on sleep duration is more recent; although not yet used by clinical manuals, it has been gaining prominence. This classification is derived from studies that demonstrate a more severe condition and worse prognosis in insomnia patients with short sleep duration (Vgontzas & Fernandez-Mendoza, 2013; Vgontzas et al., 2013). The definition of short sleep duration is still imprecise and should consider objective sleep time (determined by objective methods such as actigraphy and polysomnography) and recommendations of ideal sleep duration for each age group. Different cut-off points are reported in the literature, although a cut-off of 6 h predominates (Vgontzas & Fernandez-Mendoza, 2013).

Certainly, the classifications mentioned above are still far from encompassing all dimensions of insomnia, especially those related to cognition, mood, family history, patient experience, personality, sleep architecture, genetics, and neuroimaging. These gaps may suggest the need for establishing new phenotypes that, in turn,

Table 4.2 Already applied phenotypic classification of insomnia

Etiology:
Idiopathic/primary insomnia
Psychophysiological insomnia
Insomnia associated with poor sleep hygiene
Paradoxical insomnia
Insomnia associated with mental disorders
Behavioral insomnia of childhood
Insomnia associated with medical conditions
Physiological insomnia
Insomnia associated with substance use or withdrawal
Clinical presentation:
Time of night
Initial insomnia
Maintenance insomnia
Terminal insomnia (early morning awakening insomnia)
Course
Acute
Recurrent
Chronic
Duration of sleep
Short sleep duration
Normal sleep duration

permit to improve the way insomnia is assessed and treated. New models are being published and seek greater validation, such as the model proposed by Blanken et al. (2019) that delimits phenotypes based on life history and on affective and personality traits, and models based on genetic analysis (Stein et al., 2018; Hammerschlag et al., 2017).

4.7 Conclusions

- Insomnia is a multifaceted condition that manifests differently in different patients.
- Insomnia is an extremely common complaint in health services today and should be duly recognized and assessed.
- Insomnia disorder affects the individual globally, with a great impact on function and quality of life.

– Characterization of the patient with insomnia regarding clinical presentation and factors that modulate the condition is important. The determination of new phenotypes of insomnia depends on these features and should guide the treatment.

References

American Academy of Sleep Medicine. (2014). *International classification of sleep disorders*. American Academy of Sleep Medicine.

American Psychiatry Association. (2013). *Diagnostic and statistical manual of mental disorders*. American Psychiatric Association.

Ban, H., Kim, S., Seo, J., Kang, H., & Choi, J. (2011). Genetic and metabolic characterization of insomnia. *PLoS One, 6*(4), e18455.

Berger, A. M. (2009). Update on the state of the science: Sleep-wake disturbances in adult patients with cancer. *Oncology Nursing Forum, 36*(4), E165–E177.

Blanken, T., Benjamins, J., Borsboom, D., Vermunt, J., et al. (2019). Insomnia disorder subtypes derived from life history and traits of affect and personality. *Lancet Psychiatry, 6*(2), 151–163. https://doi.org/10.1016/s225-0366(18)30464-4

Coelho, F., & Rizzo, G. (2019). Fisiopatologia do transtorno da insônia. In A. Bacelar, L. R. Pinto Jr., & Colaboradores (Eds.), *Insônia: do diagnóstico ao tratamento* (pp. 29–36). Difusão Editora.

Conway, S. G., Muller, M. R., & Rafihi-Ferreira, R. (2019). Tratamento não farmacológico do transtorno da insônia. In A. Bacelar, L. R. Pinto Jr., & Colaboradores (Eds.), *Insônia: do diagnóstico ao tratamento* (pp. 117–138). Difusão Editora.

Espie, C., Broomfield, N., MacMahon, K., MacPhee, L., & Taylor, L. (2006). The attention-intention-effort pathway in the development of psychophysiologic insomnia: A theoretical review. *Sleep Medicine Reviews, 10*(4), 215–245. https://doi.org/10.1016/j.smrv.2006.03.002

Graci, G. (2005). Pathogenesis and management of cancer related insomnia. *The Journal of Supportive Oncology, 3*, 349–359.

Hammerschlag, A., Stringer, S., de Leeuw, C., et al. (2017). Genome-wide association analysis of insomnia complaints identifies risk genes and genetic overlap with psychiatric and metabolic traits. *Nature Genetics, 49*(11), 1584–1592. https://doi.org/10.1038/ng.3888

Hasan, R., & Brasil, I. S. P. S. (2019). Conceitos e Classificação do Transtorno da Insônia. In A. Bacelar, L. R. Pinto Jr., & Colaboradores (Eds.), *Insônia: do diagnóstico ao tratamento* (pp. 15–27). Difusão Editora.

Hertenstein, E., Feige, B., Gmeiner, T., Kienzler, C., Spiegelhalder, K., Johann, A., & Baglioni, C. (2018). Insomnia as a predictor of mental disorders: A systematic review and meta-analysis. *Sleep Medicine Reviews, 43*, 96–105. https://doi.org/10.1016/j.smrv.2018.10.006

Jansen, P., Watanabe, K., Stringer, S., Skene, N., et al. (2019). Genome-wide analysis of insomnia in 1,331,010 individuals identifies new risk loci and functional pathways. *Nature Genetics, 51*(3), 394–403. https://doi.org/10.1038/s41588-018-0333-3

Johnson, E. O., Roth, T., Schultz, L., & Breslau, N. (2006). Epidemiology of DSM-IV insomnia in adolescence: Lifetime prevalence, chronicity, and an emergent gender difference. *Pediatrics, 117*(2), e247–e256. https://doi.org/10.1542/peds.2004-2629

Morphy, H., Dunn, K., Lewis, M., Boardman, H., & Croft, P. (2007). Epidemiology of insomnia: A longitudinal study in UK population. *Sleep, 30*(3), 274–280.

Ohayon, M., & Reynolds, C. (2009). Epidemiological and clinical relevance of insomnia diagnosis algorithms according to the DSM-IV and the international classification of sleep disorders (ICSD). *Sleep Medicine, 10*(9), 952–960. https://doi.org/10.1016/j.sleep.2009.07.008

Ohayon, M. M., Carskadon, M. A., Guilleminault, C., & Vitiello, M. V. (2004). Meta-analysis of quantitative sleep parameters from childhood to old age in healthy individuals: Developing normative sleep values across the human lifespan. *Sleep, 27*(7), 1255–1273. https://doi.org/10.1093/sleep/27.7.1255

Paltiel, O., & Greenwald, R. (2008). Sleep and quality of life in cancer patients. In J. C. Verster, S. R. Pandi-Perumal, & L. Streiner (Eds.), *Sleep and quality of life in clinical medicine* (pp. 469–481). Humana Press.

Perlis, M., Posner, D., Riemann, D., Bastien, C., Teel, J., & Thase, M. (2022). Insomnia. *The Lancet, 400*(10357), 1047–1060. https://doi.org/10.1016/S0140-6736(22)00879-0

Poon, S., Quek, S., & Lee, T. (2021). Insomnia disorders: Nosology and classification past, present and future. *Journal of Neuropsychiatry and Clinical Neurosciences, 33*(3), 194–200. https://doi.org/10.1176/appi.neuropsych.20080206

Rafihi-Ferreira, R., & Soares, M. R. Z. (2012). Insônia em Pacientes com Câncer de Mama. *Estudos de Psicologia, 29*(4), 597–607.

Schutte-Rodin, S., Broch, L., Buysse, D., Dorsey, C., & Sateia, M. (2008). Clinical guideline for the evaluation and management of chronic insomnia in adults. *Journal of Clinical Sleep Medicine, 4*(5), 487–504.

Singareddy, R., Vgontzas, A. N., Fernandez-Mendoza, J., Liao, D., Calhoun, S., Shaffer, M. L., & Bixler, E. O. (2012). Risk factors for incident chronic insomnia: A general population prospective study. *Sleep Medicine, 13*, 346–353. https://doi.org/10.1016/j.sleep.2011.10.033

Spielman, A. J., Caruso, L. S., & Glovinsky, P. B. (1987). A behavioral-perspective on insomnia treatment. *The Psychiatric Clinics of North America, 10*, 541–553.

Stein, M., McCarthy, M., Chen, C., et al. (2018). Genome-wide analysis of insomnia disorder. *Molecular Psychiatry, 23*(11), 2238–2250. https://doi.org/10.1038/s41380-018-0033-5

Vgontzas, A., & Fernandez-Mendoza, J. (2013). Insomnia with short sleep duration: Nosological, diagnostic and treatment implications. *Sleep Medicine Clinics, 8*(3), 309–322. https://doi.org/10.1016/j.jsmc.2013.04.009

Vgontzas, A., Fernandez-Mendoza, J., Liao, D., & Bixler, E. (2013). Insomnia with objective short sleep time duration: The most biologically severe phenotype of the disorder. *Sleep Medicine Reviews, 17*(4), 241–254. https://doi.org/10.1016/j.smrv.2012.09.005

World Health Organization. (2018). *The International Classification of Diseases (ICD-11)*. http://www.icd.who.int. World Health Organization. Accessed 12 Oct 2022.

Chapter 5
Insomnia: Its Comorbidities and Differential Diagnosis

Daniel Guilherme Suzuki Borges

5.1 Introduction

Insomnia is a prevalent medical complaint that often coexists with other illnesses such as psychiatric disorders, neurological and medical conditions (see Boxes 5.1 and 5.2). Its diagnosis remains essentially clinical, but eventually complementary exams (e.g., labs, polysomnography, and actigraphy) are necessary when there are suspicions of concomitant medical conditions (Schutte-Rodin et al., 2008; Riemann et al., 2017).

The health provider should perform a thorough clinical interview and examination to assess both physical and mental health to address this disorder (Bonnet et al., 2014). The aim of this evaluation is to help identify comorbidities that may be contributing to the insomnia and eventually exclude medical and psychiatric conditions that may mimic it. These factors prevent patients from receiving proper treatment.

5.2 Comorbidity

Comorbidity is the term when at least two distinct diseases or disorders occur in the same patient at same time. Previously, insomnia was regarded as an accessory symptom rather than a disease itself, and it is no longer considered "primary" or "secondary" (depending on the presence or not of a comorbid disturbance). Its relationship with other illnesses is generally complex, and it is not clear if insomnia would remit once the related condition is solved (NIH, 2005).

D. G. S. Borges (✉)
Institute of Psychiatry, Faculty of Medicine, University of Sao Paulo (FMUSP), Sao Paulo, SP, Brazil

R. El Rafihi-Ferreira (ed.), *Acceptance and Commitment Therapy for Insomnia*,
https://doi.org/10.1007/978-3-031-50710-6_5

Box 5.1: Common Medical Conditions Comorbid with Insomnia

- **Neurology**: e.g., restless legs syndrome, stroke, Alzheimer disease, Parkinson disease, epilepsy, chronic pain disorders, traumatic brain injury, peripheral neuropathy, neuromuscular disorders.
- **Cardiology**: e.g., congestive heart failure, angina pectoris, cardiac arrhythmias.
- **Pulmonology**: e.g., sleep apnea, asthma, emphysema, chronic bronchitis.
- **Gastrointestinal**: e.g., gastroesophageal reflux disease, peptic ulcer disease, cholelithiasis, irritable bowel syndrome.
- **Genitourinary**: e.g., urinary incontinence, benign prostatic hypertrophy, interstitial cystitis.
- **Gynecology**: e.g., menopause, pregnancy.
- **Endocrinology**: e.g., hypothyroidism, hyperthyroidism, diabetes mellitus.
- **Musculoskeletal**: e.g., rheumatoid arthritis, osteoarthritis, fibromyalgia, disc herniation

Adapted and modified from Schutte-Rodin et al. (2008)

Box 5.2: Common Psychiatric Disorders Comorbid with Insomnia

- **Mood disorders**: e.g., major depressive disorder, bipolar mood disorder, cyclothymia dysthymia.
- **Anxiety disorders**: e.g., generalized anxiety disorder, panic disorder, posttraumatic stress disorder, obsessive compulsive disorder, phobias.
- **Psychotic disorders**: e.g., Schizophrenia, schizoaffective disorder, substance-induced psychotic disorders.
- **Others disorders**: e.g., attention-deficit/hyperactivity disorder, adjustment disorders.

Adapted and modified from Schutte-Rodin et al. (2008)

Given these facts, the preferred term is "comorbid insomnia" (APA, 2013; AASM, 2014), for example, comorbid insomnia with depressive disorder, comorbid insomnia with obstructive sleep apnea (COMISA), comorbid insomnia with chronic pain, and comorbid insomnia with substance use disorders, etc. The new status comes as a need to emphasize that insomnia should be given more attention independently of the co-occurring condition. The "secondary insomnia" approach may promote inadequate treatment when assuming the therapeutic of comorbid condition is sufficient to resolve its sleep problem.

As persistent or residual insomnia may represent a risk factor, and a poor predictor for several medical and psychiatric conditions (Hertenstein et al., 2019), both insomnia and the concomitant conditions must be assessed and treated. In addition, insomnia may be associated with new onset or relapse from major depressive disorder, as well as anxiety disorders, substance use disorders, etc.

If left untreated, insomniacs may misuse medications or alcohol to help them fall asleep and deal with anxiety, or even consume psychostimulants (e.g., caffeine) to alleviate fatigue or somnolence. This pattern of substance abuse may lead to a substance use disorder in addition to worsening insomnia (Hertenstein et al., 2019).

Regarding general medical conditions, short-sleep duration insomnia (objectively measured sleep time < 6 h) has been shown to represent a significant risk factor for numerous cardiovascular diseases (Fernandez-Mendoza, 2017), including hypertension, coronary artery disease, stroke, etc.

Therefore, it is fundamental that comorbid conditions be adequately diagnosed and treated for a successful treatment plan (Sateia et al., 2017). Consider medical or specialized referral (neurology, pneumology, ENT, psychiatry, pediatrics, sleep medicine) for a joint assessment and treatment of patients with insomnia problems.

5.3 Differential Diagnosis

5.3.1 Acute Insomnia

Acute insomnia is a common reaction to any significant (positive or negative) life status changes, just as stressful events, diseases, anticipatory anxiety, job promotion, marriage, birth of children, etc. (APA, 2013; AASM, 2014). The condition usually remits spontaneously in a few days or weeks, and symptoms are not frequent enough to meet the three-month duration criteria for chronic insomnia disorder.

Some individuals will develop maladaptive patterns of thought and behavior that will eventually result in the development of a chronic insomnia disorder.

5.3.2 Short Sleepers

Some individuals require relatively little sleep and have no daytime repercussions and symptoms (APA, 2013; AASM, 2014). They have no difficulties in falling or staying asleep, but may be worried about their sleep duration. Some of them may try to spend more time in bed, creating anxiety and conditioning that can make sleep difficult and shorter.

It is a long time characteristic remoting from childhood persisting through lifetime. If its amount is below what is expected for each age group, a "short sleeper" phenotype should be suspected (see Table 5.1).

Table 5.1 Summary of sleep duration expected during lifespan

Age group	Mean duration (hours)
Newborn	14–17
Infant (4–11 months)	12–15
Toddler (1–2 years)	11–14
Preschool (3–5 years)	10–13
School age (6–13 years)	9–11
Teenager	8–10
Adult	7–9
Older adult	7–8

Adapted and modified from Hirshkowitz et al. (2015)

5.3.3 Sleep Deprivation

Sleep deprivation refers to a persisting reduction in the sleep hours required for optimal functioning, usually an amount of time below the recommended for the age group (APA, 2013; AASM, 2014).

Individuals may experience daytime sleepiness, fatigue, reduced performance, memory and concentration deficits, increased risk of accidents, as well as detrimental effects on psychological and physical health. However, some people may not have clear daytime consequences or may have little perceived mild symptoms.

It is not easy to determine the sleep need of an individual. One method to assess this aspect could be by evaluating sleep during long periods of free time (e.g., vacations). Other approach involves determining how long a person would sleep if left to awaken spontaneously on a regular basis, including weekends and holidays. On this case, the individual must report no fatigue, somnolence, or sleep rebound.

5.3.4 Circadian Rhythm Sleep–Wake Disorder

It occurs due to desynchrony and incompatibility between the required or desired social agenda in relation to the endogenous sleep–wake rhythm (APA, 2013; AASM, 2014). Because of this, individuals may experience insomnia, daytime sleepiness, or both.

The amount of sleep is normal in periods when individuals have the opportunity to sleep freely, for example, during vacations. These patients tend to remain asymptomatic and without daytime impairment in such occasions. The specific patterns vary according to the underlying disorder:

– Delayed sleep–wake phase disorder (DSPD): This condition results in delayed sleep onset, rarely occurring before midnight. Sleep onset insomnia often occurs due to the disparity between the endogenous sleep rhythm and desired or acceptable social schedule. Sleep deprivation on workdays and rebounds on days off are commons feature.

- Advanced sleep–wake phase disorder (ASPD): It manifests as advanced sleep onset, so patients complain of somnolence early in the evening. Sleep offset arises prior to scheduled time and patients cannot get back to sleep, but its amount is normal.
- Irregular sleep–wake rhythm disorder (ISD): In ISD, there are polyphasic sleep spread across the 24-hour day. Therefore, sleep and wake times are erratic throughout the day. It's a common feature in advanced neurodegenerative disorders (e.g., Alzheimer disease, Parkinson disease).
- Non-24-hour sleep–wake rhythm disorder or free-running: Patients with this condition cannot synchronize their sleep with the external 24-hour day. Sleep onset and cessation happen later and later each day (or the opposite), so there are alternating periods of insomnia, excessive sleepiness, or both, with a short asymptomatic period.
- Shift work disorder: It occurs in shift workers with an irregular sleep and wake schedule. People usually complain of insomnia, excessive daytime sleepiness, or both (Fig. 5.1).

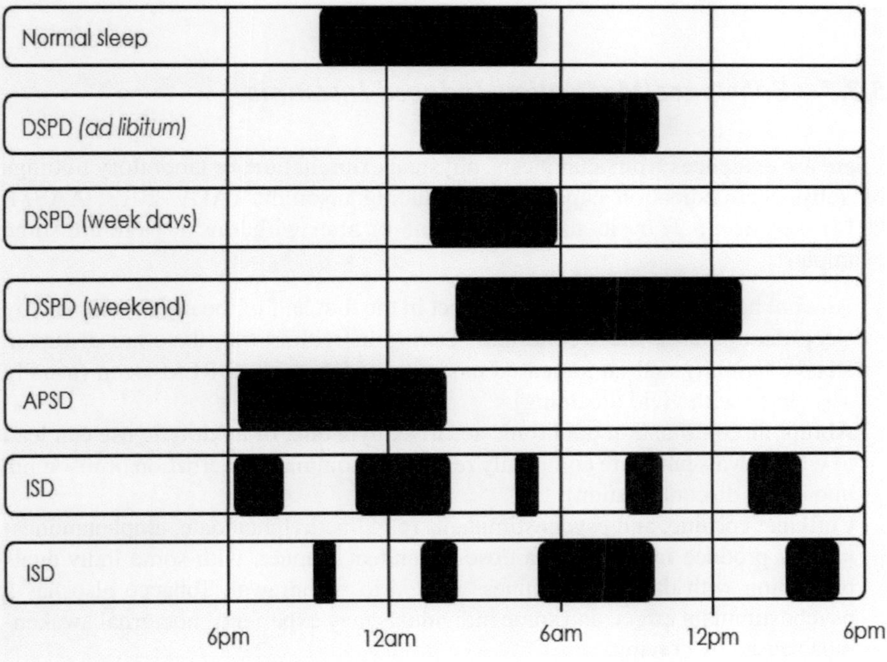

Fig. 5.1 Schematic representation of the major CRSD. Black bars represent sleep periods

5.3.5 Restless Legs Syndrome

It is a common sleep-related movement disorder characterized by an unpleasant or uncomfortable urge to move the legs. It generally occurs during periods of inactivity, particularly in the evenings, and is transiently relieved by movement (APA, 2013; AASM, 2014) and eventually spreads to other body parts such as the arms.

Because of this characteristic of nocturnal appearance or worsening, patients often complain of sleep onset insomnia and, occasionally of night awakenings. However, an urge to move the legs and any accompanying unpleasant leg sensations are features that differentiate this affection from the insomnia disorder.

5.3.6 Sleep Apnea

Most sleep apnea patients (or bed partners) report loud snoring, respiratory pauses during sleep and excessive daytime sleepiness (APA, 2013; AASM, 2014). Many of these individuals may complain of fragmented sleep, difficulty of maintaining it, and of not being restorative.

5.3.7 Substance/Medication-Induced Insomnia

There are evidences from anamnesis, physical examination, or laboratory findings of substance/medication capable of producing insomnia (APA, 2013; AASM, 2014) (see Box 5.3) by its use, intoxication or after withdrawal. Here are some examples:

- Alcohol has a short-lived sedative effect in the first half of the night, followed by sleep disruption in the second half. During its withdrawal, there are disrupted sleep continuity and an increased amount and intensity of REM sleep (usually associated with vivid dreaming).
- Abrupt discontinuation of chronic sedative, hypnotic, or anxiolytic use can lead to withdrawals but more commonly rebound insomnia (exacerbation of insomnia upon drug discontinuation).
- Caffeine, cocaine, and psychostimulants (e.g., methylphenidate, amphetamines) usually produce insomnia in a dose-dependent manner, with some individuals presenting with daytime sleepiness related to withdrawal. Tobacco also has a psychostimulant effect, and some individuals may experience nocturnal awakenings caused by craving.

Box 5.3: Common Contributing Medications and Substances to Insomnia

- **Antidepressants**: e.g., fluoxetine, paroxetine, sertraline, citalopram, escitalopram, fluvoxamine, venlafaxine, desvenlafaxine, duloxetine, moclobemide.
- **Stimulants**: e.g., caffeine, methylphenidate, d-amphetamine, lisdextroamphetamine, ephedrine, cocaine.
- **Decongestants**: e.g., pseudoephedrine, phenylephrine, phenylpropanolamine.
- **Narcotic analgesics**: e.g., oxycodone, codeine, propoxyphene.
- **Cardiovascular**: β-Blockers, α-receptor agonists and antagonists, diuretics, lipid-lowering agents.
- **Pulmonary**: theophylline, albuterol.
- **Alcohol**.

Adapted and modified from Schutte-Rodin et al. (2008)

5.3.8 Hypomania/Mania

Hypomania and mania are hallmarks for bipolar disorder. One common feature is the decreased need for sleep (APA, 2013). In these particular cases, patients report a fully refreshed sleep despite its shortening.

Abnormally elevated, expansive, or irritable mood are hallmarks to diagnose hypomania and mania. It may be accompanied by disinhibited and impulsive behaviors, engagement in excessive activities, and even features not perceived as problematic like increased productivity.

5.3.9 Anxiety Disorders

The individuals with psychophysiological insomnia have significant anxiety and fear of the sleeping process (initiating, performance, arousals, duration, and quality) and imagined (often catastrophizing) daytime repercussions (APA, 2013; AASM, 2014). These cause heightened bodily and cognitive arousals and specifically focus on sleep, unless insomnia is a comorbid condition.

5.4 Conclusions

- Insomnia is highly comorbid with medical and psychiatric conditions. Although its diagnosis is clinical and medical referral is frequently necessary.
- There are medical conditions or disorders that may mimic insomnia.
- It is essential to recognize and treat comorbid conditions for a successful insomnia therapy.

References

American Academy of Sleep Medicine (AASM). (2014). *International classification of sleep disorders* (3rd ed.). American Academy of Sleep Medicine.

American Psychiatry Association (APA). (2013). *Diagnostic and statistical manual of mental disorders*. American Psychiatric Association.

Bonnet, M. H., Burton, G. G., & Arand, D. L. (2014). Physiological and medical findings in insomnia: Implications for diagnosis and care. *Sleep Medicine Reviews, 18*(2), 111–122.

Fernandez-Mendoza, J. (2017). The insomnia with short sleep duration phenotype: An update on it's importance for health and prevention. *Current Opinion in Psychiatry, 30*(1), 56–63.

Hertenstein, E., et al. (2019). Insomnia as a predictor of mental disorders: A systematic review and meta-analysis. *Sleep Medicine Reviews, 43*, 96–105.

Hirshkowitz, M., et al. (2015). National Sleep Foundation's updated sleep duration recommendations: Final report sleep. *Health, 1*(4), 233–243.

NIH State-of-the-Science Conference Statement. (2005). Manifestations and management of chronic insomnia in adults. *NIH Consensus and State-of-the-Science Statements, 22*(2), 1–30.

Riemann, D., et al. (2017). European guideline for the diagnosis and treatment of insomnia. *Journal of Sleep Research, 26*(6), 675–700.

Sateia, M. J., Buysse, D. J., Krystal, A. D., Neubauer, D. N., & Heald, J. L. (2017). Clinical practice guideline for the pharmacologic treatment of chronic insomnia in adults: An American Academy of sleep medicine clinical practice guideline. *Journal of Clinical Sleep Medicine, 13*(2), 307–349.

Schutte-Rodin, S., et al. (2008). Clinical guideline for the evaluation and management of chronic insomnia in adults. *Journal of Clinical Sleep Medicine, 4*(5), 487–504.

Chapter 6
Hypnotic Dependence and Withdrawal

Israel Soares Pompeu de Sousa Brasil and Rosa Hasan

6.1 Hypnotics: A Story About Dependence

Insomnia is one of the most reported conditions in clinical practice and usually has substantial physical and psychological implications for patients (Avidan & Neubaner, 2017). Studies rank insomnia among the ten neuropsychiatric conditions that cause the most suffering around the world, a fact that helps explain its great treatment appeal (Collins et al., 2011). Motivated by this urgency, drug therapy with hypnotics emerged as a practical and immediate solution to the problem. However, what came next turned out to be something as or even more harmful than the disease itself—hypnotic dependence.

The title of the first "hypnotic drug" used in clinical practice can be attributed to a barbiturate, barbital, introduced in 1903, followed by phenobarbital in 1912 (Lader, 1991). Its spectrum of action was expanded by anticonvulsant and anxiolytic functions, which gave rise to other barbiturates over subsequent years. It did not take long for the first cases of dependence and overdosing to appear and benzodiazepines (BZDs) became the hypnotic drug class of choice. The first BZD, chlordiazepoxide, discovered in 1955 was followed by diazepam in 1963 (Lader, 1991). Today, there are more than 30 BZD derivatives, a number that indicates the absolute success of this drug class (Soyka, 2017). The number of people in the United States who received a BZD prescription increased by 67% between 1996 and 2013 (Lembke et al., 2018). Furthermore, most users were found not to take the medication as prescribed by the doctor or even to misuse it, a phenomenon that is more

I. S. P. de Sousa Brasil (✉)
Institute of Medical Assistance to State Civil Servants of São Paulo (IAMSPE), Sao Paulo, Brazil

R. Hasan
Institute of Psychiatry, Hospital das Clínicas, FMUSP, Sao Paulo, Brazil
e-mail: r.hasan@hc.fm.usp.br

R. El Rafihi-Ferreira (ed.), *Acceptance and Commitment Therapy for Insomnia*,
https://doi.org/10.1007/978-3-031-50710-6_6

common among young people between 18 and 25 years of age (Maust et al., 2019). The number of deaths from overdose involving BZDs consistently increased between 1999 and 2015 (Lembke et al., 2018); this fact has an even greater impact and becomes more complex by observing that opioid overdose deaths involve many individuals who also use BZDs (Jones & McAninch, 2015). Once it realized the extent of the catastrophe, in September 2020, the American health regulatory agency, the Food and Drug Administration (FDA), recognized that BZDs are associated with a risk of abuse, addiction, and other harmful effects (U.S. Food and Drug Administration, 2020).

Corroborating the maxim that history tends to be cyclical, a new drug class was launched on the market in the early 1990s with the promise of becoming a safer alternative to BZDs: the selective $GABA_A$ complex agonists, or more popularly known as "Z-drugs" (e.g., zolpidem, zaleplon, zopiclone, and eszopiclone). In fact, prescriptions of these new drugs are progressively replacing those of BZDs, with a 30-fold increase in the number of these prescriptions between 1993 and 2007 (Moloney et al., 2011), once again determining their space in the drug market. However, what has also been noticed is that many of the harmful effects of BZDs that led to the growth of the new class are also being documented among users of Z-drugs, with reports of tolerance, abstinence, cognitive effects, an association with accidents, and dependence (Schilano et al., 2019).

Once again, mankind is cornered and overcome by drugs that have not yet managed to produce the much-desired "perfect sleep", the holy grail of sleep pharmacology in clinical practice. Indeed, people continue to suffer from the side effects of these drugs and do not realize that, in fact, sleeping requires "getting back to basics". For this process to unravel, it is necessary to understand what, in fact, is happening today regarding these drugs, especially BZDs and Z-drugs.

6.2 General Concepts

6.2.1 Hypnotic Drugs and the GABA Receptor Complex

There are several commercially available drugs with hypnotic effects, although many of them have no formal indication for treating insomnia. The hypnotic effect can be due to different mechanisms depending on the medication used, and it is not uncommon that the same drug produces such effect through multiple and intricate pathways. For example, sedative antidepressants usually facilitate sleep due to their action on different neurotransmitters, but especially by antagonizing histaminergic pathways. The action of hypnotic drugs most associated with dependence (BZDs and Z-drugs), however, is based on another site: the GABA receptor complex.

Gamma-aminobutyric acid, or GABA, is one of the main inhibitory neurotransmitters in the central nervous system. It acts on receptors located on the presynaptic and postsynaptic membranes of neurons (GABA receptors), facilitating the opening of local chloride channels that results in hyperpolarization and consequent inhibition of neural transmission (Engin et al., 2018). These receptors have a complex conformation in the membrane (hence the name GABA receptor complex). They are composed of several protein subunits that determine different types of complexes. BZDs and Z-drugs bind at specific sites between the α and γ subunits of $GABA_A$ receptors (they have no effect on $GABA_B$ receptors), acting as allosteric modulators that modify the conformation of the receptor in order to facilitate the opening of chloride channels and thus potentiate the inhibitory effect of GABA (Miller & Aricescu, 2014).

The different patterns of the $GABA_A$ complex (which, as mentioned, are determined by the combination of subunits) show a varied distribution throughout the brain. Activation of a specific pattern of the $GABA_A$ complex mediates the different clinical effects of BZDs: for example, the action on α_1 subunits is associated with a sedative effect and action on α_2 and α_3 subunits with an anxiolytic effect. Z-drugs differ from BZDs exactly in terms of this feature: these drugs act more selectively, especially in complexes with α_1 subunits, which are more associated with a hypnotic effect (Sanna et al., 2002). This is exactly why Z-drugs do not exert some of the clinical effects observed for BZDs, such as anxiolytic and anticonvulsant effects.

In general, BZDs show good absorption and strong protein binding and are lipophilic (Griffin et al., 2013). Most BZDs are metabolized in the liver via microsomal oxidation or demethylation, followed by glucuronidation. Since some BZDs already possess a hydroxyl group (such as lorazepam and oxazepam), they are metabolized directly by glucuronidation and have a shorter half-life. Cytochrome P450 3A4 (CYP3A4) is involved in the metabolism of BZDs and its inhibition by other drugs can slow down the process and promote accumulation of these drugs. In addition, many BZDs have active metabolites, which further prolong the effect of the drug (Peng et al., 2022). Thus, the half-life of BZDs is highly variable and this fact must be considered in the clinical management of patients. These drugs may have a short half-life (such as triazolam, lorazepam, alprazolam, and bromazepam) or a longer half-life (such as diazepam, clobazam, and clonazepam) (Soyka, 2017).

In view of their anxiolytic, hypnotic, myorelaxant, and anticonvulsant effects, BZDs are useful in different clinical scenarios and are commonly indicated for the treatment of anxiety disorders and for the management of withdrawal syndrome such as alcohol withdrawal (Baldwin et al., 2013). The safety of BZDs is not well established when used for more than 4 weeks (Lader, 2011), and dependence has been shown to develop in half of the patients who use these drugs for more than 1 month (de las Cuevas et al., 2003). There are many side effects that can limit the use of BZDs (e.g., lethargy, dizziness, excessive sleepiness, stupor, cognitive deficits) and are often associated with accidents and falls (Gustavsen et al., 2008; Wagner et al., 2004). The concomitant use of opioids potentiates all of these effects and should be avoided. The prescription of BZDs to older adults must be discouraged since this population is known to be more susceptible to these risks (Berrymen et al., 2012). Z-drugs are specifically indicated for the treatment of insomnia but are also not formally approved for long-term use. This class has been found to have the same disadvantages as BZDs in terms of side effects and the development of tolerance and dependence (Schilano et al., 2019), although the level of evidence is not the same as that established for BZDs.

6.2.2 Mechanisms of Tolerance and Dependence

The physiological basis of the dependence process involves the mesolimbic reward system. Drugs that promote the release of dopamine in this area are potential causes of addiction (Lüscher & Ungless, 2006; Saal et al., 2003). Studies have shown that BZDs bind to $GABA_A$ receptors on interneurons in the ventral tegmental area which, in turn, triggers the activation of dopaminergic neurons (Tan et al., 2010). Physiological dependence on BZDs may even occur after a few weeks of use (Gerada & Ashworth, 1997).

Substance dependence comprises different clinical conditions that determine and characterize the pathophysiological process. Phenomena such as drug tolerance (loss of effect of the substance at a defined dose or the need to increase the dose to obtain the same effect), rebound (recurrence of the original symptoms at greater intensity after discontinuation of the drug), and withdrawal syndrome (a set of symptoms that occur after cessation or dose reduction of a substance) corroborate the diagnosis.

Tolerance to the hypnotic effects of BZDs appears to be more pronounced than tolerance to their anxiolytic effects (American Psychiatric Association, 1990). Drug tolerance can be mediated by different, not yet well-established, mechanisms such as alterations in the expression of $GABA_A$ complex subunits, compensatory activity of other neurotransmitter pathways, and less effective opening of the chlorine channels of the complex (Allison & Pratt, 2003; Bateson, 2002). Rebound involves symptoms that can be confused with withdrawal symptoms: these symptoms are usually new to the patient and include anxiety, agitation, insomnia, and sensory (e.g., paresthesia, tinnitus) and motor (e.g., tremor, spasms) alterations, in addition to more severe conditions such as epileptic seizures and delirium (Soyka, 2017). Withdrawal is due to the disinhibition of glutamatergic pathways, previously inhibited by the GABAergic effect of BZDs (Peng et al., 2022). Studies also suggest the contribution of other factors such as downregulation of BZD receptor sites in the GABA receptor complex, increased calcium flux, and elevated serotonergic activity (Baldwin, 2022). Withdrawal symptoms tend to occur earlier with the use of short half-life BZDs (within 2 to 3 days after discontinuation) compared to BZDs with a longer half-life (within 5–10 days) (Soyka, 2017); these symptoms usually start gradually, reach a peak, and subside slowly over a total period of less than 4 weeks (Baldwin, 2022).

6.2.3 Diagnostic Criteria

Many terms have been used to better characterize the phenomenon of dependence, which help delimit its different domains. Phenomena such as tolerance and withdrawal syndrome are usually listed as criteria that confirm the diagnosis.

The fourth edition of the Diagnostic and Statistical Manual of Mental Disorders (DSM-IV) employed the classification of "abuse" and "dependence" in which the first highlights social aspects (impairment of interpersonal relationships and legal problems) and the second emphasizes clinical aspects. The subsequent edition (DSM-V), in turn, eliminated this division and implemented the concept of substance use disorder, defined by 11 criteria (see Box 6.1). The severity of the condition is assigned based on the number of criteria met (2–3 criteria: mild; 4–5 criteria: moderate; 6 or more criteria: severe).

Box 6.1: Diagnostic Criteria for Substance Use Disorder According to DSM-V (American Psychiatry Association, 2013)

Substance use disorder

A problematic pattern of substance use leading to clinically significant impairment or distress, as manifested by at least two of the following criteria that must occur for a minimum period of 12 months:

- The substance is often taken in larger amounts or over a longer period of time than was intended.
- Persistent desire or unsuccessful efforts to reduce or control use of the substance.
- A great deal of time is spent in activities related to obtaining, using, or recovering from the effects of the substance.
- Craving, strong desire, or urge to use the substance.
- Recurrent use of the substance resulting in failure to fulfill roles at home, work, or school.
- Continued use of the substance despite persistent or recurrent social or interpersonal problems caused or exacerbated by its effects.
- Giving up or reducing important social, occupational, or recreational activities due to use of the substance.
- Continued use of the substance even in situations in which it poses risks to physical integrity.
- Use of the substance is continued despite knowledge of having a persistent or recurrent physical or psychological problem that tends to be caused or exacerbated by this use.
- Tolerance, defined as a markedly reduced effect with continued use of the same amount of the substance and/or the need for progressively larger amounts of the substance to achieve the same degree of intoxication.
- Withdrawal, as expressed by withdrawal syndrome characteristic of the substance used and/or use of the substance or a similar one to avoid withdrawal symptoms.

On the other hand, the 10th and the new 11th edition of the International Classification of Diseases (ICD-10 and ICR-11, respectively) adopted the expression "substance dependence" to designate this condition (see Box 6.2), in addition to establishing another clinical scenario, which would be hierarchically inferior and clinically milder than that of dependence—"harmful substance use" (ICD-10) or "harmful pattern of substance use" (ICD-11). Both classifications identify cases in which the substance causes damage to the user's health but no dependence relationship has yet been established. The latest edition adds that such harm may also be suffered by another person related to the patient (World Health Organization, 2018).

Box 6.2: Diagnostic Criteria for Substance Dependence According to ICD-10 and ICD-11

ICD-10:

The diagnosis of dependence should be made **if three or more of the following criteria have been experienced or exhibited during the previous year**:

- A strong desire or sense of compulsion to take the substance.
- Difficulties in controlling substance-taking behavior in terms of initiation, termination, or levels of use.
- A physiological withdrawal state when substance use has ceased or been reduced, as evidenced by the characteristic withdrawal syndrome for the substance, or use of the same substance (or a closely related one) with the intention of relieving or avoiding withdrawal symptoms.
- Evidence of tolerance such that increasing doses of the psychoactive substance are required to achieve effects originally produced by lower doses.
- Progressive neglect of alternative pleasures in favor of psychoactive substance use: increased amounts of time necessary to obtain or take the substance or recover from its effects.
- Persisting with substance use despite clear evidence of overtly harmful consequences, such as liver damage due to heavy drinking or depressive mood states consequent to periods of excessive consumption.

ICD-11:

The diagnosis requires **2 or all 3 criteria** described below to be present simultaneously in the individual and to occur repeatedly over a period of at least 1 year, or continuously over a period of at least 1 month:

- Loss of control over substance use—in terms of the onset, volume, circumstances, or termination of use—often, but not necessarily, accompanied by a subjective sensation of craving or urge to use the substance.
- Substance use becomes an increasing priority in life such that it takes precedence over other interests or pleasures, daily activities, responsi-

(continued)

Box 6.2 (continued)

bilities, or personal and healthcare. It assumes an increasingly central role in the individual's life and relegates other areas to a secondary plane. Substance use often persists despite the occurrence of problems.

- Physiological phenomena (indicative of neuroadaptation to the substance) manifested as: (1) tolerance; (2) withdrawal symptoms after cessation or reduction in the use of the substance, or (3) repeated use of the substance (or a pharmacologically similar one) to prevent or alleviate withdrawal symptoms. These symptoms must be characteristic for that substance and must not simply reflect a hangover effect.

6.3 Hypnotic Dependence

6.3.1 Epidemiology

Epidemiological data on hypnotic dependence are heterogeneous. The factors responsible for this variation include the diagnostic criteria chosen in each study, the geographic region studied, and the substances chosen for evaluation. In general, the use of BZDs increases with advancing age and is more frequent among women (Petitjean et al., 2007). A German population study used the abuse and dependence classification according to the DSM-IV criteria and found a prevalence of 0.8% for abusive use of sedatives in both sexes. The prevalence of dependence was 1.4% among men and 1.3% among women. A prevalence of sedative abuse of 1.1% has been reported in the United States (Huang et al., 2006). A retrospective study found that BZD use was twice as prevalent in women as in men (Olfson et al., 2015).

The following risk factors for developing BZD dependence have been described in the literature (Kan et al., 2004):

- A low educational level.
- Prescription at a young age.
- Belonging to ethnic minority groups.
- Presence of more severe depressive and anxiety symptoms.
- A history of alcoholism and dependence on other substances.
- Characteristics of BZD use: higher dosage, short half-life option, and concomitant use of other psychotropics (Okumura et al., 2016).

Patients with dependence syndrome tend to adopt certain patterns of behavior that have been documented from clinical experience and may even help identify these cases. These behavioral patterns include the following (Soyka, 2017):

- Anxiety symptoms between doses.
- Frequent return to appointments for prescription renewal.
- The patient himself/herself increasing the dose.

Table 6.1 Clinical presentation of hypnotic withdrawal

Anxiety	Tremor	Epileptic seizures
Depression	Sweating	Hyperacusis
Irritability	Nausea/vomiting	Photophobia
Delirium	Agitation	Sleepiness
Depersonalization	Dyspnea	Dysesthesia
Derealization	Headache	Cognitive deficits
Sleep disorder	Tachycardia	Involuntary movements

- "Doctor shopping" (visiting different doctors to obtain multiple prescriptions)
- Use of hypnotics during the day.
- Belief of the necessity of BZD use for daily activities.
- Reporting loss of prescription.
- Keeping pills close by for "emergencies".

Withdrawal symptoms are diverse and may vary among patients (see Table 6.1). It should be noted that the symptoms are not specific; depending on the context, it is prudent to investigate other causes of these symptoms. Differential diagnoses include hypoglycemia, stroke, electrolyte changes, and intoxication by other substances (Soyka, 2017).

6.3.2 Treatment

There are no straightforward or objective answers as to how to treat dependence syndrome or substance use disorder. No universal guidelines are available. Therapeutic alternatives are varied and each patient may require a specific management; thus, treatment should be individualized. However, there are some consensual recommendations that can guide patient management. In general, treatment covers different aspects. Care should include the adoption of measures even before the diagnosis of dependence, at the time of prescription of the hypnotic. Once the diagnosis is established, treatment can be divided into three pillars: gradual discontinuation of the drug, treatment of withdrawal symptoms, and a psychotherapeutic approach (see Fig. 6.1).

The recommendations for each item are described in the following sections.

6.3.2.1 Hypnotic Discontinuation

Once the diagnosis of dependence on a hypnotic drug (generally a BZD or Z-drug) is established and a harmful context for the patient has been determined, it is necessary to define the best strategy in order to dismantle this scenario. Before starting this process, it would be useful to reflect on the disease that led to the use of the medication in order to identify new therapeutic approaches for its resolution.

Prevention

PRIMARY

- Assessing alternatives to BZDs/Z-drugs
- Addressing psychic comorbidities
- Paying attention to risk factors for dependence
- Prescription of a lower dose with shorter effective duration

SECONDARY

- Avoiding automatic renewal of prescription
- Clinical audits
- Clinical meetings

TERTIARY

- Patient care
- Following protocols

Treatment

HYPNOTIC DISCONTINUATION

- Institutionalization and/or outpatient regimen
- Gradual dose reduction
- Switching to long half-life BZD (questionable)
- Polypharmacy → BZD monotherapy

WITHDRAWAL SYNDROME

- Symptomatic medications
- Anticonvulsants/mood stabilizers (carbamazepine, oxcarbazepine, pregabalin, gabapentin)
- Antidepressants

PSYCHOTHERAPEUTIC APPROACH

- Psychoeducation
- Cognitive behavioral therapy/acceptance and commitment therapy
- Motivational interviewing

Follow-up

- Treatment of residual/persistent insomnia
- Adequate management of mental health comorbidities
- Addressing socioeconomic risk factors
- Monitoring and patient care channel

Fig. 6.1 Summary of recommendations for the approach to hypnotic dependence

Different clinical factors, ranging from the drug taken by the patient and the duration of its use to the patient's psychic profile, must be considered when defining the best discontinuation strategy. For this very reason, there is no single protocol that could universally be recommended. Several studies using different approaches to BZD withdrawal have been published, including a Cochrane review (Darker et al., 2015) that found different levels of evidence for each of these strategies.

From a practical point of view, the first factor to be defined in the process of hypnotic discontinuation is the need for institutionalization (hospitalization or a day hospital regimen) (Peng et al., 2022). More severe cases of dependence may be better managed in a more controlled environment. The following characteristics suggest this management (Miller et al., 2018):

- A history of unsuccessful attempts to discontinue the drug.
- Use of very high doses (>100 mg diazepam or equivalent per day).
- High risk of seizures or other withdrawal complications.
- Other concomitant substance use disorders.
- Decompensated clinical or mental health comorbidities.

Institutionalization allows the simultaneous use of several approaches, a more accurate and careful dose titration of the drug, and prompt management of any complication.

There is consensus (with a high level of evidence) that slow and gradual withdrawal from hypnotics is one of the pillars of dependence treatment (Soyka, 2017). Its aim is to minimize the risk of complications during discontinuation, such as epileptic seizures and withdrawal symptoms. Several dose reduction schemes have been published; in practice, what will determine the speed of dose reduction is the patient's ability to tolerate the symptoms. Schemes can range from a 50% reduction in the BZD dose weekly to a 10–25% dose reduction every 2 weeks (Soyka, 2017). A total withdrawal period of 4 to 6 or 4 to 8 weeks seems to be sufficient in most cases and care should be taken not to prolong this period too much (Lader et al., 2009).

It is relatively common in clinical practice to switch the BZD used to another BZD with a longer half-life (clonazepam or diazepam) as part of the withdrawal strategy. This approach enables slower titration (as occurs when a drop formulation is used), which would reduce the risk of developing withdrawal symptoms. However, judging by studies in the literature, there is no clear evidence that this strategy results in good outcomes (Ashton, 2002). If the patient is using several BZDs, there is good evidence that conversion to a single BZD with a longer half-life can indeed be beneficial during the withdrawal period (Soyka, 2017).

Many patients who are dependent on hypnotics also use opioids. It is recommended that the dose of the opioid used be maintained during BZD discontinuation in order to minimize the risk of developing withdrawal symptoms (Lintzeries & Nielsen, 2010).

6.3.2.2 Pharmacological Treatment

There are no formally recommended medications (or approved by the FDA) for the specific treatment of hypnotic dependence syndrome or its withdrawal symptoms (Peng et al., 2022). Thus, pharmacological treatment becomes empirical and symptomatic. Many studies have evaluated some of these medications; however, the level of evidence is low and they are used off-label.

Anticonvulsants and mood stabilizers are often used for withdrawal treatment, especially from alcohol (Barrons & Roberts, 2010). However, the level of evidence is much lower for hypnotics. Carbamazepine/oxcarbazepine is a widely cited option (Lader, 2014); gabapentin and pregabalin are also listed but with far fewer studies (Mariani et al., 2016). The anxiolytic effect of these drugs may be useful in these cases. There are also protocols for the use of phenobarbital as prophylaxis of epileptic seizures in rapid BZD discontinuation regimens during hospitalization (Kawasaki et al., 2012). There is no evidence on the benefit of lithium, buspirone, or propranolol (Baandrup et al., 2018).

The medication may also be directed toward the treatment of sleep disorders, although an abrupt change of BZD is not recommended. Antidepressants with a hypnotic effect (e.g., trazodone, doxepin, mirtazapine), which facilitate sleep due to their predominantly antihistamine action, are recommended. Other antidepressants (such as serotonin reuptake inhibitors) may be used to treat anxiety symptoms. Studies have reported some improvement in sleep with melatonin (Baandrup et al., 2018) and flumazenil (Faccini et al., 2016) but, in general, the effect is still questionable.

6.3.2.3 Psychological/Behavioral Approach

Many types of behavioral or psychotherapeutic approaches have been studied. In fact, several models of structured intervention exist that range from short to long follow-up periods depending on the patient's needs and profile. In general, the objectives are to facilitate discontinuation of the hypnotic drug, to manage the withdrawal status, and to address both the underlying disorder and mental health comorbidities that the patient may have (Baldwin, 2022; Lader et al., 2009).

Psychoeducation is generally the first approach used (Ten Wolde et al., 2008). Presentations, texts, or letters addressed to the patients that contain information about the condition and its causes, symptoms, consequences, and treatment can provide the stimulus and initial motivation that would encourage the patient to engage in weaning from the hypnotic. Simple measures such as the doctor sending a letter to the patient encouraging treatment can have a positive prognostic effect (de Gier et al., 2011), although it is important to concomitantly invest in other approaches (Mugunthan et al., 2011).

Motivational interviewing is a counseling method that is often used in substance dependence treatments, although evidence on its use in cases involving hypnotics is still very limited. The method seeks to encourage patients to reassess their situation, analyzing the advantages and disadvantages of their behavior. By targeting the capacity to change and the expectation of improvement, motivational interviewing induces behavioral changes that may be useful for the progression of treatment (Miller & Rollnick, 2012).

Cognitive behavioral therapy (CBT) is considered the gold standard treatment for chronic insomnia disorder (Trauer et al., 2015). Although the degree of effectiveness is not the same, this therapy is also important for the management of BZD dependence (Lader et al., 2009). Among psychotherapeutic approaches, CBT has the largest number of studies in the literature and the highest level of evidence; it is also the most used approach (Darker et al., 2015). The aims of CBT are to address new behavioral repertoires, to manage dysfunctional beliefs about the condition, and to teach how to deal with expectations. For this purpose, CBT comprises different techniques that include relaxation exercises, simulations of risk scenarios, and problem-solving approaches. Measures that are usually adopted in CBT for insomnia disorder, such as sleep hygiene, stimulus control and bedtime restriction, can also be applied to these patients (Morin et al., 1994). Analysis of the evidence in the literature suggests that the therapeutic success of CBT for BZD dependence is still not guaranteed. Within this context, one study with a 15-month follow-up demonstrated that the efficacy of a controlled protocol of hypnotic withdrawal was superior to a usual approach combined with CBT (Voshaar et al., 2003). A review reported only a short-term beneficial effect, with the observation of a good response after 3 months when combined with gradual discontinuation of the hypnotic drug, but not after 6 months (Darker et al., 2015).

Acceptance and commitment therapy (ACT) is relatively new and part of the third wave of behavioral therapies. Its use in patients with chronic insomnia disorder has not been extensively documented in the literature but the results are promising (Lappalainen et al., 2019; Paulos-Guarnieri et al., 2022; El Rafihi-Ferreira et al., 2020; El Rafihi-Ferreira et al., 2022). The level of evidence on the use of ACT in patients with hypnotic dependence is even lower but a pilot trial has suggested a good response. The study found a reduction in the mean number of BZD pills and Z-drugs taken per day among patients treated with CBT combined with elements of ACT, in addition to a reduction in the number of hypnotic drug users after 6 months (Chapoutot et al., 2021).

Several other techniques can be employed, although their level of evidence is very limited. Group, couple, or family therapies are also suitable models. Psychodynamic and psychoanalytical approaches can be useful and tend to focus on the tolerance of negative emotions, problem-solving strategies, and the sense of frustration that permeates the state of substance dependence (Soyka, 2017).

6.3.3 Prognosis

In general, the prognosis of patients after treatment of hypnotic dependence is relatively good (Soyka, 2017). However, short-term outcomes can be very variable and long-term outcomes are poorly documented (Baldwin, 2022). Studies suggest that two-thirds of patients are able to remain BZD free soon after treatment but only one-third remain abstinent in the long term (Voshaar et al., 2006). The impact of simple measures such as psychoeducation on the prognosis of many of these patients should be highlighted. Studies report discontinuation of BZD use in 20–49% of patients who received this intervention (Voshaar et al., 2003; Bashir et al., 1994; Cormack et al., 1994).

The following factors have been reported to reduce the success of withdrawal (Schweizer et al., 1998; O'Connor et al., 1999, 2004):

- Clinical comorbidities: more severe symptoms of anxiety and depression, personality traits such as neuroticism, a diagnosis of panic disorder, and concomitant use of alcohol.
- A low socioeconomic level.
- Greater pharmacological complexity: higher dose of the hypnotic, prolonged duration of treatment, very fast discontinuation, and use of a short half-life BZD.

Withdrawal-associated psychological symptoms may persist in some patients even after 5 years (Golombok et al., 1987). Post-acute withdrawal syndrome is the term designated by some authors to refer to prolonged withdrawal symptoms that can include headache, paresthesia, anxiety, depression, and motor signs such as tremor and spasms (Ashton, 1991). These are more complex cases and there are no recommendations for specific formal treatment, with the same measures as mentioned above being used (Miller et al., 2018). Resolution of these symptoms is usually observed within 6–12 months but they may also persist for years in some cases (Cosci & Chouinard, 2020).

The risk of relapse or return to misuse of hypnotic drugs must be considered and monitored. Data on this phenomenon are limited but some predictive factors have been reported (Voshaar et al., 2003, 2006; Morin et al., 2005; Mol et al., 2007):

- Previous use of high BZD doses (>10 mg of diazepam or equivalent per day).
- Persistent insomnia.
- Self-perception of greater disease severity.
- Daily consumption of alcohol.
- Craving for BZD.

It should also be remembered that, in many cases, the use of BZDs is facilitated and/or perpetuated by socioeconomic factors that may not have subsided after discontinuation (unemployment, mourning, financial difficulties, abusive relationships), a context that also facilitates the return to hypnotic use (Baldwin, 2022).

6.3.4 Prevention

Knowing the complexity of hypnotic dependence, its harmful effects and treatment, preventive measures are urgently needed. A systematic review identified factors that can be fundamental for this process and highlighted that measures need to be implemented at all levels of care (Sirdifield et al., 2017). At the primary level, the aim is to avoid, if possible, the prescription of BZDs, especially to risk groups such as older adults (Schwitz, 2021). If prescribed, it is always necessary to determine the duration of medication use (which should be as short as possible), avoiding a significant dose increase. One may even suggest transient discontinuation during treatment, if clinically and pharmacologically possible. Risk factors for dependence in these patients must be identified and addressed, such as psychiatric comorbidities, chronic pain (which may be related to concomitant opioid use), alcohol abuse, sleep disorders, and risky personality traits for the condition (Sirdifield et al., 2017).

During follow-up, automatic prescription renewal of these drugs must be restricted or avoided. Integrated information systems and clinical audits carried out by care services can be useful to identify possible deviations and inappropriate prescriptions. Education campaigns and meetings on the topic among health professionals are equally important (Smith & Tett, 2010).

The patient, who is the target of all attention, must be monitored continuously from the time the hypnotic is prescribed to the post-treatment phase regarding use of the drug, possible side effects, changes in the clinical condition, and possible outcomes. Patients must have easy access to the healthcare service in order to ensure their safety and make them feel welcome.

6.4 Conclusions

- The excessive use of hypnotic drugs has been a matter of concern over the last century and has persisted until today because of the false promise of an immediate solution to sleep disorders, which are increasingly more common.
- Hypnotic drugs, especially BZDs and Z-drugs, have many adverse effects, including the risk of falls, cognitive alterations, and respiratory depression, which can culminate in the phenomena of tolerance and dependence.
- Dependence syndrome or substance use disorder associated with hypnotic drugs is a complex, heterogeneous clinical condition with an uncertain prognosis. Measures preventing the misuse of BZDs and Z-drugs should be implemented at all levels of healthcare.
- There are no universal guidelines for the treatment of hypnotic dependence but consensus recommendations exist that should guide patient management. Different clinical factors must be considered when determining the best treatment for the patient.
- The treatment generally consists of three pillars: gradual discontinuation of the hypnotic drug, the use of other drugs to relieve withdrawal symptoms, and a psychotherapeutic approach, with CBT being the technique with the highest level of evidence in the literature.
- Patient care comprises the period from before the prescription of BZD or Z-drug to follow-up after discontinuation in order to establish an objective and accurate treatment, in addition to monitoring complications and/or relapse of the disorder.

References

Allison, C., & Pratt, J. (2003). Neuroadaptive process in GABAergic and glutamatergic systems in benzodiazepine dependence. *Pharmacology & Therapeutics, 98*(2), 171–195.

American Psychiatry Association. (1990). *Benzodiazepine dependence, toxicity, and abuse: A task force report of the American Psychiatric Association*. American Psychiatric Pub.

American Psychiatry Association. (2013). *Diagnostic and statistical manual of mental disorders*. American Psychiatric Association.

Ashton, H. (1991). Protracted withdrawal syndromes from benzodiazepines. *Journal of Substance Abuse Treatment, 8*(1–2), 19–28.

Ashton, H. (2002). Benzodiazepine abuse. In W. Caan & J. de Belleroche (Eds.), *Drink, drugs and dependence: From science to clinical practice* (pp. 197–212). Routledge.

Avidan, A. Y., & Neubaner, D. N. (2017). Chronic insomnia disorder. *Continuum (Minneap Minn), 23*(4), 1064–1092.

Baandrup, L., Ebdrup, B. H., Rasmussen, J. Ø., et al. (2018). Pharmacological interventions for benzodiazepine discontinuation in chronic benzodiazepine users. *The Cochrane Database of Systematic Reviews, 3*, CD011481.

Baldwin, D. S. (2022). Clinical management of withdrawal from benzodiazepine anxiolytic and hypnotic medications. *Addiction, 117*(5), 1472–1482.

Baldwin, D. S., Aitchison, K., Bateson, A., et al. (2013). Benzodiazepines: Risks and benefits – A reconsideration. *Journal of Psychopharmacology (Oxford, England), 27*(11), 967–971.

Barrons, R., & Roberts, N. (2010). The role of carbamazepine and oxcarbazepine in alcohol withdrawal syndrome. *Journal of Clinical Pharmacy and Therapeutics, 35*(2), 153–167.

Bashir, K., King, M., & Ashworth, M. (1994). Controlled evaluation of brief intervention by general practitioners to reduce chronic use of benzodiazepines. *British Journal of General Practice, 44*(386), 408–412.

Bateson, A. (2002). Basic pharmacologic mechanisms involved in benzodiazepine tolerance and withdrawal. *Current Pharmaceutical Design, 8*(1), 5–21.

Berrymen, S. N., Jennings, J., Ragsdale, S., Lofton, T., Huff, D. C., & Rooker, J. S. (2012). Beers criteria for potentially inappropriate medication use in older adults. *Medsurg Nursing, 21*(3), 129–132.

Chapoutot, M., Peter-Derex, L., Schoendorff, B., Faivre, T., Bastuji, H., & Putois, B. (2021). Telehealth-delivered CBT-I programme enhanced by acceptance and commitment therapy for insomnia and hypnotic dependence: A pilot randomized controlled trial. *Journal of Sleep Research, 30*(1), e13199.

Collins, P. Y., Patel, V., Joestl, S. S., et al. (2011). Grand challenges in global mental health. *Nature, 475*(7354), 27–30.

Cormack, M. A., Dietze, P., Lee, N., Dunlop, A., & Taylor, D. (1994). Evaluation of an easy, cost-effective strategy for cutting benzodiazepine use in general practice. *British Journal of General Practice, 44*(378), 5–8.

Cosci, F., & Chouinard, G. (2020). Acute and persistent withdrawal syndromes following discontinuation of psychotropic medications. *Psychotherapy and Psychosomatics, 89*(5), 283–306.

Darker, C. D., Sweeney, B. P., Barry, J. M., Farrell, M. F., & Donnely-Swift, E. (2015). Psychosocial interventions for benzodiazepine harmful use, abuse or dependence. *The Cochrane Database of Systematic Reviews, 5*, CD009652.

De Gier, N., Gorgels, W., Lucassen, P., Oude Voshar, R., Mulder, J., & Zitman, F. (2011). Discontinuation of long-term benzodiazepine use: 10-year follow-up. *Family Practice, 28*(3), 253–259.

De las Cuevas, C., Sanz, E., & de la Fuente, J. (2003). Benzodiazepines: More "behavioural" addiction than dependence. *Psychopharmacology, 167*(3), 297–303.

El Rafihi-Ferreira, R., Morin, C. M., Toscanini, A. C., Lotufo, N. F., Brasil, I. S., Gallinaro, J. G., Borges, D. S., Conway, S. G., & Hasan, R. (2020). Acceptance and commitment therapy-based behavioral intervention for insomnia: A pilot randomized controlled trial. *Brazilian Journal of Psychiatry, 43*(5), 1–6. https://doi.org/10.1590/1516-4446-2020-0947

El Rafihi-Ferreira, R., Morin, C. M., Hasan, R., Brasil, I. S., Zago Ribeiro, J. H., Júnior, & Cecília Toscanini, A. (2022). A pilot randomized controlled trial (RCT) of acceptance and commitment therapy versus cognitive behavioral therapy for chronic insomnia. *Behavioral Sleep Medicine, 1–15*, 193. https://doi.org/10.1080/15402002.2022.2071272

Engin, E., Benham, R. S., & Rudolph, U. (2018). An emerging circuit pharmacology of GABAA receptors. *Trends in Pharmacological Sciences, 39*(8), 710–732.

Faccini, M., Leone, R., Opri, S., et al. (2016). Slow subcutaneous infusion of flumazenil for the treatment of long-term, high-dose benzodiazepine users: A review of 214 cases. *Journal of Psychopharmacology, 30*(10), 1047–1053.

Gerada, C., & Ashworth, M. (1997). ABC of mental health: Addiction and dependence – I: Illicit drugs. *BMJ, 315*(7103), 297–300.

Golombok, S., Higgitt, A., Fonagy, P., Dodds, S., Saper, J., & Lader, M. (1987). A follow-up study of patients treated for benzodiazepine dependence. *The British Journal of Medical Psychology, 60*(2), 141–149.

Griffin, C. E., 3rd., Kaye, A. M., Bucno, F. R., et al. (2013). Benzodiazepine pharmacology and central nervous system-mediated effects. *The Ochsner Journal, 13*(2), 214–223.

Gustavsen, I., Bramness, J. G., Skurtveit, S., Engeland, A., Neutel, I., & Mϕrland, J. (2008). Road traffic accident risk related to prescriptions of the hypnotics zopiclone, zolpidem, flunitrazepam and nitrazepam. *Sleep Medicine, 9*(8), 818–822.

Huang, B., Dawson, D. A., Stinson, F. S., et al. (2006). Prevalence correlates and comorbidity of nonmedical prescription drug use and drug use disorders in the United States. *The Journal of Clinical Psychiatry, 67*(07), 1062–1073. https://doi.org/10.4088/JCP.v67n0708

Jones, C. M., & McAninch, J. K. (2015). Emergency department visits and overdose deaths from combined use of opioids and benzodiazepines. *American Journal of Preventive Medicine, 49*(4), 493–501.

Kan, C. C., Hilberink, S. R., & Breteler, M. H. (2004). Determination of the main risk factors for benzodiazepine dependence using a multivariate and multidimensional approach. *Comprehensive Psychiatry, 45*(2), 88–94.

Kawasaki, S. S., Jacapraro, J. S., & Rastegar, D. A. (2012). Safety and effectiveness of a fixed-dose phenobarbital protocol for inpatient benzodiazepine detoxification. *Journal of Substance Abuse Treatment, 43*(3), 331–334.

Lader, M. (1991). History of benzodiazepine dependence. *Journal of Substance Abuse Treatment, 8*(1–2), 53–59.

Lader, M. (2011). Benzodiazepines revisited – Will we ever learn? *Addiction, 106*(12), 2086–2109.

Lader, M. (2014). Benzodiazepines harm: How can it be reduced? *British Journal of Clinical Pharmacology, 77*(2), 295–301.

Lader, M., Tylee, A., & Donaghue, J. (2009). Withdrawing benzodiazepines in primary care. *CNS Drugs, 23*(1), 19–34.

Lappalainen, P., Langrial, S., Oinas-Kukkonen, H., Muotka, J., & Lappalainen, R. (2019). ACT for sleep – Internet-delivered self-help ACT for subclinical and clinical insomnia: A randomized controlled trial. *Journal of Contextual Behavioral Science, 12*, 119–127.

Lembke, A., Papac, J., & Humphreys, K. (2018). Our other prescription drug problem. *The New England Journal of Medicine, 378*(8), 693–695.

Lintzeries, N., & Nielsen, S. (2010). Benzodiazepines, methadone and buprenorphine: Interactions and clinical management. *The American Journal on Addictions, 19*(1), 59–72.

Lüscher, C., & Ungless, M. A. (2006). The mechanistic classification of addictive drugs. *PLoS Medicine, 3*(11), e437.

Mariani, J. J., Malcolm, R. J., Mamczur, A. K., et al. (2016). Pilot trial of gabapentin for the treatment of benzodiazepine abuse or dependence in methadone maintenance patients. *The American Journal of Drug and Alcohol Abuse, 42*(3), 333–340.

Maust, D. T., Lin, L. A., & Blow, F. C. (2019). Benzodiazepine use and misuse among adults in the United States. *Psychiatric Services (Washington, D.C.), 70*(2), 97–106.

Miller, P. S., & Aricescu, A. R. (2014). Crystal structure of a human $GABA_A$ receptor. *Nature, 512*(7514), 270–275.

Miller, W. R., & Rollnick, S. (2012). *Motivational interviewing: Helping people change* (3rd ed.). Guilford.

Miller, S. C., Fiellin, D. A., Rosenthal, R. N., et al. (2018). *The ASAM principles of addiction medicine* (6th ed., pp. 797–803). ASAM.

Mol, A. J., Oude Voshaar, R. C., Gorgels, W. J., Breteler, M. H., van Balkom, A., van de Lisdonk, E., et al. (2007). The role of craving in relapse after discontinuation of long-term benzodiazepine use. *Journal of Clinical Psychiatry, 68*(12), 1894–1900.

Moloney, M. E., Konrad, T. R., & Zimmer, C. R. (2011). The medicalization of sleeplessness: A public health concern. *American Journal of Public Health, 101*(8), 1429–1433.

Morin, C. M., Culbert, J. P., & Schwartz, S. M. (1994). Nonpharmacological interventions for insomnia: A meta-analysis of treatment for insomnia: A meta-analysis of treatment efficacy. *The American Journal of Psychiatry, 151*(8), 1172–1180.

Morin, C. M., Belánger, L., Bastien, C., & Vallières, A. (2005). Long-term outcome after discontinuation of benzodiazepine for insomnia: A survival analysis of relapse. *Behaviour Research and Therapy, 43*(1), 1–14.

Mugunthan, K., McGuire, T., & Glasziou, P. (2011). Minimal interventions to decrease long-term use of benzodiazepines in primary care: A systematic review and meta-analysis. *The British Journal of General Practice, 61*(590), e573–e578.

O'Connor, K., Belánger, L., Marchand, A., Dupuis, G., Elie, R., & Boyer, R. (1999). Psychological distress and adaptational problems associated with discontinuation of benzodiazepines. *Addictive Behaviors, 24*(4), 537–541.

O'Connor, K., Marchand, A., Belánger, L., Mainguy, N., Landry, P., Savard, P., et al. (2004). Psychological distress and adaptational problems associated with benzodiazepine withdrawal and outcome: A replication. *Addictive Behaviors, 29*(3), 583–593.

Okumura, Y., Shimizu, S., & Matsumoto, T. (2016). Prevalence, prescribed quantities, and trajectory of multiple prescriber episodes for benzodiazepines: A 2-year cohort study. *Drug and Alcohol Dependence, 158*, 118–125.

Olfson, M., King, M., & Schoenbaum, M. (2015). Benzodiazepine use in the United States. *JAMA Psychiatry, 72*(2), 136–142.

Paulos-Guarnieri, L., Linares, I. M. P., & El Rafihi-Ferreira, R. (2022). Evidence and characteristics of Acceptance and Commitment Therapy (ACT)-based interventions for insomnia: A systematic review of randomized and non-randomized trials. *Journal of Contextual Behavioral Science, 23*, 1–14. https://doi.org/10.1016/j.jcbs.2021.11.001

Peng, L., Morford, K. L., & Levander, X. A. (2022). Benzodiazepines and related sedatives. *The Medical Clinics of North America, 106*(1), 113–129.

Petitjean, S., Ladewig, D., Meier, C. R., Amrein, R., & Wiesbeek, G. A. (2007). Benzodiazepine prescribing to the Swiss adult population: Results from a national survey of community pharmacies. *International Clinical Psychopharmacology, 22*(5), 292–298.

Saal, D., Dong, Y., Bonci, A., & Malenka, R. C. (2003). Drugs of abuse and stress trigger a common synaptic adaptation in dopamine neurons. *Neuron, 37*(4), 577–582.

Sanna, E., Busonero, F., Talani, G., Carta, M., Massa, F., Peis, M., Maciocco, E., & Biggio, G. (2002). Comparison of the effects of zaleplon, zolpidem and triazolam at various GABAA receptor subtypes. *European Journal of Pharmacology, 451*(2), 103–110.

Schilano, F., Chiappini, S., Corkery, J. M., et al. (2019). An insight into Z-drug abuse and dependence: An examination of reports to the European Medicines Agency Database of suspected adverse drug reactions. *The International Journal of Neuropsychopharmacology, 22*(4), 270–277.

Schweizer, E., Rickels, K., de Martinis, N., Case, G., & García-España, F. (1998). The effect of personality on withdrawal severity and taper outcome in benzodiazepine dependent patients. *Psychological Medicine, 28*(3), 713–720.

Schwitz, A. (2021). Benzodiazepines: The time for systematic change is now. *Addiction, 116*(2), 219–221.

Sirdifield, C., Chipcase, S. Y., Owen, S., & Siriwardena, A. N. (2017). A systematic review and meta-synthesis of patients' experiences and perceptions of seeking and using benzodiazepines and Z-drugs: Towards safer prescribing. *The Patient, 10*(1), 1–15.

Smith, A. J., & Tett, S. E. (2010). Improving the use of benzodiazepines – Is it possible? A non-systematic review of interventions tried in the last 20 years. *BMC Health Services Research, 10*(1), 1–12.

Soyka, M. (2017). Treatment of benzodiazepine dependence. *The New England Journal of Medicine, 376*(12), 1147–1157.

Tan, K. R., Brown, M., Labouèbe, G., et al. (2010). Neural bases for addictive properties of benzodiazepines. *Nature, 463*(7282), 769–774.

Ten Wolde, G. B., Dijkstra, A., van Empelen, P., van den Houit, W., Neven, A. K., & Zitman, F. (2008). Long-term effectiveness of computer-generated tailored patient education on benzodiazepines: A randomized, controlled trial. *Addiction, 103*(4), 662–670.

Trauer, J. M., Qlan, M. Y., Doyle, J. S., et al. (2015). Cognitive-behavioral therapy for chronic insomnia: A systematic review and meta-analysis. *Annals of Internal Medicine, 163*(3), 191–204.

U.S. Food and Drug Administration. (2020). *FDA requiring boxed warning updated to improve safe use of benzodiazepine drug class*. Available at: https://www.fda.gov/drugs/drug-safety-and-availability/fda-requiring-boxed-warning-updated-improve-safe-use-benzodiazepine-drug-class. Accessed 9 Dec 2022.

Voshaar, R. O., Gorgels, W., Mol, A., van Balkom, A., Breteler, M., van de Lisdonk, E., et al. (2003). Predictors of relapse after discontinuation of long-term benzodiazepine use by minimal intervention: A 2-year follow-up study. *Family Practice, 20*(4), 370–372.

Voshaar, R. C., Gorgels, W. J., Mol, A. J., van Balkom, A. J., Mulder, J., van de Lisdonk, E. H., Breteler, M. H., & Zitman, F. G. (2006). Predictors of long-term benzodiazepine abstinence in participants of a randomized controlled benzodiazepine withdrawal program. *Canadian Journal of Psychiatry. Revue Canadienne de Psychiatrie, 51*(7), 445–452. https://doi.org/10.1177/070674370605100706

Wagner, A. K., Zhang, F., Soumerai, S. B., et al. (2004). Benzodiazepine use and hip fractures in the elderly: Who is at greatest risk? *Archives of Internal Medicine, 164*(14), 1567–1572.

World Health Organization. (2018). *The International Classification of Diseases (ICD-11)*. http://www.icd.who.int. World Health Organization. Accessed 12 Oct 2022.

Part II
Assessment of Insomnia

Chapter 7
Initial Interview in the Therapeutic Setting

Ila Marques Porto Linares and Renatha El Rafihi-Ferreira

Satisfactory therapeutic results depend on a careful assessment that considers the client as a whole. Thus, the first step in starting an intervention is to assess the complaint and gather the variables that may be associated with its development and maintenance. The data collection process begins with the initial contact with the client. Based on the collected information, it is then possible to formulate the case. These points are discussed in this chapter, which also explores elements present in the first therapeutic contact such as format and environment for conducting the interview and treatment, the professional qualified to apply ACT, clinical interview, determination whether the client is a candidate for ACT-based therapies, course of treatment, and other treatment options, if necessary.

Case Formulation

The process of case formulation in ACT is essential for the development of intervention strategies that meet the needs of each client. ACT is an approach that is based on functional contextualism; therefore, the case formulation in ACT consists of analysis of the complaints reported by the client considering not only the frequency and type of the complaint but above all its function, context, and history.

Functional contextualism views events as continuous actions of the organism within a historically and situationally defined context and aims to predict and influence these events. The philosophical perspective on functional contextualism is the pragmatic and functional view of radical behaviorism, emphasizing the functional analysis of behavior as the main methodological tool (Hayes et al., 2006; Oshiro & Ferreira, 2021). Based on its theoretical foundation and psychotherapeutic model,

I. M. P. Linares (✉)
Faculty of Medicine, University of São Paulo, São Paulo, Brazil

R. El Rafihi-Ferreira
Department of Clinical Psychology, University of São Paulo, São Paulo, Brazil
e-mail: rerafihi@usp.br

R. El Rafihi-Ferreira (ed.), *Acceptance and Commitment Therapy for Insomnia*,
https://doi.org/10.1007/978-3-031-50710-6_7

ACT does not consist of a combination of procedures and techniques but determines parameters for explanation, intervention, and evaluation of its clinical effectiveness.

Case formulation using a contextual approach considers functional analysis, the identification of processes, intervention planning, and assessment (Ferreira, 2021). The aim of case formulation is to identify relationships between events that occur in the environment and actions of the organism. Investigation of the function of behavior is the main target of case formulation. In this analysis, the antecedents and consequences of which the behavior is a function are sought in the environment. In other words, all behavior must be analyzed considering the context in which it occurs. To investigate the function of a behavior, the occasion when the response occurs is identified, that is, the antecedent, the response, and subsequent consequences. During treatment by the clinician, assessment and intervention are intertwined processes that occur throughout the therapeutic process. Case formulation provides the basis for treatment planning. Identification of the variables of which the behavior is a function is the key step in case formulation.

Case formulation in ACT is structured using the model of psychological flexibility. This model was described in the chapter "Acceptance and Commitment Therapy" of this book. Based on the delimitation of the complaint reported by the client, we seek to identify how the complaint is connected to psychological inflexibility processes (experiential avoidance, cognitive fusion, dominance of the conceptualized past and future, self as content, lack of values, and inaction) and psychological flexibility (acceptance, cognitive defusion, contact with the present moment, self as context, values, and committed actions) (Ferreira, 2021; Sandoz, 2021).

The first step in the formulation or conceptualization of a case is to gather information about the client such as his/her life story, complaint, and expectations. The data collection or evaluation process, which includes the initial interview, is essential to obtain detailed information about the complaint and its context. Based on the case formulation, treatment planning is performed, which requires structuring interventions, the format and frequency of sessions, and therapeutic directions. It is worth noting that treatment planning comprises the strategies and techniques that will be used throughout the intervention.

The process of case formulation and treatment planning in ACT for insomnia complaints does not differ from the case formulation for other complaints described above. In the context of insomnia, careful data collection is necessary and must include objective information on sleep patterns such as sleeping and waking times, time needed to fall asleep, time in bed, and the number and duration of awakenings. These data can be collected based on retrospective and prospective measurements using questionnaires, diaries, and actigraphy. A complete description of these measurements can be found in the chapters "Evaluation and Retrospective Measurements" and "The role of actigraphy and sleep diaries in assessing sleep in adults with insomnia" of this book. In addition to the information about the sleep complaint, data on the individual's context, including how he/she relates to the insomnia complaint and his/her thoughts and feelings, as well as life values, goals, and psychological processes that interfere with the pursuit of these values, are collected.

To understand the complaint of insomnia, the professional must investigate the function of the complaint within the individual's context and to what extent the six processes of psychological inflexibility (experiential avoidance, cognitive fusion, dominance of the conceptualized past and feared future, self as content, lack of values, and inaction) are responsible for maintaining the complaint. Next, once the clinician understood what triggered and might be perpetuating insomnia, the professional is able to better structure the treatment plan and to select strategies and techniques that will be implemented throughout the intervention. During therapy, behavior change occurs based on the progression of the six processes of psychological flexibility. It should be noted that a direct relationship and interconnection exist between assessment, case formulation, and treatment. Thus, neglecting or reducing the relevance of each of these steps will compromise the effectiveness of the proposed treatment.

7.1 Format and Environment for Conducting the Interview and Treatment

The format of the interview and treatment of the sleep complaint can be face-to-face or virtually, individually and in groups, since many studies on CBT-I have confirmed the effectiveness of different formats (Boness et al., 2020). It is worth noting that virtual therapy will permit access to specialized professionals. Although there are no studies that compared online versus face-to-face application of ACT, which does not permit to state categorically how the format interferes with the outcome, studies using different intervention formats with favorable results are available (e.g., individual or group modalities, remote, face-to-face, or self-administered) (Paulos-Guarnieri et al., 2022).

Regarding the therapeutic environment, regardless of the treatment modality adopted, it is important that its structure and conditions provide sufficient comfort, safety, and acceptance. In a virtual environment, the clinician must guide clients to look for a reserved space so that they have privacy to talk about their issues without being interrupted; good quality internet and a screen with an adequate size that allows to visualize psychoeducation and session activities that often require screen sharing are necessary. In a physical environment, the clinician can use a space with a table, blackboard or notebook for psychoeducation and armchairs for the client, professional, and a family member who may accompany the client to a session.

The clinical environment can be located in a sleep center or in an independent clinic/office. Offices within a sleep center complex can provide access to a multidisciplinary team of sleep physicians, neurologists, and psychiatrists. Affiliation of the clinic with a sleep center or association can facilitate client access. The aim of disseminating ACT for insomnia is to make the treatment accessible in private clinics and in public health institutions, including primary care and health services and psychology teaching schools at universities, among others.

Whether in a virtual or physical environment, the clinician must reserve a space to store client records, questionnaires, scales, and materials used in the session.

7.2 Qualified and Appropriate Professional to Apply ACT-Based Therapies for Insomnia

The best qualified professional to apply ACT-based therapy for insomnia is a psychologist trained in ACT who has in-depth knowledge of sleep and its intervention strategies in order to ensure that a duly prepared person with a theoretical and practical basis performs the interventions. It is, therefore, extremely important that professionals invest in their training in terms of both knowledge about sleep and contextual approaches. The therapist's training must consider the constant updating of the scientific literature in the area. In addition to theoretical updates, supervision is essential to improve the quality of clinical care, especially for beginners. Contact with the multidisciplinary team that attends the population with sleep problems is important and can contribute to the evolution of cases.

7.3 First Contact with the Client

The first contact with the client is a critical moment in the establishment of a bond between the professional and client and consequently in the continuation of psychotherapeutic follow-up. Establishing a therapeutic bond is also important for the client to feel comfortable in reporting the necessary information and thus to enable data collection, as well as case formulation and development of a treatment plan.

Some therapist behaviors can favor establishment of the bond, such as an empathetic and understanding attitude, non-judgmental acceptance, authenticity, self-confidence, flexibility, commitment, tolerance, and interest. Gestural behaviors, maintaining eye contact, verbalizing thoughts and feelings, a non-directive attitude, and occasional guidance are also important elements that should be included in the therapist's repertoire (Bandeira et al., 2006).

It is important that the therapist takes care in building this bond, which will contribute to greater adherence and more effective results regarding the client's complaint. Also seeking to establish a good therapeutic relationship and to gather information for case formulation, clinicians must observe their own reactions during the initial interview and throughout the therapeutic process. Within this context, thoughts, feelings, associations, memories, and physical sensations experienced during contact with the client can be relevant data. It is during the first meeting that the professional informs the client about the rules and conditions of therapy, including confidentiality, schedules, absences, session replacement, and session fee.

7.4 Clinical Interview

The diagnosis of insomnia is essentially clinical and requires a careful anamnesis. The initial clinical interview or anamnesis is composed of several elements, including the client's identification (name, age, sex, marital status, profession, religion), cultural and contextual aspects, main complaint (onset of symptoms and triggering and perpetuating factors), personal and family history, medications used, and clinical and psychiatric history. In the field of sleep, the clinical interview also needs to contain some specific elements in order to obtain relevant information for understanding the current presentation.

Therapist

> *When did this problem start?*
> *Was there a time when insomnia was significantly less pronounced?*
> *Does your insomnia have the same intensity, frequency, and duration as when it started?*
> *Do you recognize the complaint or does your partner recognize it?*

Other sleep disorders

Other sleep disorders whose symptoms resemble those of insomnia, but arise from another cause, must be ruled out. These conditions include obstructive sleep apnea, restless legs syndrome, circadian rhythm disorders (phase advance and delay), insomnia secondary to medication use, and poor sleep hygiene.

Therapist

> *Do you snore at night?*
> *Do you have any type of sleep-related discomfort other than insomnia?*

Nocturnal symptoms

Symptoms as difficulty falling asleep, nocturnal awakenings, early morning awakening, and perception of poor sleep quality can occur alone or simultaneously. Additionally, the progression of symptoms and their duration, frequency, and severity are also part of this evaluation step.

Therapist

> *Have you been feeling sleepy during the day?*
> *Do you fall asleep easily during the day?*

Daytime impairments

According to the International Classification of Sleep Disorders (AASM, 2014), symptoms such as fatigue, malaise, impairment in attention, concentration or memory, daytime sleepiness, proneness for errors and accidents, mood disturbance, social and vocational dysfunction, and reduced motivation make up the diagnosis of insomnia.

Therapist

Are the negative impacts of the problem broadening or restricting your life?
Are you finding yourself less attentive or struggling to memorize information that you used to be able to memorize before?

Daytime routine

Considering that sleep is a 24-hour activity, it is necessary to obtain information about daytime habits, work and/or study routine and hours, practice of physical activity (time, frequency, and type of exercise), and napping. It is also extremely important to investigate the use of stimulants such as caffeine and eating habits, including the times and type of food usually consumed.

Therapist

What activities do you usually perform during the day?
What time do you eat your meals?
At what time of day do you perform physical activity?

Sleep routine

Regarding sleep routine, investigation of the sleeping environment is necessary, that is, the conditions of the room (luminosity, noise, temperature). It is also important to identify everything the client does before going to sleep, including activities that take place in the bed/room such as reading and use of electronic devices. The presence of animals in the bed and whether alcohol is consumed close to bedtime must also be investigated.

It is also important to assess which client behaviors are perpetuating factors of insomnia, that is, behaviors that may contribute to the maintenance of insomnia such as going to bed earlier than recommended, napping during the day, increased use of stimulants and use of an inappropriate type/amount, and avoidance of physical activity.

The combination of retrospective and prospective measurements is fundamental. These measurements are part of the initial assessment (see chapter "Evaluation and Retrospective Measurements") and substantially contribute to the direction of decisions and evaluation of the effectiveness of the intervention during the course of treatment.

Therapist

What time do you sleep and wake up during the week and on weekends?
How long does it take you to fall asleep after going to bed?
How long does it take you to get up after waking up?
What activities do you perform before going to bed? What effects do these activities have on your sleep?
In case you use a hypnotic drug to sleep, what is the dosage, amount, and type of medication?

What do you do to try to improve insomnia and what are the effects of these behaviors?
What thoughts about sleep and insomnia run through your head throughout the day and night?
What do you do when you wake up in the middle of the night?

In addition to the questions suggested in this chapter, the professional can use the retrospective and prospective measurements described in the next chapters, which provide data and information that will help with the clinical interview and the understanding of the case.

7.5 Determination if the Client Is a Candidate for ACT-Based Therapies for Insomnia

The association between psychological inflexibility and sleep problems suggests that psychological inflexibility contributes to the maintenance of insomnia (Daly-Eichenhardt et al., 2016). Most of the insomnia-associated problems are related to the attempt to control symptoms and to an exaggerated effort to fall asleep. ACT-based interventions can be useful to reduce the effort to fall asleep by accepting physiological and bodily arousal. These therapies may also increase adherence to stimulus control and sleep restriction techniques, which aim to increase the willingness to experience short-term discomfort produced by behavioral techniques (Dalrymple et al., 2010).

Thus, treating insomnia using an ACT-based intervention is indicated for any population, that is, there are no populations for which ACT for insomnia could be harmful. Regarding this theoretical approach, from the time that a certain complaint produces suffering for the individual, it must become a therapeutic target.

7.6 Course of Treatment

ACT can be applied as monotherapy or in combination with stimulus control and time-in-bed restriction techniques. For this purpose, the sessions should involve the revision of tasks and of the sleep diary, psychoeducation about sleep, and behavioral strategies, as well as the development of psychological flexibility based on the six processes of ACT.

The ACT protocol for insomnia generally comprises 4–14 weeks, with a duration of 60–120 min per session (Paulos-Guarnieri et al., 2022). It is important to mention that ACT addresses complaints beyond sleep; thus, the number of sessions is not necessarily tied to a fixed protocol and it is up to the clinician to determine the number of sessions based on the case formulation. Performing assessments throughout the intervention is important so that the therapist obtains elements as to how the intervention affects sleep and the relationship that the client has with sleep.

7.7 Determination of Other Treatment Options, If Necessary

The set of techniques that compose the CBT-I protocol have the greatest empirical support for the treatment of insomnia and are a treatment option for clients with this complaint. Recently, third-generation behavioral therapies such as mindfulness- and ACT-based therapies have also provided beneficial results. If the combination of these therapies does not show benefits, it is important to reassess the variables involved in the maintenance of the complaint.

The duration of treatment varies from individual to individual and more complex cases may require a longer duration, with results being obtained in the medium and long term. In all cases, an inter- and multidisciplinary approach is recommended along with behavioral therapies for insomnia. Therefore, referral to sleep science professionals, such as a sleep physician in cooperation with a psychologist, is necessary. In cases in which pharmacotherapy is indicated by the sleep physician, non-pharmacological interventions in combination with the medication are recommended. In addition to the psychotherapeutic approach, other interventions such as physical activity and Tai Chi that have shown benefits for insomnia can be part of the list of multidisciplinary care and can contribute positively to quality of life and sleep (Yang et al., 2012; Irwin et al., 2014).

7.8 Conclusion

ACT represents a shift in the insomnia paradigm since it does not focus solely on the sleep complaint and symptom control but on the client as a whole. Hence, the focus of ACT is to promote psychological flexibility and quality of life. To intervene in these aspects and in the variables directly related to sleep, the clinician must invest in the initial contact with the client, exploring the individual's life history and the context of his/her interaction with the complaint. The initial interview is extremely important since case formulation and therapeutic management will be established based on the collection of initial information. Therefore, a careful assessment of the case will improve the therapeutic process.

References

American Academy of Sleep Medicine. (2014). International classification of sleep disorders. 3rd ed. Darien: American Academy of Sleep Medicine.

Bandeira, M., Quaglia, M. A. C., Freitas, L. C., de Sousa, A. M., Costa, A. L. P., Gomides, M. M. P., & Lima, P. B. (2006). Habilidades interpessoais na atuação do psicólogo. *Interação, 10*(1), 139–149.

Boness, C. L., Hershenberg, R., Kaye, J., Mackintosh, M. A., Grasso, D. J., Noser, A., et al. (2020). An evaluation of cognitive behavioral therapy for insomnia: A systematic review and application of Tolin's criteria for empirically supported treatments. *Clinical Psychology (New York), 27*(4), e12348. https://doi.org/10.1111/cpsp.12348

Dalrymple, K. L., Fiorentino, L., Politi, M. C., & Posner, D. (2010). Incorporating principles from acceptance and commitment therapy into cognitive-behavioral therapy for insomnia: A case example. *Journal of Contemporary Psychotherapy, 40*(4), 209–217. https://doi.org/10.1007/s10879-010-9145-1

Daly-Eichenhardt, A., Scott, W., Howard-Jones, M., Nicolaou, T., & McCracken, L. M. (2016). Changes in sleep problems and psychological flexibility following interdisciplinary acceptance and commitment therapy for chronic pain: An observational cohort study. *Frontiers in Psychology, 7*, 1326. https://doi.org/10.3389/fpsyg.2016.01326

Ferreira, T. A. S. (2021). Avaliação e formulação de caso na Terapia de Aceitação e Compromisso. In C. K. B. Oshiro & T. A. S. Ferreira (Eds.), *Terapias Contextuais Comportamentais: análise funcional e prática clínica* (pp. 120–131). Manole.

Hayes, S. C., Luoma, J. B., Bond, F. W., Masuda, A., & Lillis, J. (2006). Acceptance and commitment therapy: Model, processes and outcomes. *Behaviour Research and Therapy, 44*(1), 1–25. https://doi.org/10.1016/j.brat.2005.06.006

Irwin, M. R., Olmstead, R., Carrillo, C., Sadeghi, N., Breen, E. C., Witarama, T., Yokomizo, M., Lavretsky, H., Carroll, J. E., Motivala, S. J., Bootzin, R., & Nicassio, P. (2014). Cognitive behavioral therapy vs. Tai Chi for late life insomnia and inflammatory risk: A randomized controlled comparative efficacy trial. *Sleep, 37*(9), 1543–1552. https://doi.org/10.5665/sleep.4008

Oshiro, C. K. B., & Ferreira, T. A. S. (2021). *Terapias Contextuais Comportamentais: análise funcional e prática clínica*. Manole.

Paulos-Guarnieri, L., Linares, I. P. M., & El Rafihi-Ferreira, R. (2022). Evidence and characteristics of Acceptance and Commitment Therapy (ACT)-based interventions for insomnia: A systematic review of randomized and non-randomized trials. *Journal of Contextual Behavioral Science, 23*, 1–14. https://doi.org/10.1016/j.jcbs.2021.11.001

Sandoz, E. K. (2021). Terapia de aceitação e compromisso: o processo e a prática da mudança consciente [recurso eletrônico]. In S. C. Hayes, K. D. Strosahl, & K. G. Wilson (Eds.), *Tradução: Sandra Maria Mallmann da Rosa; revisão técnica: Mônica Valentim* (2nd ed.). Artmed.

Yang, P. Y., Ho, K. H., Chen, H. C., & Chien, M. Y. (2012). Exercise training improves sleep quality in middle-aged and older adults with sleep problems: A systematic review. *Journal of Physiotherapy, 58*(3), 157–163. https://doi.org/10.1016/S1836-9553(12)70106-6

Chapter 8
Evaluation and Retrospective Measurements

Ila Marques Porto Linares and Marwin do Carmo

8.1 Assessment Strategies for Insomnia

Assessment is essential to clinical practice and should be implemented at different stages throughout insomnia treatment. The assessment must take place before starting treatment for diagnostic purposes; to identify predisposing, precipitating, and perpetuating factors and to survey the harm associated with insomnia. It is also necessary to evaluate during the treatment to examine the course of the implemented intervention and, after the treatment, to reveal the results obtained with the intervention and provide data that support its effectiveness. In this sense, the assessment serves as a compass to guide clinicians in making decisions.

Pre- and post-treatment assessments of insomnia can be performed retrospectively and prospectively. The retrospective format uses instruments that collect complaints and markers within a time interval before the assessment, that is, the presence of markers and complaints in recent months. The prospective format refers to the daily estimates that occur during a specific period, such as using a sleep diary throughout the intervention.

Although there is no standardized assessment format for complaints related to insomnia, like any investigative process, it must be composed of different tools to better track possible elements that outline the complaint in question. Thus, in addition to anamnesis or clinical history, questionnaires, and scales about sleep specific to insomnia and other possible clinical conditions and self-registration usually make up for sleep assessment.

Clinical history characterizes the complaint, whether insomnia is related to difficulties initiating or maintaining sleep, early awakenings, and mixed conditions. Additionally, it seeks to understand the impacts and losses resulting from insomnia and its course, whether continuous, intermittent, or progressive. Comorbidities,

I. M. P. Linares (✉) · M. do Carmo
Faculty of Medicine, University of São Paulo, Sao Paulo, Brazil

R. El Rafihi-Ferreira (ed.), *Acceptance and Commitment Therapy for Insomnia*,
https://doi.org/10.1007/978-3-031-50710-6_8

different clinical conditions, medications, day and night activities, pre-sleep routine, diet, quality of life, and sleep-wake schedules are also essential elements that should be surveyed (Schutte-Rodin et al., 2008).

Measurement scales for assessing insomnia should not be used as the sole diagnostic criteria. Nonetheless, the data obtained using these tools can contribute to this investigation. The remainder of this chapter describes some scales used to assess the severity of insomnia, sleep quality, and general sleep complaints. Scales that investigate chronotypes and other sleep disorders can also be helpful tools at the beginning of an investigative process (the scales described here do not exhaust instruments available in the literature). A summary of the instruments presented in this chapter is displayed in Table 8.1.

8.1.1 A Note on Validity[1]

It is beyond the scope of this chapter to delve into the theoretical and technical aspects of psychological measurement, as they are thoroughly covered in books such as Borsboom (2005). However, it is important to note that when choosing a measurement tool for clinical practice, especially in high-stake settings, it is crucial to exercise caution and thoughtfulness in the selection process. Despite the simplicity and practicality of self-report instruments, it is not sufficient to simply create or translate items on the fly to have a valid tool. Instead, there should be evidence that the instrument can effectively measure the intended construct, as defined by Cronbach and Meehl (1955) as construct validity. Furthermore, it is essential to note that validity is not obtained through a single quantitative index but rather through the accumulation of evidence from various sources that justify the test's uses and interpretations (American Educational Research Association, American Psychological Association, & National Council on Measurement in Education [AERA, APA, and NCME], 2014).

Unfortunately, not all scales published in scientific journals have undergone rigorous construct validation (Flake et al., 2017). Clinicians must make well-informed decisions when choosing a measurement tool by thoroughly examining the chosen instrument. Moreover, it helps to clearly understand the construct you want to assess and its relationship to other variables. To aid in this process, we suggest considering the following points, inspired by Flake and Fried's (2020) questions to increase transparency and avoid questionable measurement practices.

1. Determine whether the authors have clearly defined the measured construct and all relevant variables and processes.

[1] Note that the scales presented in this chapter were not selected *because* of their validity evidence quality but by popularity or innovation in clinical and research settings. Readers should judge the quality matter on their own.

Table 8.1 Instruments for assessment of sleep and complementary variables

Test	Reference	Assesses	Number of items	Components	Validation sample
Sleep assessment instruments					
Insomnia Severity Index (ISI)	Bastien et al. (2001)	Patient's perception of their insomnia	7	Unidimensional	Adults (36–52 years) with insomnia complaints
Pittsburgh Sleep Quality Index (PSQI)	Buysse et al. (1989)	Sleep quality	19	Subjective sleep quality, sleep latency, sleep duration, habitual sleep efficiency, sleep disturbances, use of sleeping medications, and daytime dysfunction.	Adults (24–83 years) with and without sleep problem complaints
Epworth Sleepiness Scale (ESS)	Johns (1992)	Level of daytime sleepiness or sleep propensity	8	Unidimensional	Adults (36–52 years) with and without sleep disorders
Stanford Sleepiness Scale (SSS)	Hoddes et al. (1972)	Sleepiness	7	Unidimensional[a]	Adults over 18 years old
Dysfunctional Beliefs and Attitudes About Sleep Scale (DBAS-16)	Morin et al. (2007)	Beliefs, attitudes, expectations, evaluations, and attributions about sleep	16	Consequences of insomnia; Worry about sleep; sleep expectations; medication	Adults (20–71 years) with insomnia symptoms
Sleep Problem Acceptance Questionnaire (SPAQ)	Bothelius et al. (2015)	Acceptance in insomnia	8	Activity engagement and willingness	Adults (mean age of 42 years and SD = 15) with insomnia complaints
Sleep Acceptance Scale (SAS)	Rafihi-Ferreira et al. (2023)	Sleep acceptance	6	Avoidance and distress	Adults (18–59 years) with and without insomnia complaints
Sleep-Related Behaviours Questionnaire (SRBQ)	Ree and Harvey (2004)	Safety behaviors in insomnia	32	Unidimensional[b]	Adults (18–63 years) with and without insomnia complaints

(continued)

Table 8.1 (continued)

Test	Reference	Assesses	Number of items	Components	Validation sample
Psychological and psychiatric instruments					
Acceptance and Action Questionnaire-II (AAQ-II)	Bond et al. (2011)	Psychological flexibility	10	Unidimensional	Adults over 18 years old across six samples
Brief Experiential Avoidance Questionnaire (BEAQ)	Gámez et al. (2014)	Experiential avoidance	15	Behavioral avoidance, distress aversion, procrastination, distraction/ suppression, repression/denial, and distress endurance	Undergraduate students, psychiatric outpatients, and community adults (age range of 18–62 years)
Multidimensional psychological flexibility inventory (MPFI-24)	Grégoire et al. (2020)	Psychological flexibility and psychological inflexibility	24	Flexibility and inflexibility	Adults with a mean age of 34.2 (SD = 12.4)
Beck Anxiety Inventory (BAI)	Beck et al. (1988)	Anxiety severity	21	Somatic symptoms and subjective anxiety and panic symptoms	Adults with an average of 35 years with affective and anxiety disorders
Beck Depression Inventory (BDI-II)	Beck et al. (1996)	Depression severity	21	Unidimensional	College students and adult and adolescent psychiatric outpatients
Depression Anxiety Stress Scales (DASS-21)	Lovibond and Lovibond (1995) and Antony et al. (1998)	Depression, anxiety, and stress	14	Depression, anxiety, and stress	Adult psychiatric outpatients and nonclinical (age range of 18–65 years)
The Hospital Anxiety and Depression Scale (HADS)	Zigmond and Snaith (1983)	Anxiety and depression	14	Anxiety and depression	Outpatients with ages between 16 and 65 years

(continued)

Table 8.1 (continued)

Test	Reference	Assesses	Number of items	Components	Validation sample
Patient Health Questionnaire (PHQ)	Kroenke et al. (2001)	Depression severity	9	Unidimensional	Adults (18 years or older), primary care and obstetrics-gynecology patients

[a]MacLean et al. (1992) suggested a two-factor structure for the SSS, although their analysis was conducted using a modified version of the scale

[b]Ree and Harvey (2004) did not attempt to find a factorial structure in their paper, so the one-dimensionality of the scale was untested

2. Evaluate the quality of the validity evidence provided and consider its applicability in a specific context.
3. Verify that the instrument appears to measure what you intend to measure, as measures with the same construct name may assess different constructs.
4. Although different versions of the same scale may seem to tap the same construct, differences in item wording, the number of items, or the response format may convey distinct information.
5. Review the scoring rules provided by the authors and exercise caution if an interpretation of the scores is not provided. Usually, the authors suggest how the responses should be scored, such as summing the raw scores, averaging the total score over the number of items, calculating separate component scores, or calculating a standardized score.
6. If modifying an existing scale, ensure that there is a justification for doing so and be aware that any further interpretation will have only qualitative value.

It is also important to note that when using an existing psychological instrument in a distinct context from its original development, it is vital that studies attest to the construct's existence and similarity in the new context (Flake et al., 2017). This process, known as cross-cultural adaptation, requires more than simply translating the test items and instructions. Herdman et al. (1998) proposed a model that assesses five types of equivalence in a cross-cultural adaptation study: conceptual equivalence, item equivalence, semantic equivalence, operational equivalence, and measurement equivalence. The absence of such equivalence evidence seriously threatens the scale validity.

8.2 Sleep-Related Assessment

8.2.1 Sleep Assessment Instruments

- *Insomnia Severity Index* (Bastien et al., 2001): The Insomnia Severity Index (ISI) is a self-reported questionnaire used to measure the severity of insomnia symptoms. It consists of seven items that assess the individual's difficulty initiating sleep, difficulty maintaining sleep, early morning awakening, dissatisfaction with sleep, perception of sleep problems by others, impairment of daytime functioning, and the degree of distress caused by insomnia. Each item is rated on a scale of 0 (no problem) to 4 (very severe problem). The total score ranges from 0 to 28, with scores greater than or equal to 15 indicating the presence of clinically significant insomnia: absence of insomnia (0–7); sub-threshold insomnia (8–14); moderate insomnia (15–21); and severe insomnia (22–28). The ISI is a widely used tool in both research and clinical settings to evaluate the severity of insomnia and monitor changes in symptoms over time.
- *Pittsburgh Sleep Quality Index* (Buysse et al., 1989): The Pittsburgh Sleep Quality Index (PSQI) is a self-reported questionnaire used to measure an individual's sleep quality and patterns. It consists of 19 items that assess 7 components of sleep quality: subjective sleep quality, sleep latency, sleep duration, habitual sleep efficiency, sleep disturbances, use of sleeping medication, and daytime dysfunction. Each component is scored on a scale of 0 to 3, and the total score ranges from 0 to 21. Scores greater than or equal to 5 indicate poor sleep quality, and scores higher than 11 indicate a possible sleep disorder. Examples of questions from the Pittsburgh Sleep Quality Index (PSQI) include the following: (1) *During the past month, how long (in minutes) has it usually take you to fall asleep each night?* (2) *During the past month, how many hours of actual sleep did you get at night?* (3) *During the past month, how would you rate your sleep quality overall?* (4) *During the past month, how often have you taken medicine to help you sleep?*

8.2.2 Sleepiness and Fatigue Instruments

- *Epworth Sleepiness Scale* (Johns, 1992): The Epworth Sleepiness Scale (ESS) is a self-reported questionnaire used to measure an individual's level of daytime sleepiness. It consists of eight items that assess the likelihood of dozing off or falling asleep in different situations, such as sitting and reading, watching television, or sitting inactive in a public place. Each item is rated on a scale of 0 (would *never* doze) to 3 (*high* chance of dozing), with higher scores indicating greater daytime sleepiness. The total score ranges from 0 to 24, with higher scores indicating more severe daytime sleepiness.

– *Stanford Sleepiness Scale* (Hoddes et al., 1972): The Stanford Sleepiness Scale (SSS) is a seven-point subjective measure of the perception of sleepiness, with each level representing a different degree of sleepiness. The levels range from 1 (Feeling active and vital, awake) to 7 (No longer fighting sleep, sleep onset soon). It is a momentary assessment scale and can detect sleepiness as it waxes and wanes over a day.

8.2.3 Sleep Cognitions and Sleep-Related Behavior Instruments

– *Dysfunctional Beliefs and Attitudes About Sleep Scale* (Morin et al., 2007): The Dysfunctional Beliefs and Attitudes About Sleep Scale (DBAS-16) measures sleep-disruptive cognitions, such as beliefs, attitudes, expectations, evaluations, and attributions. Its 16 items were derived from the original 30-item scale and are rated on an 11-point scale ranging from 0 (strongly disagree) to 10 (strongly agree). Similar to the original version, the DBAS-16 assumes a four-factor structure: (a) consequences of insomnia, (b) worry about sleep, (c) sleep expectations, and (d) medication. Examples of items are as follows: (1) *When I sleep poorly on one night, I know it will disturb my sleep schedule for the whole week.* (2) *Without an adequate night's sleep, I can hardly function the next day.* (3) *I have little ability to manage the negative consequences of disturbed sleep.* (4) *I am worried that I may lose control over my abilities to sleep.*
– *Sleep Problem Acceptance Questionnaire* (Bothelius et al., 2015): The Sleep Problem Acceptance Questionnaire (SPAQ) is a self-assessment tool designed to evaluate individuals' acceptance of their sleep issues. As a relatively new measure, it comprises eight items that assess two factors—Activity Engagement and Willingness. Activity Engagement pertains to the extent of an individual's persistence in carrying out routine activities despite dissatisfaction with their sleep quality. On the other hand, Willingness captures the individual's ability to give up the struggle to control and overcome sleep problems. Each item is rated on a 7-point Likert scale, with 0 indicating "Disagree" and six signifying "Completely agree." The total score ranges from 0 to 48, with Willingness items scores being reversed. A higher score implies a lower acceptance of sleep problems. The SPAQ can provide insight into how acceptance of sleep problems may affect treatment outcomes and overall quality of life. The SPAQ includes items such as (1) *Although things have changed, I am living a normal life despite my sleeping problems.* (2) *My life is going well, even though I have sleeping problems.* (3) *I need to concentrate on getting rid of my sleeping problems.* (4) *It's important to keep on fighting these sleeping problems.*
– *Sleep Acceptance Scale* (Rafihi-Ferreira et al., 2023): The Sleep Acceptance Scale (SAS) is a brief self-assessment tool for adults to measure their acceptance of sleep problems. It comprises six items, rated on a scale that ranges from 1

(never) to 7 (always), where higher scores indicate lower acceptance of sleep problems. The questionnaire is divided into two dimensions: Avoidance (two items) and Distress (four items). Some of the SAS items are as follows: (1) *I avoid making plans or doing things I enjoy or need to do because of my sleep*. (2) *The thought of going to sleep makes me uneasy*. (3) *I have negative feelings towards my sleep*. (4) *I am scared of not being able to fall asleep*.

– *Sleep-Related Behaviours Questionnaire* (Ree & Harvey, 2004): The Sleep-Related Behaviours Questionnaire (SRBQ) is a self-report measure comprised of 32 items assessing safety and avoidance behaviors related to sleep problems. Each item is rated on a scale of 0 (Almost never) to 4 (Almost always), where higher scores indicate a greater frequency of sleep-related safety behaviors. The following items are a sample of the behaviors to cope with tiredness or improve sleep assessed by the SRBQ: (1) *I spend time considering ways to improve sleep*. (2) *I reduce my expectations of what I can achieve*. (3) *I give up trying to work*. (4) *I keep busy to stop thinking about my sleep*.

8.2.4 Complementary Instruments for Psychological and Psychiatric Assessment

Psychological and psychiatric aspects, such as anxiety and depression, are recurrently present in the diagnosis of insomnia, acting as part of the cause or by-product of the sleep disorder in question. Therefore, to effectively assess insomnia, it is important to investigate impairments associated with daytime functioning and other relevant factors related to the reported sleep complaint. The following instruments are presented as examples. We describe tools to assess anxiety, depression, and ACT processes, such as psychological inflexibility, flexibility, and acceptance. However, it should be noted that they do not encompass the entirety of the literature; for example, measures such as the State-Trait Anxiety Inventory (STAI) and the Quality of Life Scale (SF-36) are not mentioned.

8.2.4.1 Psychiatric Instruments

– *Beck Anxiety Inventory* (Beck et al., 1988): The Beck Anxiety Inventory (BAI) is a self-report inventory that assesses the severity of anxiety symptoms in adults. The inventory consists of 21 items, each of which asks the individual to rate the intensity of a specific symptom or feeling of anxiety during the past week on a 4-point scale (0–3) where 0 = not at all, 1 = mildly, 2 = moderately, 3 = severely. The items assess common anxiety symptoms such as numbness or tingling, trembling hands, fear of dying, and indigestion. The total score ranges from 0 to 63, with higher scores indicating greater severity of anxiety symptoms. The BAI manual recommends the classification of anxiety levels as minimal anxiety (0 to

7), mild anxiety (8 to 15), moderate anxiety (16 to 25), and severe anxiety (26 to 63).

- *Beck Depression Inventory* (Beck et al., 1996): Similar to the BAI, the Beck Depression Inventory (BDI) is also a 21-question multiple-choice self-report, rated on a Likert scale from 0 to 3, using the same anchors. The BDI is designed to assess the severity of depression symptoms in individuals older than 13 years. Its total score ranges from 0 to 63, with higher scores indicating greater severity of depression symptoms. A recommended cut-off point is 0–13 for minimal depression, 14–19 for mild depression, 20–28 for moderate depression, and 29–63 for severe depression. The items assess symptoms such as sadness, pessimism, loss of pleasure, and suicidal thoughts.
- *Depression Anxiety and Stress Scales* (Lovibond & Lovibond, 1995; Antony et al., 1998): The Depression Anxiety Stress Scales (DASS) is a set of three self-report measures designed to measure the three related negative emotional states of depression, anxiety, and stress. Each of the three scales contains 14 items, rated on a four-point Likert scale from 0 (did not apply to me at all) to 3 (applied to me very much or most of the time), in which respondents rate the frequency and severity of psychological distress experienced in the last week. The DASS is also available in a shorter version with 21 items, referred to as DASS21, that assesses the same constructs but with seven items per scale. The DASS was developed with nonclinical samples with participants 17 or older. The following items are a sample of each DASS scale: *I found it hard to wind down* (stress), *I was aware of dryness of my mouth* (anxiety), and *I couldn't seem to experience any positive feeling at all* (depression).
- *Hospital Anxiety and Depression Scale* (Zigmond & Snaith, 1983): The Hospital Anxiety and Depression Scale (HADS) is a self-reported questionnaire used to measure anxiety and depression symptoms. It consists of 14 items, seven assessing anxiety symptoms and the other seven assessing depression symptoms. All its 14 items refer exclusively to the emotional state and do not reflect somatic symptoms. Participants rate each item on a 4-point Likert scale, with higher scores indicating greater symptom severity. The global score in each subscale ranges from 0 to 21, and scores greater or equal to 9 may reveal the presence of anxiety/depression. Two Depression items are *I still enjoy the things I used to enjoy,* and *I have lost interest in my appearance*, whereas two Anxiety items are *Worrying thoughts go through my mind* and *I feel tense or "wound up."*
- *Patient Health Questionnaire* (Kroenke et al., 2001): The Patient Health Questionnaire (PHQ) is a self-reported questionnaire used to assess the severity of depression symptoms over the last 2 weeks. Each of its nine items assesses a specific symptom of depression, such as loss of interest or pleasure, feelings of hopelessness, and difficulty sleeping. Items are rated on a 4-point Likert scale (0 = Not at all, 4 = Nearly every day), with higher scores indicating greater symptom severity. The suggested classification of depression severity based on the total score is 0–4 = None-minimal, 5–9 = Mild, 10–14 = Moderate, 15–19 Moderately Severe, and 20–27 = Severe. The items request the respondent to rate

the frequency of problems such as *Little interest or pleasure in doing things*, *Feeling tired or having little energy*, or *Trouble concentrating on things*.

8.2.4.2 Psychological Instruments

- *Acceptance and Action Questionnaire-II* (Bond et al., 2011): The Acceptance and Action Questionnaire-II (AAQ-II) is a self-report measure that assesses an individual's level of psychological flexibility. The measure comprises ten items, rated on a 7-point Likert scale (1–7) where one represents "never true," and seven represents "always true." The items are designed to assess an individual's ability to accept painful experiences, memories, feelings, and worries without getting caught up in them and to take action that is consistent with their values. The scores for each question are then added together to obtain a total score. A higher total score indicates a lower level of psychological flexibility. It should be noted that the AAQ-II has a unidimensional structure, meaning that it only yields general scores and does not provide specific scores for different dimensions of psychological flexibility.
- *Brief Experiential Avoidance Questionnaire* (Gámez et al., 2014): The Brief Experiential Avoidance Questionnaire (BEAQ) is a measure of experiential avoidance assessing avoidance of pain, uneasiness, effort, upset, unpleasantness, discomfort, emotions, painful emotions, feelings, bad feelings, upsetting feelings, fear/anxiety, unpleasant memories, and doubts in 15 items. The items are rated using a 6-point Likert scale from 1 (strongly disagree) to 6 (strongly agree). It was developed as a brief alternative to the Multidimensional Experiential Avoidance Questionnaire (MEAQ; Gámez et al., 2011) to be used in situations where the length of the 62-item version could be an issue. The brief version was shown to replicate the good psychometric properties found in the MEAQ.
- *Multidimensional Psychological Flexibility Inventory Short Form* (Grégoire et al., 2020): The Multidimensional Psychological Flexibility Inventory (MPFI-24) is a self-reported assessment tool that evaluates psychological flexibility and psychological inflexibility. It was first conceived with 60 items (Rolffs et al., 2016) and later adapted as a 24-item scale to help clinicians and researchers assess the full complexity of the Hexaflex model with a shorter but comprehensive tool. The MPFI-24 has two general factors of flexibility and inflexibility, each assessing 12 distinct processes.

8.3 Conclusion

As previously described, qualitative and quantitative methods for assessing sleep, such as scales, questionnaires, and sleep self-reports, are very important for directing clinical interventions. Endorsing their relevance are the low cost, their non-invasive nature, and the possibility of detailing the complaint. However, the choice of elements that compose the assessment requires analysis of what is sought to be investigated in each case; therefore, an individualized view of each patient is essential. In this sense, it is necessary to understand why, for what, and how to use assessment instruments.

It is worth mentioning that scales, questionnaires, and self-registration also have limitations, such as the lack of continuity, recall bias, subjectivity, and lack of well-validated measures. In turn, objective tools such as actimetry offer greater precision in the data collected; however, they cost significantly more and require professional specialization. Additionally, in isolation, these assessment tools are insufficient to understand the variables that precipitate and perpetuate insomnia.

Finally, developing more assessment tools can improve and optimize the process of understanding the sleep pattern, diagnosing possible disorders, and enhancing the accuracy of the choice of intervention based on a particular complaint. In any case, these tools only contribute to the data collection, which must be duly analyzed by the clinician.

References

American Educational Research Association, American Psychological Association, & National Council on Measurement in Education. (2014). *Standards for educational and psychological testing*. American Educational Research Association.

Antony, M. M., Bieling, P. J., Cox, B. J., Enns, M. W., & Swinson, R. P. (1998). Psychometric properties of the 42-item and 21-item versions of the depression anxiety stress scales in clinical groups and a community sample. *Psychological Assessment, 10*(2), 176–181. https://doi.org/10.1037/1040-3590.10.2.176

Bastien, C. H., Vallières, A., & Morin, C. M. (2001). Validation of the insomnia severity index as an outcome measure for insomnia research. *Sleep Medicine, 2*(4), 297–307. https://doi.org/10.1016/s1389-9457(00)00065-4

Beck, A. T., Epstein, N., Brown, G., & Steer, R. A. (1988). An inventory for measuring clinical anxiety: Psychometric properties. *Journal of Consulting and Clinical Psychology, 56*(6), 893–897. https://doi.org/10.1037/0022-006x.56.6.893

Beck, A. T., Steer, R. A., & Brown, G. (1996). *Beck depression inventory–II (BDI-II) [Database record]*. APA PsycTests. https://doi.org/10.1037/t00742-000

Bond, F. W., Hayes, S. C., Baer, R. A., Carpenter, K. M., Guenole, N., Orcutt, H. K., Waltz, T., & Zettle, R. D. (2011). Preliminary psychometric properties of the acceptance and action questionnaire-II: A revised measure of psychological inflexibility and experiential avoidance. *Behavior Therapy, 42*(4), 676–688. https://doi.org/10.1016/j.beth.2011.03.007

Borsboom, D. (2005). *Measuring the mind: Conceptual issues in modern psychometrics*. Cambridge University Press.

Bothelius, K., Jernelöv, S., Fredrikson, M., McCracken, L. M., & Kaldo, V. (2015). Measuring acceptance of sleep difficulties: The development of the sleep problem acceptance questionnaire. *Sleep, 38*(11), 1815–1822. https://doi.org/10.5665/sleep.5170

Buysse, D. J., Reynolds, C. F., Monk, T. H., Berman, S. R., & Kupfer, D. J. (1989). The Pittsburgh sleep quality index: A new instrument for psychiatric practice and research. *Psychiatry Research, 28*(2), 193–213. https://doi.org/10.1016/0165-1781(89)90047-4

Cronbach, L. J., & Meehl, P. E. (1955). Construct validity in psychological tests. *Psychological Bulletin, 52*(4), 281–302. https://doi.org/10.1037/h0040957

Flake, J. K., & Fried, E. I. (2020). Measurement Schmeasurement: Questionable measurement practices and how to avoid them. *Advances in Methods and Practices in Psychological Science, 3*(4), 456–465. https://doi.org/10.1177/2515245920952393

Flake, J. K., Pek, J., & Hehman, E. (2017). Construct validation in social and personality research: Current practice and recommendations. *Social Psychological and Personality Science, 8*(4), 370–378. https://doi.org/10.1177/1948550617693063

Gámez, W., Chmielewski, M., Kotov, R., Ruggero, C., & Watson, D. (2011). Development of a measure of experiential avoidance: The multidimensional experiential avoidance questionnaire. *Psychological Assessment, 23*(3), 692–713. https://doi.org/10.1037/a0023242

Gámez, W., Chmielewski, M., Kotov, R., Ruggero, C., Suzuki, N., & Watson, D. (2014). The brief experiential avoidance questionnaire: Development and initial validation. *Psychological Assessment, 26*(1), 35–45. https://doi.org/10.1037/a0034473

Grégoire, S., Gagnon, J., Lachance, L., Shankland, R., Dionne, F., Kotsou, I., Monestès, J., Rolffs, J. L., & Rogge, R. D. (2020). Validation of the english and french versions of the multidimensional psychological flexibility inventory short form (MPFI-24). *Journal of Contextual Behavioral Science, 18*, 99–110. https://doi.org/10.1016/j.jcbs.2020.06.004

Herdman, M., Fox-Rushby, J., & Badia, X. (1998). A model of equivalence in the cultural adaptation of HRQoL instruments. *Quality of Life Research, 7*, 323–335.

Hoddes, E., Dement, W., & Zarcone, V. (1972). Abstracts of papers presented to the eleventh annual meeting of the Association for the Psychophysiological Study of Sleep: The development and use of the Stanford Sleepiness Scale (SSS). *Psychophysiology, 9*(1), 150.

Johns, M. W. (1992). A new method for measuring daytime sleepiness: The Epworth sleepiness scale. *Sleep, 14*(6), 540–545. https://doi.org/10.1093/sleep/14.6.540

Kroenke, K., Spitzer, R. L., & Williams, J. B. (2001). The PHQ-9: Validity of a brief depression severity measure. *Journal of General Internal Medicine, 16*(9), 606–613. https://doi.org/10.1046/j.1525-1497.2001.016009606.x

Lovibond, P. F., & Lovibond, S. H. (1995). The structure of negative emotional states: Comparison of the depression anxiety stress scales (DASS) with the Beck depression and anxiety inventories. *Behaviour Research and Therapy, 33*(3), 335–343.

MacLean, A. W., Fekken, G. C., Saskin, P., & Knowles, J. B. (1992). Psychometric evaluation of the Stanford Sleepiness Scale. *Journal of Sleep Research, 1*(1), 35–39. https://doi.org/10.1111/j.1365-2869.1992.tb00006.x

Morin, C. M., Vallières, A., & Ivers, H. (2007). Dysfunctional beliefs and attitudes about sleep (DBAS): Validation of a brief version (DBAS-16). *Sleep, 30*(11), 1547–1554. https://doi.org/10.1093/sleep/30.11.1547

Rafihi-Ferreira, R. E., Carmo, M., Paulos-Guarnieri, L., & Pires, M. L. N. (2023, January 26). *Development of the Sleep Acceptance Scale (SAS)*. Retrieved from psyarxiv.com/3gqp4

Ree, M. J., & Harvey, A. G. (2004). Investigating safety Behaviours in insomnia: The development of the sleep-related behaviours questionnaire (SRBQ). *Behaviour Change, 21*(01), 26–36. https://doi.org/10.1375/bech.21.1.26.35971

Rolffs, J. L., Rogge, R. D., & Wilson, K. G. (2016). Disentangling components of flexibility via the Hexaflex model: Development and validation of the multidimensional psychological flexibility inventory (MPFI). *Assessment, 25*(4), 458–482. https://doi.org/10.1177/1073191116645905

Schutte-Rodin, S., Broch, L., Buysse, D., Dorsey, C., & Sateia, M. (2008). Clinical guideline for the evaluation and management of chronic insomnia in adults. *Journal of Clinical Sleep Medicine: JCSM: Official Publication of the American Academy of Sleep Medicine, 4*(5), 487–504.

Zigmond, A. S., & Snaith, R. P. (1983). The hospital anxiety and depression scale. *Acta Psychiatrica Scandinavica, 67*(6), 361–370. https://doi.org/10.1111/j.1600-0447.1983.tb09716.x

Chapter 9
The Role of Actigraphy and Sleep Diaries in Assessing Sleep in Adults with Insomnia

Maria Laura Nogueira Pires

9.1 Actigraphy: Basic Concepts

When individuals are awake, they are frequently moving. When individuals are sleeping, movements are almost absent and they are characterized by low level of activity. Actigraphy is a technology that allows the objective quantification of movement level continuously over time by means of acceleration sensors built in a small watch-like device called actigraphy. The device is frequently worn on the wrist while the person behaves in its natural environment over an extended period of days, as one week or even longer depending on the clinical.

In an updated report by the American Academy of Sleep Medicine, actigraphy in patients with insomnia showed to be consistent with polysomnography and more sensitive than sleep logs which supported its use in insomnia evaluation (Smith et al., 2018). The experts recognize that, although objective monitoring is not required in daily practice, actigraphy may be a useful tool in various clinical contexts, such as differential diagnosis from suspect case of circadian rhythm sleep disorders or paradoxical insomnia, in order to objectively evaluate treatment response and when self-records are unreliable or burdensome.

9.2 Actigraphy: Basic Technological Features

There are several types of commercial monitors available on the market and Fig. 9.1 show an actigraphy by Condor Instruments which record motion in three axes (*x*-, *y*-, and *z*-axis are illustrated in Fig. 9.1). Current models of monitors are equipped

M. L. N. Pires (✉)
São Paulo, Brazil
e-mail: laurapires@uol.com.br

R. El Rafihi-Ferreira (ed.), *Acceptance and Commitment Therapy for Insomnia*,
https://doi.org/10.1007/978-3-031-50710-6_9

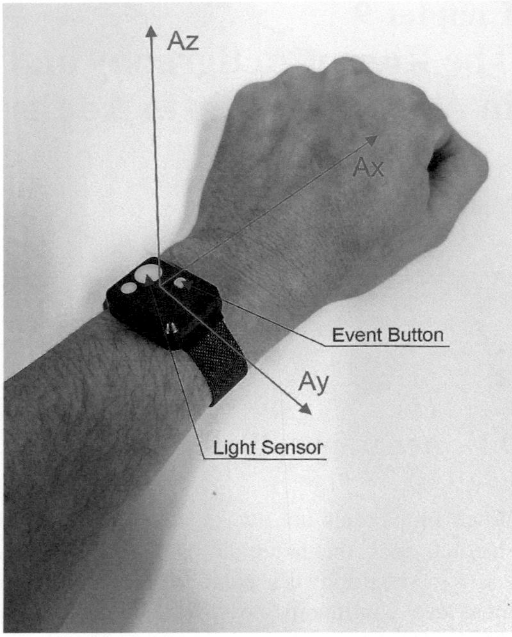

Fig. 9.1 Actigraphy model by Condor Instruments. (Source: Author)

with memory with the ability to record motor activity over extended periods of time, such as weeks and months. Movement data are saved after they are processed with filters to remove the gravity bias on each axis and raw accelerometer output is expressed in arbitrary units referred to as "counts". The activity counts are usually stored in 1-min epochs and a reader device is used to transfer data from actigraphy to computer for analysis using the manufacture's software algorithm.

Most actigraphy devices have an event marker button on their surface and patients can be instructed to press it to inform when specific events happened during the day such as to mark bedtime, wake time and night awakenings (Fig. 9.1). The event marker is thought to have higher accuracy than the sleep diary since the last requires the patient to check the time and remember it in the following morning. Light sensors are also available in current models and can be used to identify light exposure levels during the day and night (Fig. 9.1).

9.3 Clinically Relevant Actigraphic Measures

The inference of sleep and wakefulness states from the activity is done using an algorithm available in proprietary software. The Cole–Kripke (Cole et al., 1992) is a well-established and validated algorithm used to score actigraphy data collected in the adult population and it classifies each epoch as "sleep" or "wake" based on activity counts of that epoch of interest and nearest epochs.

It is from the rest period segment (the sleep period) that the proprietary-automated software derives multiple sleep variables corresponding to the measurements

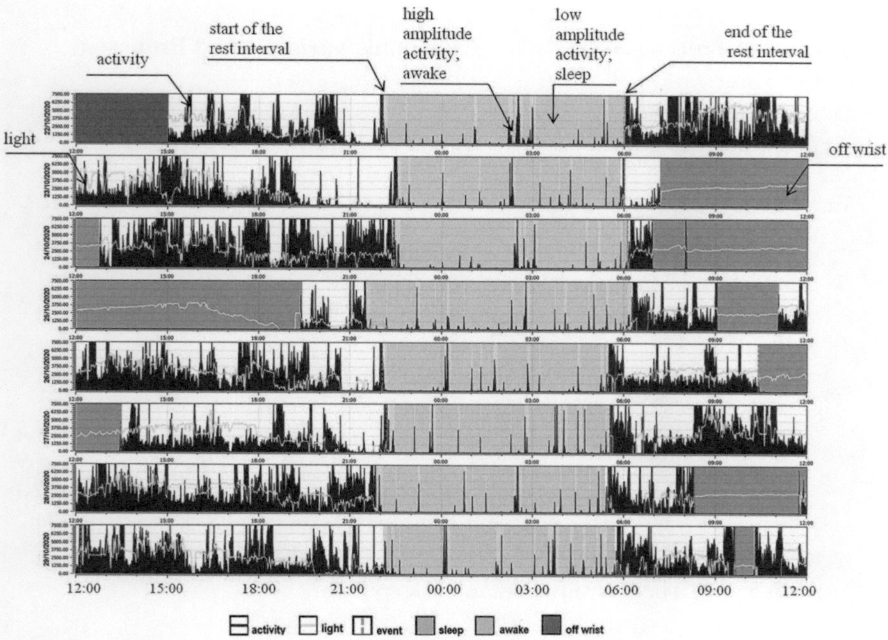

Fig. 9.2 Example actogram of a patient with insomnia. The record was made with ActTrust actigraphy (Condor Instruments) and analyzed with ActStudio software. (Source: Author)

obtained by polysomnography, the gold standard of sleep assessment (Fekedulegn et al., 2020). The software automated identification of the start and end of the rest interval, however, may be imprecise since it is based solely on activity data. It can be improved by manual adjustments made by the scorer using the light sensor and the event button (Ancoli-Israel et al., 2015). The end points of the rest interval can be more accurate when manually demarcated by the abrupt and sustained changes in activity levels (when the wearer lie down in bed attempting to sleep and when he gets out of bed to start the day) and light exposure (lights are turned off/turned on) combined with the time stamps from the event button signalizing the patient's intention to sleep or when he gets out of bed to start the day (see Fig. 9.2). Supplemental information can also be obtained from sleep diary and questions about non-wear periods, bedtime and get up time and day issues (e.g., if it was a typical day/night or not) can assist the scorer to data editing, such as manual trimming, defining rest interval, and excluding off-wrist periods from analyses.

Actigraphic estimates have been used to objectively assess the multi-dimensional construct of "sleep health" (Chung et al., 2021), including sleep timing (when patient typically had his major sleep episode), duration (how long the patient sleep during the day), regularity (day-to-day variability in sleep timing and/or sleep duration), efficiency (sleep quality), and alertness/sleepiness (wakefulness during daytime). Definitions of the main sleep and rhythmicity variables derived from actigraphy are shown in Box 9.1 together with their proposed cutoff values (Natale et al., 2014; Fekedulegn et al., 2020; Chung et al., 2021).

Box 9.1: Definitions of the Main Actigraphic Variables and Proposed Cutoff Values

1) Sleep timing

When the patient typically sleeps?

Variables

Bedtime: hour and minute when the patient lies down in bed with the intention of sleeping and turns the light out.
Get up time: hour and minute when the patient gets out of bed to start the day.
Time in bed (TIB): time from bedtime to get up time.

2) Sleep duration and efficiency (quality)

Does the patient have difficulty falling asleep? Does the patient have difficulty to maintain sleep, with frequent and/or long awakenings? There is a significant variability in awakenings from night to night? Does the patient spend too much time in bed relative to time spend sleeping? There is sufficient total sleep time?

Variables

Sleep onset latency: time between bedtime and sleep onset, usually defined as the first epoch scored as asleep by the algorithm. Cutoff value: less than 15 min.
Total sleep time (TST): time scored as sleep during time in bed (TIB minus sleep latency + WASO). Cutoff value: 6–8 h/night.
Sleep efficiency: proportion of time in bed spent asleep (TST/TIB, expressed as %). Cutoff value: greater than or equal to 85%.
Wake after sleep onset (WASO): time spent awake between sleep onset and sleep offset. Cutoff value: equal or less than 20 min.

3) Sleep regularity and rhythmicity:

There is a significant variability in bedtime/wake time from one day to another?

Variables

Sleep onset and offset regularity: standard deviation calculated across days of less than 30 min.
Sleep duration regularity: standard deviation calculated across days of less than 60 min.
Interdaily stability (IS): estimates the stability of the rest-activity rhythm across days. Scores range from 0 to 1, and higher values indicate better synchronization and a more stable rhythm.

(continued)

Box 9.1 (continued)

4) Alertness/sleepiness

Naps can be defined as sleep intervals longer or equal to 20 min in duration within a 24-h day. Are naps frequent? How long they usually last? Do they typically occur at certain time during the day or they are more frequently on weekends? Is there an association between naps and nocturnal sleep quality or duration?

Variables

Frequency of days napped; frequency of naps on a given day(s) or week, duration, and timing (evening and/or day).

Source: Author

9.4 Actogram

An actogram is the graphic representation of the activity over time and Fig. 9.2 shows the sleep pattern of a 60-year-old patient. Consecutive days are plotted on the vertical and time of day is plotted on the horizontal axis. Sleep was assessed with the ActTrust actigraphy (Condor Instruments) and analyzed with ActStudio software, Cole-Kripke algorithm. The patient wore the actigraphy on the nondominant wrist for 8 consecutive days. He was instructed to press the event button when getting into bed with the intention to sleep, when got up in the morning, and during the watch removal. The end points of the nocturnal rest interval were manually selected taking in account data from activity and light sensors and event marker. Each vertical line indicates the activity level on the 1-minute epoch (higher the activity level, higher the amplitude of the line). Nocturnal rest intervals are identified in light blue and segments of watch removal in purple color.

Visual inspection of this recording shows a stable timing of sleep periods and sleep interrupted by awakenings. No naps. His usual bedtime is 22:08 (SD of 18 minutes; ranging from 21:32 to 22:34), he had no difficulty in falling asleep, taking an average of 7 min to fall asleep, and wake time is typically at 05:46 (SD of 17 minutes; ranging from 05:23 to 06:15), with a mean time in bed of 07:38. The interdaily stability index (IS) was 0.62, indicating stability of the sleep-wake cycle.

However, sleep was characterized by activity of high amplitude and fragmented by awakenings (mean WASO of 58 minutes, ranging from 00:39 to 01:26), average sleep efficiency of 85% (ranging from 79% to 90%), and total sleep time of 06:29 (SD of 27 minutes, ranging from 05:51 to 07:30).

Together, these findings are compatible with low day-to-day variation in sleep duration and timing, adequate sleeping time and insomnia characterized by difficulties of maintaining sleep and low sleep quality.

9.5 Clinical Actigraphy Report

The clinical actigraphy report is the document that describe the patient's characteristics, reasons for the exam, technical specifications, and data interpretation. When actigraphy is used for clinical purposes as assessing sleep of patients with insomnia (and other sleep disorders), the report should ideally be elaborated and signed by health professionals who have qualification in mental health care, such as psychologists and physicians, with expertise in sleep science and tools for insomnia diagnosis and evaluation. Basic reporting guidelines for actigraphy report is shown in Box 9.2.

Box 9.2: Basic Guidelines for Elaborating an Actigraphy Report

1) Identification and reasons

- Patient data: name, sex, age; local.
- Identification of the requesting professional; reasons for the examination (complementary to the diagnosis, treatment planning, follow-up, etc.)
- Identification of the health professional who analyzed the record.

2) System information

- Actigraph manufacturer and model; software used; scoring algorithm.

3) Data collection and processing

- Site of use: dominant/nondominant wrist.
- Record duration: start and end date; number of days analyzed; number of days excluded from analysis and reasons.
- Quality of the record: removals from the device, presence of events that influenced the quality of the record, technical failures of the device, presence of artifacts.
- Description of data cleaning/editing.

4) Scoring procedures

- Procedure for determining rest intervals (manual and/or automated by the software).
- Definition of sleep and circadian measures and cutoff values, when applicable (bedtime, wake time, time in bed, sleep onset latency, WASO, sleep efficiency, total sleep time, and interdaily index).

5) Analysis

- Description of results by measures of central tendency (mean; median) and variability (standard deviation; range); when necessary, consider separated analyzes for work and non-working days.

(continued)

Box 9.2 (continued)

- Inform main findings in light of the reasons for the examination and patient specificities; duration, quality, and regularity of sleep; daytime activity pattern and rhythmicity; additional considerations; limitations.
- Summary.

Source: Author

9.6 Instructions for Use

The overall quality of the exam depends heavily on the instructions given to the patient. The starting point is to explain, in clear and context-appropriate language, the general technical aspects of actigraphy and the objectives of the exam. A basic characteristic to be clarified is that it is fundamentally a device equipped with an accelerometer that will measure movements during continuously and with that it will be possible to estimate the timing, duration, and quality of sleep and the sleep pattern across consecutive days.

The patient should be instructed to wear the device on the nondominant wrist, like a watch, in a comfortable way, without looseness or tightness. The precautions to be taken are the same as with any watch and, as they are expensive equipment, care must be taken to ensure that they are not damaged or lost. Thus, patients should be instructed not to use the device in risk situations such as during vigorous activities as is the case of running, gym training, and similar situations.

Most devices are water resistant. Thus, the patient must be aware that it is okay to use it during everyday activities such as washing hands or while showering. However, if the device is not waterproof, it must be removed in case of immersion, as is the case of swimming pools, bathtubs, and similar situations.

Current devices have light and body temperature sensors. In these cases, the patient must be informed that the light sensor will help to know the pattern of light exposure throughout the day. As the light sensor is located on the external surface of the device, it is important to guide the patient to avoid covering it with clothing. The body temperature sensor, in turn, is located at the bottom, in contact with the skin, with no need for specific guidance beyond explaining its function.

Some models have an event button on their surface that, when pressed, makes a mark in the record. This functionality is valuable to inform the moments that certain events happen during the day (bedtime, wake time, naps, medication time, etc.). Instructions should be provided in writing so that the patient can refer to them when needed. Finally, it is important to guide how to proceed in case of doubts (Box 9.3).

Box 9.3: Basic Instructions on How to Wear an Actigraphy

Actigraphy is an easy way to know the pattern and quality of your sleep.

The actigraph is a device that measures movement and you should wear it on your nondominant wrist like a watch, day and night, for _____ days.

The actigraph wristband should fit snugly around the wrist, without being loose or tight.

The device is water-resistant, so it doesn't matter if it gets wet when you wash your hands or while showering. But it must be removed when you go swimming or bathing.

This device is expensive. Be careful not to lose it and do not use it in places where there is such a risk.

Remove the device during vigorous physical activity such as jogging, sports, or when going to the gym.

On the surface of the device there is a sensor that measures the ambient light. Avoid covering the sensor with clothing. You can pull or fold the sleeve.

When to push the button?

The actigraph has a button on its surface and when pressed it makes a mark on the record. Press the button:

1. When to go to bed, turn off the light and try to sleep.
2. Upon waking up in the morning and getting out of bed.
3. When napping.

If you forget to press the button, don't worry. Press the button on the next occasion.

If you have any questions, please contact: ______________

Source: Author

9.7 Sleep Diaries

Sleep diaries have been extensively used as a valuable and low-cost tool in research and clinical practice to gather subjective sleep to help with diagnosis and treatment of insomnia. The use of smartphone is now widespread and this paved the way for electronic sleep diaries. Digital sleep diaries have gained popularity over the pen-and-paper diaries: they are less time-consuming for filling, the format prevent input errors, data from several days or weeks are calculated automatically by the application (app), and the clinician have access to visual representation of data which facilitates an accurate interpretation of the patient's sleep. Nowadays there is a variety of apps options in the market (i.e., Apple Store and Google Play Store), but models that do not display the sleep estimates to users (patients) seems to be preferred for use in clinical settings.

In order to help with sleep monitoring, a standardized sleep diary, termed Consensus Sleep Diary (CSD), was suggested by an international panel of insomnia experts (Carney et al., 2012). The expanded version of the CSD also asked the patient to give his best estimate about how long did he sleep. Although the CSD generates two different total sleep time values, indicated by the patient and calculated, total sleep time has been shown to be a more accurate measure to distinguish patients with insomnia from normal sleepers when indirectly calculated from a set of items (time in bed, sleep onset latency, wake after sleep onset, and terminal awakening) rather by a single item (Natale et al., 2015). However, there may be clinical situations where comparisons between values can be useful as in case of patients who have difficulties in identifying their own sleep pattern.

Initially developed to be used in clinical research with adults with insomnia at Institute of Psychiatry, University of São Paulo, Brazil (Renatha Rafihi-Ferreira, personal communication), a digital sleep diary based on CSD from Condor Instruments (Condorinst.com) also have additional items about naps, use of sleeping medication and if a given day is working day or not that is highly useful for clinical purposes (Fig. 9.3 and Table 9.1).

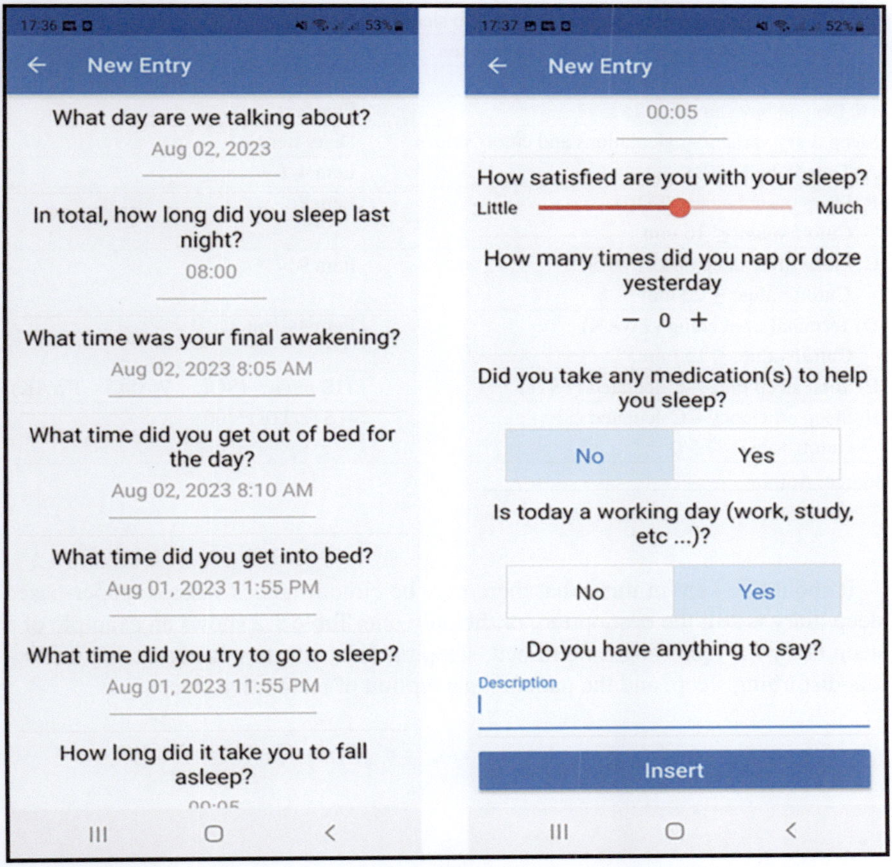

Fig. 9.3 Screenshot of digital sleep diary from Condor Instruments. (Source: Author)

Table 9.1 Digital sleep diary by Condor Instruments: items, response format, sleep diary variables calculations and cutoff values proposed by Natale et al. (2015)

Sleep diary items	Response format
1. What day are we talking about?	Month/day/year
2. In total, how long did you sleep last night?	hh:mm
3. What time was your final awakening?	hh:mm
4. What time did you get out of bed for the day?	hh:mm
5. What time did you get into bed?	hh:mm
6. What time did you try to go to sleep?	hh:mm
7. How long did it take you to fall asleep?	hh:mm
8. How many times did you wake up, not counting your final awakening?	Number
9. In total, how long did these awakenings last?	hh:mm
10. How satisfied are you with your sleep?	Rating scale ranging from "little" to "much"
11. How many times did you nap or doze yesterday?	Number
12. How long did the naps or dozes last?	hh:mm
13. Did you take any medication(s) to help you sleep?	Number
14. If so, list medication(s), dose, and time taken	Free text
15. Is today a working day (work, study, etc.)?	No/yes
16. Do you have anything to say?	Free text
Sleep diary variables calculations and cutoff values	Diary item
A) Time in bed (TIB)	Item 4–6
B) Sleep onset latency (SOL) Cutoff value: ≤ 16 min	Item 7
C) Wake after sleep onset (WASO) Cutoff value: ≤ 20 min	Item 9
D) Terminal awakening (TWAK) Cutoff value: ≤ 15 min	Item 4–item 3
E) Total sleep time—Calculated (TSTc)	TIB *minus*–(SOL + WASO + TWAK)
F) Sleep efficiency—Calculated (SEc) Cutoff value: 87.5%	(TSTc/TIB)*100

Source: Author

It should be kept in mind that there may be circumstances where a paper-based sleep diary is still the best option, or the only one. Table 9.2 shows an example of a sleep diary for recording time in bed, sleeping difficulties, presleep activities, factors disturbing sleep, and the patient's perception of restorative sleep.

Table 9.2 Example of paper-based sleep diary

	Day 1	Day 2	Day *x*
	dd/mo	dd/mo	dd/mo
Write down the date and day of the week	....	....	......
1. What time did you get out of bed for the day?	hh:mm	hh:mm	hh:mm
2. What time did you turn off the light and try to sleep last night?	hh:mm	hh:mm	hh:mm
3. Did you have difficult falling asleep last night?	( ) no	( ) no	( ) no
	( ) yes	( ) yes	( ) yes
4. Did you have difficult staying asleep last night?	( ) no	( ) no	( ) no
	( ) yes	( ) yes	( ) yes
5. Did you wake up earlier than planned and you were unable to fall back to sleep?	( ) no	( ) no	( ) no
	( ) yes	( ) yes	( ) yes
6.What activities you did during the two hours before going to sleep last night? Tick all that apply	( ) alcohol	( ) alcohol	( ) alcohol
	( ) caffeine	( ) caffeine	( ) caffeine
	( ) heavy meal	( ) heavy meal	( ) heavy meal
	( ) exercise	( ) exercise	( ) exercise
	( ) other:..........	( ) other:..........	( ) other:..........
7. What activities you did shortly before turning off the light and trying to sleep last night? Tick all that apply	( ) paper reading	( ) paper reading	( ) paper reading
	( ) cell phone	( ) cell phone	( ) cell phone
	( ) computer	( ) computer	( ) computer
	( ) work/study	( ) work/study	( ) work/study
	( ) watch TV	( ) watch TV	( ) watch TV
	( ) sleeping med	( ) sleeping med	( ) sleeping med
	( ) other:...........	( ) other:...........	( ) other:...........
8. Did you nap yesterday? Tick all that apply	( ) no nap	( ) no nap	( ) no nap
	( ) morning nap	( ) morning nap	( ) morning nap
	( ) afternoon nap	( ) afternoon nap	( ) afternoon nap
	( ) night nap	( ) night nap	( ) night nap
9.Was your sleep disturbed last night? Write down the mental/physical/environmental reasons (noise, brightness/temperature, snoring, pain, nightmare, stress, worries, anxiety, restlessness, etc.)			
10. How rested did you feel when you get up and start the day?	1 = not at all	1 = not at all	1 = not at all
	2 = a little bit	2 = a little bit	2 = a little bit
	3 = somewhat	3 = somewhat	3 = somewhat
	4 = very much	4 = very much	4 = very much
	5 = completely	5 = completely	5 = completely

Source: Author

9.8 Final Considerations

Actigraphy and sleep diaries have been proven as useful tools in clinical practice for longitudinal assessment of sleep in patients with insomnia with benefits for diagnosis formulation and monitoring treatment response. The choice should rely on the balance between several factors including patient's preference, less cumbersome alternative, patient's ability to give accurate information and costs.

References

Ancoli-Israel, S., Martin, J. L., Blackwell, T., Buenaver, L., Liu, L., Meltzer, L. J., et al. (2015). The SBSM guide to actigraphy monitoring: Clinical and research applications. *Behavioral Sleep Medicine, 13*(Suppl 1), S4–S38.

Carney, C. E., Buysse, D. J., Ancoli-Israel, S., Edinger, J. D., Krystal, A. D., Lichstein, K. L., & Morin, C. M. (2012). The consensus sleep diary: Standardizing prospective sleep self monitoring. *Sleep, 35*, 287–302.

Chung, J., Goodman, M., Huang, T., Bertisch, S., & Redline, S. (2021). Multidimensional sleep health in a diverse, aging adult cohort: Concepts, advances, and implications for research and intervention. *Sleep Health, 7*, 699–707.

Cole, R. J., Kripke, D. F., Gruen, W., Mullaney, D. J., & Gillin, J. C. (1992). Automatic sleep/wake identification from wrist activity. *Sleep, 15*, 461–469.

Fekedulegn, D., Andrew, M. E., Shi, M., Violanti, J. M., Knox, S., & Innes, K. E. (2020). Actigraphy-based assessment of sleep parameters. *Annals of Work Exposures and Health, 64*(4), 350–367. https://doi.org/10.1093/annweh/wxaa007

Natale, V., Léger, D., Martoni, M., Bayon, V., & Erbacci, A. (2014). The role of actigraphy in the assessment of primary insomnia: A retrospective study. *Sleep Medicine, 15*, 111–115.

Natale, V., Léger, D., Bayon, V., Erbacci, A., Tonetti, L., Fabbri, M., & Martoni, M. (2015). The consensus sleep diary: Quantitative criteria for primary insomnia diagnosis. *Psychosomatic Medicine, 77*, 413–418.

Smith, M. T., McCrae, C. S., Cheung, J., Martin, J. L., Harrod, C. G., Heald, J. L., & Carden, K. A. (2018). Use of actigraphy for the evaluation of sleep disorders and circadian rhythm sleep-wake disorders: An American Academy of Sleep Medicine systematic review, meta-analysis, and GRADE assessment. *Journal of Clinical Sleep Medicine, 14*(7), 1209–1230.

Part III
Behavioral Treatment for Insomnia

Chapter 10
Sleep Hygiene

Renatha El Rafihi-Ferreira and Andrea Cecilia Toscanini

10.1 Sleep Environment

The bedroom, that is, the environment where individuals sleep, must be their place of physical and emotional recovery. Therefore, factors such as comfort, lighting, temperature, and sounds and noise must be considered when preparing the sleeping environment. Box 10.1 reports guidelines that address these factors.

Box 10.1 Guidelines on the Sleep Environment

Comfort

The bedroom should be comfortable, making it a sleep sanctuary. Thus, the room should be clean, airy, and organized. All these recommendations should be adapted to each patient's socioeconomic reality.

- The mattress needs to be suitable for the patient's needs and medical conditions such as pain, rheumatological diseases, or any other clinical or orthopedic condition.
- Bed linens must also provide comfort and must be appropriate for seasonal temperatures.
- Pillow height should be equal to the distance from neck to shoulder in order to ensure that the spine is aligned during sleep.

Lighting

(continued)

R. El Rafihi-Ferreira (✉)
Department of Clinical Psychology, University of São Paulo, Sao Paulo, Brazil
e-mail: rerafihi@usp.br

A. C. Toscanini
Sleep Ambulatory (ASONO) at the Clinics Hospital of the University of São Paulo, Sao Paulo, Brazil

R. El Rafihi-Ferreira (ed.), *Acceptance and Commitment Therapy for Insomnia*,
https://doi.org/10.1007/978-3-031-50710-6_10

Box 10.1 (continued)

The sleep environment must be bright and airy during the day and dark at night.

- To keep the room dark, blackout curtains and a closed door can help maintain adequate lighting. When adjusting room light is not possible, sleep masks could be an effective option to reduce light exposure.
- The use of electronic devices such as cell phones, tablets, notebooks, computers, and TVs before going to bed should be discouraged. Light emission, especially blue light, from the screen of these devices can compromise sleep onset latency. Thus, we recommend avoiding their use at least 1 hour before going to bed and preferentially keep them out of the bedroom.

Important: If the person commonly gets up during the night, night lights may be used to avoid accidents.

Temperature

The room should have a pleasant temperature to avoid thermal discomfort during sleep. High or very low temperatures compromise central thermoregulation that occurs during sleep, triggering nocturnal arousals that could result in sleep fragmentation with daytime and nighttime consequences. Hence, precautions are necessary such as the use of appropriate pajamas for the season and expected temperature, as well as appropriate bed linens. If there is disagreement between bed partners, separate bedding is an option, keeping the global temperature neutral in the case of air conditioning, a fan, or similar.

Sounds and noise

A quiet environment contributes to the quality of sleep. Sounds and noises can cause microarousals with daytime consequences. Closing the door and wearing earplugs can help maintain silence.

10.2 Eating Habits

Food and substance consumption can also affect sleep. Guidelines on eating habits and substance use are shown in Box 10.2.

Box 10.2 Food Consumption and Substance Use Guidelines

Food

- Going to bed after overeating or feeling hungry can interfere with adequate rest. Choose a light dinner and easily digestible foods such as fruits and cereal bars before going to bed.
- Hard-to-digest or high-fat foods may be associated with circadian rhythm disruptions. Trying to sleep after eating large portions of fatty foods can be uncomfortable and also interfere with rest. Excess protein, especially red meat, can slow digestion and consequently compromise the rapid response to sleep. Thus, avoid high-fat and hard-to-digest foods at dinner.

Fluids

- Although water consumption is always encouraged, drinking water before going to bed can increase nocturnal awakenings due to the need to go to the bathroom. Thus, reduce fluid intake 1–2 hours before going to bed.

Stimulants

- Nicotine is a stimulant that compromises sleep quality. Avoid smoking at night and nicotine consumption at least 4–6 hours before going to bed.
- Caffeine acts on the central nervous system, remaining in the body for a few hours, and promotes a state of mental alertness and influences psychomotor and cognitive performance. Products containing caffeine can increase sleep latency causing difficulty in initiating and maintaining sleep, compromising overall sleep quality.

Thus, avoid the consumption of caffeinated products at least 6 hours before going to bed. Products containing caffeine include coffee, soft drinks, and chocolate. Caffeine is also present in white tea, yellow tea, green tea, black tea, and other dark teas. Hence, choose a relaxing beverage before going to bed.

Alcohol

- Avoid consuming alcohol, especially at night. Although alcohol causes muscle relaxation, which can lead to a feeling of sleepiness, its activity on the central nervous system is stimulating and can inhibit an adequate sleep rhythm. Alcohol consumption before going to bed is associated with fragmented sleep, including microarousals during the night.

10.3 Routine

Daytime routine is key to achieve quality sleep. The activities we perform during the day can also influence our night. Therefore, having regular times for these activities is fundamental and helps our body to understand that the time for relaxation will come soon. Routine guidelines are presented in Box 10.3.

Box 10.3 Daytime Routine Guidelines

Regular schedules

- Consistent bedtime and wake-up times contribute positively to circadian rhythm regularity. Set the alarm to go off at the same time every day, preferably including weekends.
- Eat meals at the same times and also have regular schedules for work, study, and other activities.
- Perform mental and physical activities on a regular basis.

Physical activity

- Practice physical activity preferably in the morning (except if you have a late chronotype). Physical activity induces an increase in cortisol secretion. Thus, in the morning, it can favor a state of alertness to spend the day without sleepiness. However, physical activity close to bedtime can affect the ability to fall asleep. Avoid exercising during the hours before going to bed.

Sunlight

- Sunlight is an important regulator of the biological clock and we can use it to our advantage if we regularly expose ourselves to light in the morning. Therefore, reserve at least 30 minutes daily for sun exposure in the morning.

Naps

- Daytime naps can lower sleep pressure by delaying the nighttime sleep schedule. Hence, avoid daytime napping. Staying awake throughout the day can make it easier to fall asleep at night.

10.4 Sleep Ritual

A sleep ritual consists of a set of activities that precede sleep and should be composed of elements that give you pleasure and peace of mind. The activities must occur every day so that the body understands that it is time to sleep based on these activities. It is important that the pre-sleep ritual starts about 40–60 minutes before bedtime and that it occurs in the same order. The activities that make up the pre-sleep ritual should be calm and relaxing and should be finalized in the bedroom. An example of a pre-sleep ritual is taking a shower, putting on pajamas, having a cup of tea, disconnecting from daily activities, and reading. Box 10.4 lists some guidelines on pre-sleep activities, that is, the sleep ritual.

Box 10.4 Sleep Ritual Guidelines

Pre-sleep activities

- A warm to hot shower 1 hour before going to bed can favor sleep since it provides a temperature that contributes to the process of falling asleep.
- It is important that the pre-sleep ritual excludes stimulating physical and mental activities. Try to disconnect from daily activities and choose readings not related to work or study. Dedicate yourself to reading poetry, novels, fiction, or other content that encourages relaxation. Give preference to physical books. Electronic books must not be part of the pre-sleep routine and must be kept at a distance!
- Hearing classical music or sounds of nature can help with the relaxation process.

10.5 Worries

Worries and problems before going to bed can affect the process of falling asleep. Therefore, in the case of excessive worries, write them down in a notebook. Transfer worries, anguish, and thoughts to the paper. This can help to "empty the mind". Identify what bothers you when you go to bed and, if possible, write it down on a piece of paper to deal with those thoughts, problems, and worries only on the next day. Box 10.5 shows a model of a thought diary.

Box 10.5 Thought Diary

Write in this space your thoughts, feelings, or worries. For this, answer the following question "What bothers you when go to bed?"

To-do-list for the next day:

- 1
- 2
- 3
- 4
- 5

Thoughts on the day gone by

Thoughts about problems

Random thoughts

Fear of not being able to sleep

Vent in your diary

In conclusion, the elements of sleep hygiene can be addressed in a psychoeducation session and can be discussed during the course of the intervention. It is important to mention that, due to individual variability, not all guidelines have the same impact on different patients. The guidelines must be personalized considering demand, context, and individual characteristics of the patient.

Bibliography

Perlis, M. L., Aloia, M., & Kuhn, B. (2011). *Behavioral treatment for sleep disorders: A comprehensive primer of behavioral sleep medicine*. Elsevier.

Perlis, M. L., Jungquist, C., Smith, M. T., & Posner, D. (2005). *Cognitive behavioral treatment of insomnia: A session-by-session guide*. Springer.

Chapter 11
Stimulus Control Therapy for Insomnia

Maria Laura Nogueira Pires and Ksdy Maiara Moura Sousa

11.1 The Falling Asleep Process

Recognizing that sleep is not a behavior but a state of the organism leads behavior analysts to focus on the transition from waking to sleep. As conceptualized by Bootzin (1972), falling asleep is an operant behavior that is reinforced by sleep. Under this perspective, sleep initiation is a behavioral chain that is under control of various discriminative stimuli, including interoceptive stimuli such as sleepiness and reduced mental alertness, proprioceptive cues such as sleeping posture, and external cues such as pre-bed preparation behaviors that signal that a reinforcer, sleep, is available.

The period of behavioral quietude that precedes sleep onset—low physiological and mental arousal—is the consummatory response for sleep, and when it is under appropriate stimulus control (e.g., dark and quiet room, comfortable temperature and bedding clothes, bedtime routine), the transition into sleep is highly likely to be short and smooth.

Motivating operations will affect the value of sleep as a reinforcer. The sleep-wake cycle is understood to be regulated by the interaction of two biological mechanisms known as a homeostatic factor (Process S), which posits that the pressure to sleep increases with the time awake, and a circadian factor (Process C), which posits that there is a time of day that the probability to fall asleep is higher (Borbely, 1982). In this context, motivating operations that alter the motivational state toward sleep,

M. L. N. Pires (✉)
Private Practice in Sleep Psychology, Sao Paulo, Brazil
e-mail: laurapires@uol.com.br

K. M. M. Sousa
Private Practice in Sleep Psychology, Sao Paulo, Brazil

SleepUp Tecnologia em Saúde, Sao Paulo, Brazil

R. El Rafihi-Ferreira (ed.), *Acceptance and Commitment Therapy for Insomnia*,
https://doi.org/10.1007/978-3-031-50710-6_11

such as a consistent sleep-wake schedule, an appropriate time of day for trying to sleep, and enough time awake since previous sleep, will facilitate the falling asleep process by increasing the reinforcement value of sleep and the emission of the sleep consummatory response (Blampied & Bootzin, 2013).

Classical conditioning can also play a role in insomnia when cues associated with pre-bed activities or the bedroom become associated with negative emotions such as anxiety, worries, and frustration about not falling asleep. Under these circumstances, a conditioned response of arousal is elicited, and the sleeping process is disrupted. This explains why insomniacs may fall asleep easily in other places than the bedroom, such as on a couch, chair, or even away from home (Bootzin & Nicassio, 1978).

The perspective of falling asleep as an operant behavior that is reinforced by sleep and, as such, must be under the control of discriminative stimuli is the basis of stimulus control therapy for insomnia, an effective treatment for insomnia as a stand-alone treatment or when associated with other interventions (Bootzin et al., 1991).

11.2 Stimulus Control Therapy for Insomnia

The stimulus control therapy for insomnia involves five orientations (Bootzin et al., 1991), and the choice of strategy to be carried out is part of the psychoeducation process that seeks to teach the patient the relationship between the applied method and the objectives to be achieved. Below are the main guidelines given to the patient during the psychotherapeutic process:

1. *Go to bed only when sleepy*: This instruction aims to help the patient identify signs that he is drowsy and, therefore, increase the chance of falling asleep quickly when he goes to bed. It is common for insomniacs to report tiredness and go to bed without sleep, either because they believe they need to sleep at a certain time or because they believe they need to be in bed for sleep to come. Thus, this guidance should be directed to the patient who is going to bed without sleep and is waiting for sleep to arrive in bed. These habits can often lead to feelings of frustration or anxiety, increase alertness, and make it difficult to fall asleep. When we guide the patient to go to bed only when they feel sleepy, this ensures that excessive time in bed and anxiety about falling asleep are reduced, favoring a quick onset of sleep.
2. *Getting out of bed when unable to sleep*: Patients are advised to get out of bed if they cannot sleep after 20 or 30 minutes by going to another part of the house, avoiding activities that wake them up, and returning to bed only when sleepy. This guideline can be used both for sleep onset and for patients who usually wake up in the middle of the night and are no longer able to fall asleep. The

mechanism here is the same as mentioned above, as the time spent in bed without sleeping can be a factor in maintaining wakefulness due to the hyperalert state generated.

3. *Using the bed only for sleeping or sexual activity*: This instruction aims to associate the bed with sleeping behavior and thus facilitate the onset of sleep. This instruction should be given when the patient uses the bed for activities other than sleep, such as watching television, eating, working, using electronic devices, making plans, or solving problems. In this case, there may be an aversive conditioning between the sleeping environment and the bed, as it turns out to be a place of stress, tiredness, anxiety, and wakefulness.
4. *Have a regular wake-up time, regardless of the number of hours slept*: The purpose of this instruction is to strengthen the regularity of the sleep rhythm. Many patients usually extend their time in bed with the intention of restoring nighttime sleep. This behavior, which is more commonly observed on weekends, leads to irregularities in schedules, making it difficult to fall asleep. Regularity in sleeping and waking times facilitates the process of falling asleep.
5. *Avoid daytime naps*: Naps lasting 30 minutes or more can lead to impairments in daytime functioning and alteration of the circadian rhythm, impairing the onset of nocturnal sleep. Therefore, patients should be instructed to avoid napping during the day, and, if this is not possible, this nap should last approximately 20 minutes. Naps should be avoided at night since they can impair the sleeping process.

Some adaptations are necessary for specific cases, in particular the guidance on getting out of bed and the bedroom, which should be adapted for the elderly, patients using hypnotics, and patients who share the sleeping environment or live in environments with low privacy.

Sleep undergoes changes in its structure, course, and duration throughout development. Elderly people tend to have a shorter and more fragmented sleep time, with an increase in the time awake after sleeping, to nap more during the day, often in places outside the bedroom, and to sleep and wake up earlier (Cooke & Ancoli-Israel, 2011; Hughes & Martin, 2022).

Several factors may be involved in the association between bed and sleep in the elderly. The aging process can be associated with the presence of chronic diseases such as cardiovascular changes, depression, neurodegenerative diseases and insomnia (Edwards et al., 2010; Fillenbaum et al., 2000). Elderly people can also have low mobility and frailty, as well as being bedridden or living in long-term institutions. Also, the instruction for the elderly to get out of bed if they are not sleepy can lead to changes in their caregivers' sleep. Thus, it is important to choose safe alternatives that patients with limited mobility and increased risk of falling can do in bed instead of struggling to sleep (Hughes & Martin, 2022). Also, the chronic use of sedative hypnotics is frequent among patients with insomnia, with a North American estimate indicating that half of the patients use sleep medication for a period longer than 2 years (Kaufmann et al., 2018). It is well recognized that sedative hypnotics are associated with dependence and a range of important adverse effects that include the risk of falls and fractures. The counter control technique can be useful for these patients. This technique involves keeping the patient in bed when awake during the night with relaxing activities unrelated to falling asleep. Instead of trying to fall asleep or worrying about the consequences of not sleeping well, the patient is motivated to read, meditate, and listen to quiet music, among other activities (Bootzin & Epstein, 2000; Hughes & Martin, 2022).

Stimulus control technique can also be challenging for the patient who lives in a house with little private space preventing him from using the bedroom only for sleep and sex. Based on the literature (Bootzin & Epstein, 2000; Hughes & Martin, 2022; Simpson & Manber, 2022), some suggestions for adaptations for this and other situations are shown in Table 11.1.

Table 11.1 Conventional and adapted stimulus control instructions

Conventional strategy	Adapted strategy	Indications
Leave the bed/bedroom if unable to fall asleep within 20 minutes	*Older people and users of sedative-hypnotic drugs* Consider the counter control strategy to reduce the risk of falling.	If there is a risk of falling and/or physical limitations that restrain the individual getting out of bed by themselves and safely.
Avoid naps	*Older people* Naps should be limited to 30 minutes and taken in a sleeping environment with open windows and natural light. Incorporate strategies to increase alert activities. Examples of such activities include walking outside, standing at regular intervals, or engaging in social interactions such as playing cards with others.	Elderly people who nap in places other than their sleeping environment, such as on the couch or armchair while watching TV.
	Users of sedative-hypnotic drugs Avoid the use of hypnotics during daytime naps, as this is the first step in tapering off medication.	Patients using sedative hypnotic during naps.
Go to bed only when sleepy	*Users of sedative-hypnotic drugs* Instruct the patient to take the medication 30 minutes or immediately before going to bed.	
Use the bed only for sleep and sex	*Older people* Avoid staying awake while in bed during the day; avoid sleeping in places other than bed.	Older adults that are used to sleep in other places than bed, such as a sofa or chair.
	Individuals that share the sleeping environment or live in a single-room house Consider an additional mattress; consider room dividers, folding screens or curtains.	Where the *sleeping* accommodation is not individual; there is no room division to add privacy.

Source: Authors

11.3 Final Considerations

When approaching patients with insomnia, it is necessary to clarify and understand how the maladaptive behaviors that interfere with the process of falling asleep were established. Any behavior change requested from the patient must be systematically monitored and followed up until the objectives are achieved. Furthermore, the implementation process of the behavioral stimulus control strategy must be based on a detailed assessment of important variables such as the patient's motivation, the patient's understanding of the method, the patient's context, including their living conditions, the feasibility of carrying out the activity in their own environment, and even the presence of social support as such from their family members.

References

Blampied, N. M., & Bootzin, R. R. (2013). Sleep: A behavioral account. In *APA handbook of behavior analysis, Vol. 2: Translating principles into practice* (pp. 425–453). American Psychological Association. https://doi.org/10.1037/13938-017

Bootzin, R. (1972). Stimulus control treatment for insomnia. *Proceedings of the American Psychological Association, 1972*, 395–396.

Bootzin, R. R., & Epstein, D. R. (2000). Stimulus control. In K. L. Lichstein & C. M. Morin (Eds.), *Treatment of late-life insomnia* (pp. 167–184). Sage Publications, Inc.

Bootzin, R. R., & Nicassio, P. M. (1978). Behavioral treatments for insomnia. *Progress in Behavior Modification, 6*, 1–45. https://doi.org/10.1016/B978-0-12-535606-0.50007-9

Bootzin, R. R., Epstein, D., & Wood, J. M. (1991). Stimulus control instructions. In *Case studies in insomnia* (pp. 19–28). Springer US. https://doi.org/10.1007/978-1-4757-9586-8_2

Borbely, A. A. (1982). A two process model of sleep regulation. *Human Neurobiology, 1*, 195–204.

Cooke, J. R., & Ancoli-Israel, S. (2011). Normal and abnormal sleep in the elderly. *Handbook of Clinical Neurology, 98*, 653–665. https://doi.org/10.1016/B978-0-444-52006-7.00041-1

Edwards, B., O'Driscoll, D., Ali, A., Jordan, A., Trinder, J., & Malhotra, A. (2010). Aging and sleep: Physiology and pathophysiology. *Seminars in Respiratory and Critical Care Medicine, 31*(5), 618–633. https://doi.org/10.1055/s-0030-1265902

Fillenbaum, G. G., Pieper, C. F., Cohen, H. J., et al. (2000). Comorbidity of five chronic health conditions in elderly communityresidents: Determinants and impact on mortality. *The Journals of Gerontology Series A: Biological Sciences and Medical Sciences, 55*(2), M84–M89. https://doi.org/10.1093/gerona/55.2.M84

Hughes, J. M., & Martin, J. L. (2022). CBT-I for older adults. In *Adapting cognitive behavioral therapy for insomnia* (pp. 347–366). Elsevier. https://doi.org/10.1016/B978-0-12-822872-2.00005-0

Kaufmann, C. N., Spira, A. P., Depp, C. A., & Mojtabai, R. (2018). Long-term use of benzodiazepines and nonbenzodiazepine hypnotics, 1999–2014. *Psychiatric Services, 69*(2), 235–238. https://doi.org/10.1176/appi.ps.201700095

Simpson, N., & Manber, R. (2022). CBT-I in patients who wish to reduce use of hypnotic medication. In *Adapting cognitive behavioral therapy for insomnia* (pp. 437–456). Elsevier. https://doi.org/10.1016/B978-0-12-822872-2.00014-1

Chapter 12
Sleep Restriction

Silvia Gonçalves Conway and Bárbara Araújo Conway

12.1 Introduction

Sleep Restriction Therapy (SRT) is an established treatment for insomnia that has been used in clinical practice for over 30 years (Maurer et al., 2021). It was first described and tested in 1987 by Spielman and colleagues (1987a). It is commonly delivered as part of a multicomponent cognitive-behavioral therapy for insomnia (CBT-I) but has also been linked to beneficial effects as a stand-alone intervention (Edinger & Means, 2005; Buysse et al., 2011). It has been shown to be the most effective technique to reduce insomnia symptoms and to consolidate sleep (Epstein et al., 2012; Kalmbach et al., 2019). The theoretical perspective of SRT derives from circadian sleep–wake concepts and physiologic sleep–wake regulation models, which postulate that regular sleep schedule and full wakefulness throughout day and evening reinforce circadian sleep–wake rhythm and potentialize homeostatic drive for sleep. Its goal is sleep consolidation and abolition of arousal during sleep period.

Figure 12.1 illustrates the sleep model proposed by Borbély and Achermann (1999), Borbély et al. (2016). SRT is a structured and standardized protocol that involves restricting and regularizing a patient's time in bed to prime and strengthen it. The protocol reviews weekly progress and promotes adjustment on the sleep schedule to match it with sleep needs. The time in bed restriction in a regular schedule is a way to anticipate and sustain the sleep deprivation effects, potentiating the sleep drive and reflecting on an alleviation of sleep efforts. The results achieve the diminishing cognitive and physiological arousal and enhance the consolidation and predictability of sleep.

S. G. Conway (✉) · B. A. Conway
Psychiatry Institute, Faculty of Medicine at the University of São Paulo, São Paulo, Brazil
e-mail: silvia.conway@hc.fm.usp.br; barbara.conway@hc.fm.usp.br

R. El Rafihi-Ferreira (ed.), *Acceptance and Commitment Therapy for Insomnia*,
https://doi.org/10.1007/978-3-031-50710-6_12

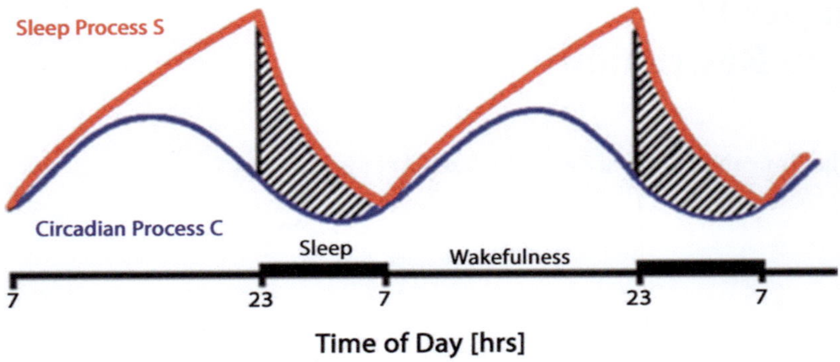

Fig. 12.1 Borbély sleep modelBorbély sleep model (1999, 2016) posits two processes involved in sleep homeostasis: Sleep Process and Circadian Process. Sleep Process (red line) represents the homeostatic sleep drive, which increases the longer a person is awake. Circadian Process (blue line) involves timing information, derived from the suprachiasmatic nucleus (SCN). Mediated by *zeitgebers*, mainly light, meal, and sleep schedule, the SCN synchronizes with the daylight and stimulates arousal networks that promote and sustain wakefulness, modulating the enhancement of performance and alertness. When the sun goes down, the weakening of light information triggers melatonin production and secretion, which is believed to decrease the alerting signal from the SCN and synchronize the tendency of sleeping with the night, when the circadian drive exhibits its oscillatory output in opposite direction from the day, favoring the homeostatic sleep drive to be expressed and discharged, represented by the scratched line. (Source and adaptation: Borbély and Achermann (1999), Borbély et al. (2016))

12.2 Habits and Behaviors Associated to Sleep Homeostatic Drive Dysregulation

Pre-sleep anticipatory anxiety is a common feature of insomnia patients. The focus on sleep became the axis of patients' attention during day and night. Caffeine consumption, for example, is commonly used to contour sleep deprivation effects, as well as alcohol consumption is adopted by some patients to induce sleep. During the night, insomnia behavior usually comprehends excessive time in bed, irregular sleep–wake schedule, control of clock timing during sleep time, concern about the harmful effects of sleep deprivation, and a set of inadequate tasks and behaviors undertaken inadvertently in an awake mode in bed.

The alteration of sleep schedules used to be adopted as an ineffective coping strategy to obtain more sleep, that is, a way to offer more opportunity of time to sleep: going to bed earlier, canceling morning appointments and or implementing naps during the day—all behaviors adopted to try to compensate sleep deprivation effects of previous insomnia nights or to avoid it in hypothetical awakenings that can occur in the following sleep period. This endeavor is related to the sleep loss complaint hyper focus that grounds an obsessive behavior of sleep searching, offering more opportunity to repair or alleviate the tiredness from sleep loss. These behaviors impair the nocturnal sleep pattern, increase the sleep effort, decrease the sleep efficiency, and enhance the cognitive and physiological arousal, reinforcing the cognitive vicious cycle of insomnia, including pre-sleep anticipatory anxiety, concerns about harmful effects of sleep deprivation on daily activities, interpersonal relationships, and health damages in the long term.

Insomnia disorder does not begin instantly. In most cases, the first symptoms are closely related to problems in real life. It is anguish in the form of insomnia. As long as the symptoms persist, the difficulties with sleep can complicate, becoming the focus of a patient's attention. That is the changing point, when the person abandons the core of the problem and tries desperately to recover the sleep loss by a series of strategies throughout day and night.

Figure 12.2a illustrates the sum of these strategies transformed on a strength resistance against sleep. That's why people with insomnia disorder usually experience a series of poor nights of sleep followed by a good and satisfactory night of sleep, after which the series of poor nights begin again and so on (Fig. 12.2b). It illustrates the strong power of the vicious cycle of insomnia against the homeostatic sleep drive. As long as the sequence of poor nights of sleep happens, the sleep deprivation increases, enhancing the sleep homeostatic drive. When it exceeds the sleep resistance condition of insomnia, the sleep pressure imposes a full night of recovery sleep. However, as soon as the sleep homeostatic drive is discharged, the conditioned behaviors and beliefs around insomnia play its strength, intercepting the natural expression of sleep–wake cycle and the insomnia nights return as protagonist (Fig. 12.2c). That is, although there is preservation of sleep physiology conditions, the psychological conditions make resistance against it—such as unconscious resistance, fears of sleep loss consequences, and obsessive thoughts and behaviors in search of recovery sleep loss or contour tiredness.

Insomnia disorder does not begin abruptly, nor will it disappear magically. The compendium of CBT-I techniques, as well as other psychological approaches, such as Acceptance Commitment Therapy (ACT), aims to crack and melt each one of the sleep resistance elements. SRT targets some of these sustaining factors, mainly excessive time in bed and disorganized sleep schedule, but it also addresses excessive concern about the harm caused by sleep deprivation the next day and pre-sleep anticipatory anxiety. SRT anticipates and sustains the expression of the homeostatic sleep drive power. The effects surpass the physiological response to sleep deprivation, such as the organization of sleep schedules and the consolidation of sleep. They also extend to psychological aspects associated with insomnia, including pre-sleep arousal (Maurer et al., 2022), which leads to a reduction in the frequency and intensity of fear-related thoughts, control behaviors, and pre-sleep expectations (Fig. 12.2d). This indicates that when combined, all strategies mutually reinforce one another.

12.3 Sleep Restriction Therapy Components and Efficacy

SRT is composed of two central behavioral techniques that aim to reduce variability in sleeping time and wakefulness during sleep period:

a

b

c

d

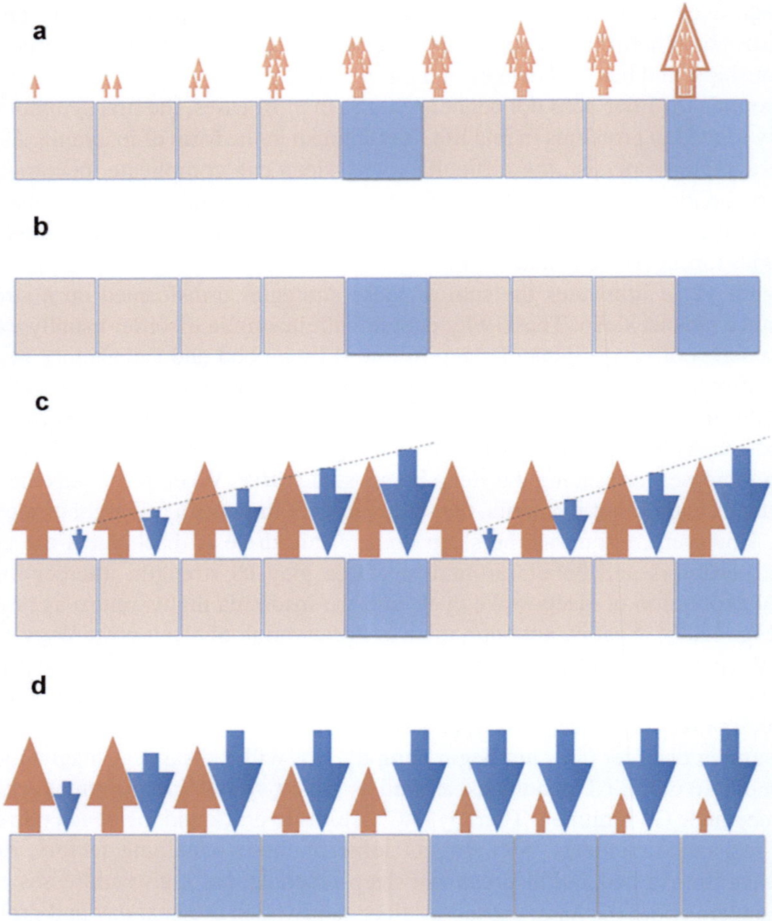

Fig. 12.2 Insomnia resistance drive versus homeostatic sleep drive
Orange arrow represents the insomnia resistance to sleep. Blue arrow represents the homeostatic sleep drive. The dimension of each arrow represents the strength of resistance or drive. Orange square represents an insomnia night. Blue square represents a restful night. Each little orange arrow exhibited on Figure (**a**) illustrates each one of the strategies that patients usually adopt to contour sleep deprivation or to control sleeping, such as caffeine consumption during the day, or alcohol during the night; clock watch all over night; canceling commitments at the end or at the beginning of the day to guarantee sleep; time in bed extension to compensate for sleep deficits, etc. The sum of these behaviors become a strength that makes resistance against sleep, being represented by the large orange arrow, consolidating the difficulties with sleep as an insomnia disorder. Figure (**b**) illustrates the typical sleep pattern of insomnia: a sequence of poor nights of sleep followed by a good and satisfactory night of sleep, after which the series of poor nights begin again and so on. Figure (**c**) illustrates the strength fight between the insomnia resistance drive and homeostatic sleep drive. As the resistance to sleep plays its strength night by night, the homeostatic sleep drive grows each night, becoming strong enough to impose over the psychological resistance, that is when the insomnia pattern gives in and the patient experiences a restful night. The dashed line represents the homeostatic sleep drive increase tendency. As soon as the sleep homeostatic

- Time in Bed Regularization (TBR): patients are asked to keep a fixed bed and rise time.
- Time in Bed Restriction (TIBR): patients are asked to keep a fixed sleep period.

The sleep period is defined based on the total sleep time (TST) estimates informed by a self-reported sleep diary. It represents the opportunity for sleep that should be reduced in accordance with the current exercise of sleep. Bed and rise time will be defined according to the sleep period definition and patient routine. The coupled reference values (bed and rise time that fits the sleep period) are nicknamed as "sleep window," which will be gradually adjusted to reach the need for sleep of each patient. The full application and adjustments of SRT are better described, step by step, on the "Sleep Restriction Therapy application: step by step" topic.

SRT efficacy shows reduction on sleep onset latency (SOL) and wake after sleep onset (WASO) and improvement on sleep efficiency (SE) in the short term (Miller et al., 2014; Maurer et al., 2021; Belfer et al., 2021) and better outcome on the Insomnia Severity Index (Maurer et al., 2021), with no effects for TST. Even though insomnia patients complain of insufficient sleep time, it is not usual to observe that. What happens is that they have a poor sleep experience when they often try to recover from sleep loss by spending a longer TIB. This behavior yields too much effort to get and/or resume sleep. The avoidance of sleep deprivation and its consequences stress the patient, potentializes the attention over sleep and perpetuates insomnia in the long term, leading to poor sleep efficiency, not very well consolidated and, very often, sleep misperception. That is why the effects of SRT are not necessarily a huge increment in TST, but a change in sleep pattern that is correlated to an increased sleep depth (Belfer et al., 2021), improving and correcting the perception of sleep that leads to an improvement of patients' satisfaction.

Maurer et al. (2020) dismantled SRT and compared sleep measures between TIBR (+ sleep hygiene) versus TBR (+ sleep hygiene). Based on self-reported sleep diaries and actigraphy, they demonstrated that TIBR technique shows better sleep outcomes than TBR when taken isolated on SOL, WASO, SE in the short and long terms. Moreover, TIBR technique promoted improvement in sleep-related quality of life in the long term. Even though weaker, TIBR also demonstrated better sleep outcomes by polysomnography than TBR (Maurer et al., 2020). It highlights TIBR as the key component of SRT intervention. The fit of sleep ability onto sleep opportunity is the principal factor to enhance the sleep homeostatic drive. As the sleep efficiency is achieved in accordance to the stabilization of sleep ability, periods of sleep opportunity are extended (titration) in order to reach sleep needs (Fig. 12.3). Among insomniacs, it is very difficult to maintain a good sleep efficiency when it is

Fig. 12.2 (continued) drive is discharged, the insomnia sleep pattern returns by its conditioned behaviors and consolidated beliefs. Figure (**d**) illustrates SRT effects: as soon as the sleep window is implemented, the homeostatic sleep drive is anticipated, exerting its strength. As the sleep window keeps steady, the homeostatic sleep drive keeps its fast expression night by night, provoking the weakening of the insomnia resistance. Night after night, each element of resistance gets weaker, diminishing the pre-sleep anticipatory anxiety and concerns around insomnia. This process facilitates the return of restful sleep till the settling of insomnia disorder

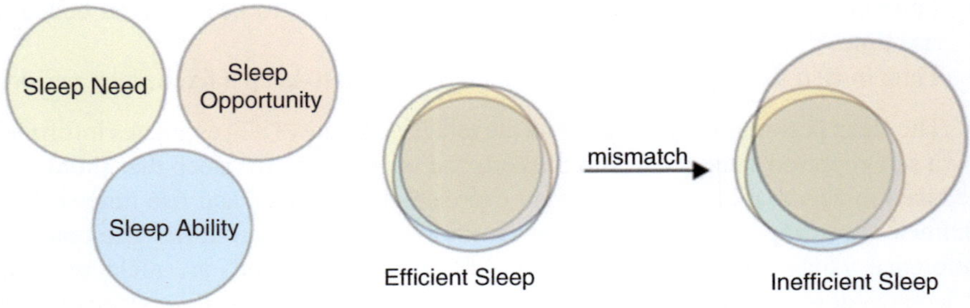

Fig. 12.3 Sleep opportunity extension impairs sleep efficiencySleep opportunity restriction aligns with sleep opportunity and sleep ability, leading to efficient sleep. The overabundance of sleep opportunity in a scenario of low sleep ability produces poor sleep efficiency and perpetuates insomnia in the long term. (Figure source: Belfer et al., (2021))

given an overabundance of sleep opportunity. The amount of it, more than the timing, determines the response (Maurer et al., 2020; Belfer et al., 2021). Nevertheless, worse sleep quality has also been associated with irregular bedtimes (Kang & Chen, 2009), which regularization corroborates to the reduction of daytime sleepiness and SE increment (Manber et al., 1996). So, sleep opportunity applied in a regular schedule potentializes sleep drive and sleep–wake circadian rhythm, both involved in sleep homeostasis. For that, it is recommended to implement both strategies together, seven nights a week with only small variations over successive weeks of treatment, well described on the following topic.

12.4 Sleep Restriction Therapy Application: *Step by Step*

SRT initiates with the definition of sleep window: sleep opportunity in accordance to sleep ability defined based on a regular bedtime. The initial amount of sleep restriction is determined based on an individual's TST extracted from at least 2 weeks of self-report sleep diaries and, eventually, actigraphy register. Usually, the beginning of SRT application promotes the greatest restriction of sleep opportunity, that is expected to enhance sleep drive and stabilize sleep ability during the bedtime period. Improved sleep can take days to manifest, as homeostatic sleep drive builds (Fig. 12.4). The titration of sleep opportunity consists of a slow process used to increase it as sleep is consolidated and becomes more efficient. It depends on the match of: (a) the stabilization of sleep inside the sleep window; (b) with at least 90% of SE (85% for the elderly); and (c) patient's reports of insufficient TST. This report means, as expected, that the sleep ability achieved the sleep opportunity in a stable

Fig. 12.4 (continued) oriented not to sleep before or after the sleep window: 7 h of sleep opportunity to happen between 00 and 7 AM. The conditioned sleep pattern persists as the homeostatic sleep drive builds. For that, improved sleep can take days to manifest. Responses to SRT may vary from faster SOL (**c**), lower WASO (**d**), diminishing the frequency of nocturnal awakenings (**e**) or mixed responses such as is described, usually accompanied by better sleep satisfaction

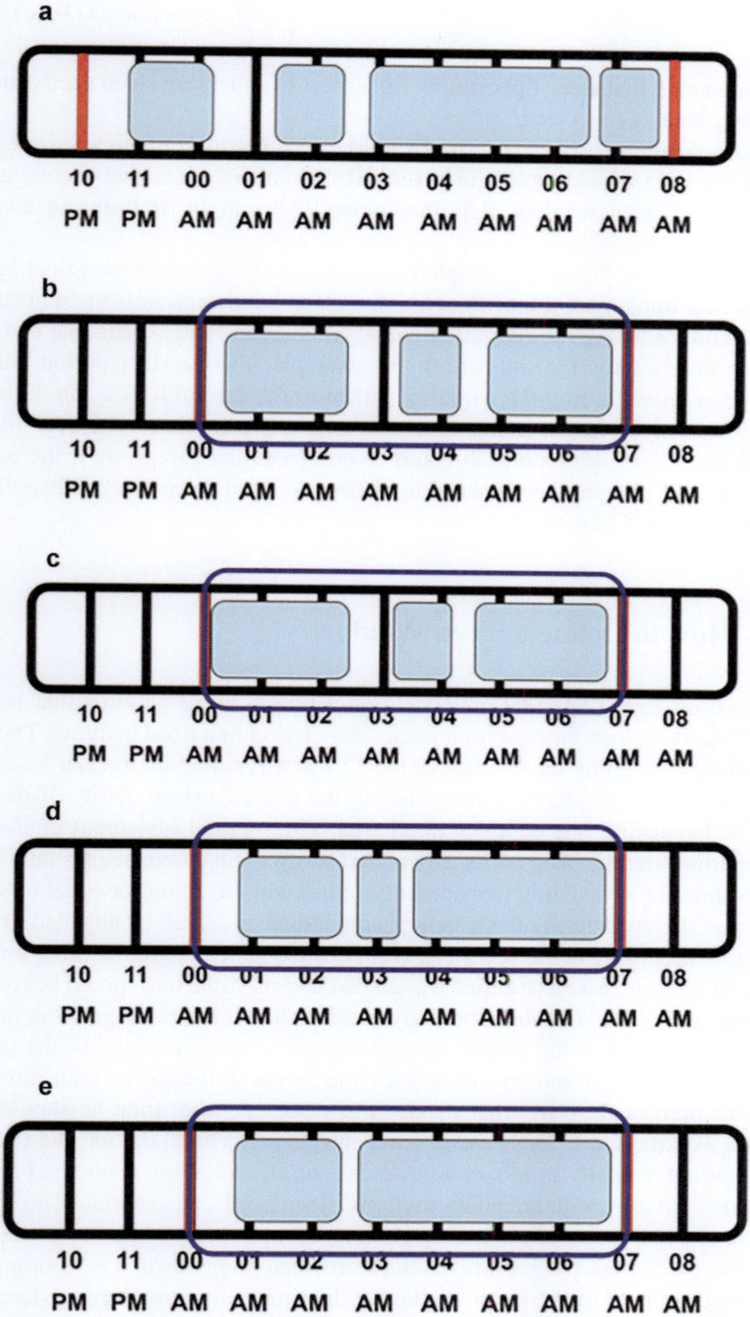

Fig. 12.4 SRT effects on a schematic example of difficulty in initiating and maintaining sleep Red dash corresponds to the bed and rise time, respectively. Blue blocks correspond to sleep bouts. Blue dash corresponds to the sleep window. (**a**) illustrates a typical night of a patient with difficulty in initiating and maintaining sleep, in which the sleep opportunity (total time in bed = 10 h) is very superior to the total sleep time (7 h) that usually happens in four bouts of sleep. (**b**) The sleep window was defined based on sleep diaries collected by 2 consecutive weeks and the patient was

way, evidencing that sleep opportunity falls short of satisfying sleep needs and that more sleep time is requested.

SRT applications used to last over *8 weeks*. In order to promote adjustments on sleep needs and to avoid prolonging eventual sleep deprivations that encompass the setting of the sleep window, it is recommended to apply SRT during consecutive weeks.

The *sleep diary* should be completed as long as the insomnia treatment lasts. It consists of a fundamental tool to define the sleep window, points the adjustments needed on it, as well as to suggest situations, behaviors, and beliefs that can interfere with sleep expression and pattern. For example, a worse sleep period linked to bad news received during the workday, linked to the care of a sick son during the night, followed by higher consumption of alcohol, etc. Moreover, SRT titration depends on sleep diary reports. It could be completed by caregivers if the patients are physically or cognitively incapable of completing a sleep diary. Sleep diary is well described in Chap. 9.

12.5 How to Define a Sleep Window?

As shown on Fig. 12.4, SRT involves prescribing a sleep window that matches patient-reported sleep duration to a fixed sleep period in a fixed bedtime. The sleep duration is obtained by the average of the TST self-reported on the last 2 weeks of sleep diaries. This reference corresponds to the patient's sleep ability. If the sleep ability is happening late at night (increased SOL—initial insomnia) and/or with awake periods during sleep period (increased WASO—maintenance insomnia) and/or early morning awakening (terminal insomnia) with SE minor or equal to 80%, it means that the opportunity to sleep is overabundant and must be adjusted to a narrow period according to the real sleep ability of the patient. After defining the sleep period, patients are asked to define a fixed bed and rise time that should be followed seven nights a week. For that, the daily routine should be investigated in order to consider the time that the patient arrives at home—what he does till the time he decides to lie down, if and how he relaxes, the period of the day he feels more alert and more tired or drowsy, what makes him wake up, what time he should leave home on workdays, etc. This investigation aims to understand routine and circadian preferences, eventually proposes adjustments on it, and helps define bed and rise times that fits better with circadian rhythms, sleep needs, and routine. The bed and rise time also has to consider the sleep pattern description, for example: if the patient has an increased SOL and reports feeling alert when lying down, it is recommended to fix the beginning of the sleep window at the time he reports starting sleep time; on the other hand, if sleep is well consolidated until 4:30 AM, becoming fragmented after that, it could be suggested to consider the rise time at 4:30 AM.

Consider the following example to illustrate the SRT application step by step:

James (male, 41 years old) complains about difficulties in initiating and maintaining sleep. He reported as always having more nocturnal habits that conflicts with the early work time. Since the time to wake up should be at a maximum of 7 AM, he decided to sleep earlier than his preference in order to have more sleep opportunity. In the beginning of his work life, he started having trouble in initiating sleep. As he assumed more responsibilities in work, he began to experience difficulties in maintaining sleep. It started 10 years ago, exactly when he was promoted as manager. As the insomnia symptoms intensified, James became more concerned with the amount of sleep he was able to get and, in order to guarantee sleep time and ease the sleep deprivation, he decided to extend the sleep period to 8 AM and go to bed earlier (at 10 PM), turning off all the lights and forcing relaxation in order to get to sleep. He reported being very disappointed with himself because he is always late to work, tired, and afraid of losing control over work performance. Moreover, he avoids social meetings to preserve these sleep habits. He filled up 2 weeks of sleep diaries, which sleep measures averages are shown in Table 12.1.

As shown in Table 12.1, James' sleep ability is happening late at night (increased SOL—initial insomnia) and with awake periods all night long (increased WASO—maintenance insomnia) with SE equal to 70%. As the frequency of nocturnal awakening is three times per night, it means that the sleep ability used to occur in four bouts of sleep comprehending 7 h of TST. Figure 12.4a illustrates the schematic sleep pattern of James. The sleep period should be defined according to TST. In this case, a sleep period of 7 h. The investigation of James' circadian preferences and routine demonstrated that the later he lies down, the easier he could initiate sleep. Moreover, he referred to having a sensation of deepest sleep at the last bout of sleep, after 3 or 4 AM. However, he should leave home for work at 7:40 AM, meaning the need to get up at 7 AM. Discussing the many pros and cons of evening and morning routine, James decided to fix bedtime between 00 AM to 7 AM. That is the James' sleep window: a sleep period of 7 h fixed to occur only between 00 AM to 7 AM.

After defining the sleep window, patients are oriented to respect it seven nights a week and to avoid napping during daytime or in the evening. The sleep window defines the period that the patient can go to sleep, not before or after that. Moreover, they are oriented to follow sleep hygiene orientations, avoiding use of electronic equipment that emits light (mobile, tablet, television, computer) at least 1 hour

Table 12.1 James' sleep measures prior to SRT intervention

Sleep measure	Value
Initial sleep period	10 PM
Terminal sleep period	08 AM
Sleep onset latency (SOL)	55 min
Frequency of nocturnal awakenings	3 times a night
Wake time after sleep onset (WASO)	125 min
Early morning awakening (EMA)	15 min
Total sleep time	7 h
Total time in bed	10 h
Total awake time (SOL + WASO + EMA)	195 min
Sleep efficiency	70%

before the beginning of the sleep window and along all sleep period. If they awaken during the sleep period, they are oriented to leave bed and bedroom (if possible) and engage in some refreshing activity, such as reading a book, writing personal issues, painting a mandala, knit, crochet, or any other pleasure activity that does not provoke alertness. These orientations follow the Sleep Hygiene basements and Stimulus Control Therapy, previously described in Chaps. 10 and 11, respectively.

Attention!

- The sleep diary should be completed as long as the insomnia treatment lasts.
- To define the sleep window, consider collecting at least two consecutive weeks of sleep diaries.
- To avoid severe drowsiness, the sleep window should never last less than 5 h.
- Patients should be encouraged not to nap during daytime or in the evening.
- Besides definition of sleep window and how to deal with it, SRT includes orientations based on sleep hygiene and stimulus control therapy.

12.6 How to Titrate the Sleep Window?

For the following weeks of the treatment, it is advisable to see patients every week. The adherence to the sleep window may provoke sleep deprivation, especially for the first and second weeks of the treatment. The weekly segment may offer opportunities for adjustments, clarifications, and orientations. In terms of SRT, the goal of the following encounters should be to promote total adherence to the sleep window in order to make sleep initiation faster (SOL decrease) and sleep consolidated (decrease in awakenings frequency and in WASO), meaning a better sleep pattern that achieves patients' sleep and wakefulness satisfaction. For that, Spielman et al. (2011) proposed and revised some rules to evaluate sleep measures obtained by the self-report sleep diary:

- If SE was ≥90% (85% in seniors), sleep window should be increased by 15–30 min.
- If SE was <85%(80% in seniors), sleep window should be reduced by 15–30 min.
- If SE was between 85% and 90%, no changes should be made on sleep window.

Beyond the rules above, in some cases, patients may suffer from severe drowsiness. In such cases, 20 or 30 min should be added to the sleep window in order to alleviate the effects of sleep deprivation. However, it should be clinical and critically analyzed, since insomnia patients refer to the sleepiness, tiredness, inattention, and other immediate sleep deprivation effects to avoid leaving the "comfort zone," represented by the challenge of the sleep window strategy.

Improvements in sleep with SRT require ongoing restriction of sleep opportunity. It means that the immediate suspension of restricted sleep opportunity after

SRT provokes a regression of nocturnal sleep efficiency back to baseline (Belfer et al., 2021).

When patients achieve SE ≥90% and sleep pattern changes to a more consolidated sleep, indicating sleep satisfaction—feeling well throughout the day and not being vulnerable to insomnia episodes—the SRT should be suspended. Nevertheless, patients should be oriented to keep the bedtime and rise time defined during the treatment as the main reference to keep a good sleep homeostasis and a healthy sleep–wake circadian rhythm.

Back to James' example, the sleep window was defined as a sleep period of 7 h fixed to occur only between 00 AM to 7 AM. Table 12.2 synthesizes the sleep window and the titration segments of SRT. During the session that followed the first week of SRT implementation (Week 1), James reported difficulty in rising at the agreed time, arguing tiredness and sleep deprivation. Because of that, he decided by himself to change the alarm clock to 7:30 AM. As the bedtime was fixed at 00 AM, even above the pre-sleep anticipatory anxiety, the sleep homeostasis started to play its strength night after night, turning SOL faster than baseline and diminishing the awakening frequency (from 2 to 3) and WASO (from 125 to 100 min). TST decreased from 7 h to 6.5 h because of the persistence of the main insomnia features (awakenings and higher WASO) beneath TIB restriction. The intervention focused on reinforcing the principles of sleep homeostasis and James was strongly oriented to respect the sleep window. For the second week, as he followed the orientations properly, WASO decreased. The observed increment of SOL was an anxiety answer, precisely the fear of sleep deprivation effects. Although tired, during this week, he realized that the respect to the sleep window led to a more consolidated sleep, nurturing hopes to get a better sleep pattern in the following weeks. James now adhered to SRT 100%. From week 3 to 5, as soon as the SRT effects became more prominent, he became more confident, relaxing more day by day, night after night. It helped him to diminish pre-sleep anxiety, turning faster the SOL (from 40 to 25 min) and diminishing awakening frequency (from 2 to 1) and WASO (from 80 to 40 min). These sleep measures reflected on the SE growing (from 68.9% to 82.5%), representing a growing conquest of sleep consolidation. Although SE was <85%, James reported increased self-confidence, marked by total adherence to the strategies and acknowledgment of their effects. Concurrently, features of his insomnia, such as SOL, awakenings, and WASO, began to subside. This improvement indicates that there was no need to modify his sleep window. So, the conversion to a better sleep pattern was proved by week 6 to 8, when faster SOL was consolidated along with WASO decrement week by week (from 40 to 0 min) and total abolishment of awakenings during the night (week 8) and, SE increment (from 82.3% to 93.0%). At the session that followed the 8th week of treatment, James demonstrated total satisfaction with the results: consolidated sleep pattern, faster SOL, and absence of pre-sleep anticipatory anxiety. Nevertheless, he reported the need for more sleep, especially at the end of the sleep period. At week 8, the TST achieved was below from the one collected at baseline (6h40 versus 7 h, respectively). As SE was 93.0%, it was proposed an increase of 20 min to the sleep window for the next week. Considering the work time, James decided to distribute 10 min before and 10 min

Table 12.2 James' sleep window and the titration segments of SRT

	References		Sleep measure post sleep restriction therapy (week by week)										
	SM prior to SRT	Sleep window	W 1	W 2	W 3	W 4	W 5	W 6	W 7	W 8	W 9	W 10	W 11 F-up
Initial sleep period	10 PM	00 AM	00 AM	00 AM	00 AM	00 AM	00 AM	00 AM	00 AM	00 AM	23:50 PM	23:40 PM	23:30 PM
Terminal sleep period	8 AM	7 AM	7:30 AM	7 AM	7 AM	7 AM	7 AM	7 AM	7 AM	7 AM	7:10 AM	7:10 AM	7:15 AM
Sleep onset latency (SOL)	55 min	NA	30 min	40 min	30 min	25 min	25 min	20 min	20 min	20 min	20 min	15 min	20 min
Frequency of nocturnal awakenings	3	NA	2	2	2	1	1	1	1	0	0	0	1
Wake time after sleep onset (WASO)	125 min	NA	100 min	80 min	60 min	60 min	40 min	20 min	10 min	NA	NA	NA	2 min
Early morning awakening (EMA)	15 min	NA	15 min	15 min	10 min	10 min	10 min	10 min	10 min	10 min	5 min	5 min	5 min
Total sleep time	7h00	NA	6h30	5h00	5h30	5h35	5h55	6h20	6h30	6h40	7h00	7h15	7h30
Total time in bed	10h00	7h00	7h45	7h15	7h10	7h10	7h10	7h10	7h10	7h10	7h25	7h35	7h50
Total awake time (SOL + WASO + EMA)	195 min	NA	145 min	135 min	100 min	95 min	75 min	50 min	40 min	30 min	25 min	20 min	27 min
Sleep efficiency	70.0%	NA	83.9%	68.9%	76.7%	77.9%	82.5%	88.3%	90.7%	93.0%	94.4%	95.6%	95.7%
Subjective sleep quality (0–10)	5	NA	4.5	3	4.0	5.0	6.0	6.0	7.0	7.5	8.5	9.0	9.2

Legend: *SM* Sleep measure, *SRT* Sleep restriction therapy, *NA* not applicable, *W* week, *min* minutes, *F-up* Follow up (2 weeks after week 9)

after the bedtime and rise time, defining a new sleep window of 7h20 (between 23:50 PM and 7:10 AM). At week 9, the results observed were a correspondent increment in TST and SE, with sleep pattern preserved, indicating the possibility to enhance the sleep window by 10 min more (between 23:40 PM and 7:10 AM). As James answered well (week 10), with faster SOL, higher SE, reporting much more relaxed, with no fear about the returning of insomnia symptoms but still needing an alarm clock to wake up, it was hypothesized that the TST at baseline was below his real necessity of sleeping time, probably representing a feature of hypervigilance. For that, it was proposed to increase the sleep window by 15 min. In order to attend to his routine needs and preferences, it was settled between 23:30 PM and 7:15. At week 11, TST achieved 7h30 (30 min more than baseline) with sleep consolidated and SE preserved above 95%. Finally, James reported waking up totally restored, with no somnolence residue. The suspension of SRT was done with orientations regarding the importance of sleep hygiene and the bedtime regular habits.

12.7 What to Do When Patients Are Medicated with Pharmacotherapy Agents to Promote Sleep?

When patients are medicated with sleep inductors, anxiolytic, or other sedative agents, the treatment length could be prolonged, following the same references and logic of the procedure defined for 8 weeks. However, it is recommended to first adjust sleep patterns and only after that dishabituate pharmacotherapy agents, following recommendations and advice by a sleep physician.

12.8 Actigraphy Register—When to Use and When Not to Use

Actigraphy is a noninvasive and validated method of objectively measuring motor activity and rest over a period of days to weeks. Through a mathematical algorithm, these measures can estimate the sleep–wake pattern and rhythm. The International Classification of Sleep Disorders (American Academy of Sleep Medicine, 2014) suggests actigraphy to evaluate insomnia and circadian rhythm alterations. As well described in this chapter and illustrated by Fig. 12.3, insomnia patients tend to spend long periods of wakefulness in bed, which may compromise sleep estimates obtained by actigraphy (Rösler et al., 2023). Nevertheless, actigraphy may be considered for patients who are very resistant to completing a sleep diary or those who are physically or cognitively incapable to complete a sleep diary. In SRT, the TST estimated by actigraphy will be adopted to define the sleep window.

In cases of sleep misperception, those who have a huge sleep duration underestimation, the use of actigraphy is controversial. On the one hand, the comparison of the different amounts of TST (actigraphy versus own perception) may help the patient to realize his underestimates of TST, demystifying his worse expectations and equivocal comprehension about his hypothetical poor sleep, providing relaxation and better sleep routine. On the other hand, for other patients, the establishment of a sleep window based on TST derived by actigraphy may weaken the strength of SRT intervention. It happens because sleep misperception is commonly found on a very fragmented sleep mixed with hypervigilance, meaning a kind of consciousness state that takes place as long as the sleep period happens, rendering difficult the perception of sleep and promoting a perception of permanent wakefulness. When actigraphy measures detect a TST almost equal to TIB (e.g., SE ≥90%), the sleep window based on that will not have the strength to change the sleep pattern, not even the hypervigilance, since TST taken objectively (actigraphy) is much more extended than that perceived by the patient report. In terms of cognition, changes will be hardly promoted, since TIB will be maintained almost the same as before the intervention. In such cases, the subjective TST must be taken into account in order to promote homeostatic sleep drive and provoke cognitive changes, especially perception. Consider the following example to illustrate it:

Rachel (female, 48 years, married, advertising professional) complains of insomnia symptoms for 18 years. She reported a TST of 4 h. She doesn't refer to sleepiness during the day and any other symptom of sleep deprivation. However, she reports difficulties to "turn the mind off" during day and night. As she resisted to complete the sleep diary, arguing anxiogenic effects, actigraphy monitoring over 14 days was offered alternatively. The analysis parameters evidenced a normal SOL (varying from 20–35 min), TST of 7 h on average, WASO very reduced (5–15 min) and high SE (~ 90%). The sleep pattern occurs in a unique sleep bout, however, full of very brief fragmentations. The SRT intervention based on the TST of 7 hours obtained by actigraphy defined a sleep window of 7 hours, very proximal to her TIB of 7h45. Since the hypervigilance persisted occurring in parallel to sleep bout, almost equal to that before SRT intervention, the sleep misperception persisted, impairing the results in terms of subjective complaints. After 3 weeks of failure of this strategy, the sleep psychologist decided to reduce the sleep opportunity. As she reported a subjective TST of 4 h, the professional decided to be more conservative, as recommended by SRT experts, and asked her to define a sleep window based on 5 h. The results appeared soon after the last approach. Rachel described sleepiness and tiredness in the morning, after lunch and dinner on the days following the new sleep window. Moreover, she began to report having a restorative sleep, consolidated and deep, nevermore hearing the noises around the neighborhood. For the following weeks of the treatment, the sleep psychologist titrated the sleep window as described in this chapter, and Rachel finished the SRT intervention very satisfied, referring to 7h30 of TST, very refreshed, with no insomnia symptoms.

Rachel's example illustrates that even sleep misperception can be corrected by SRT. Nevertheless, objective measures, such as that obtained by actigraphy, cannot be taken as reference when there is a huge discordance with subjective measures, especially when objective WASO is almost absent. It means that hypervigilance must be abolished and should be a goal of the intervention. Besides relaxation strategies and analytical approach, homeostatic sleep drive plays an important role in that, helping to promote sleepiness, and so clarifying the real perception of sleep. It highlights the importance of physiological challenges to promote cognitive change among insomnia patients with sleep misperception.

12.9 Effect-Size of SRT Intervention and Difficulties in SRT Adherence

The main effect-size of SRT is sleep deprivation (Kyle et al., 2014; Maurer et al., 2020, 2021, 2022), especially increased daytime sleepiness, and objective performance impairment (Kyle et al., 2014; Maurer et al., 2022) These effects tend to be more accentuated in the beginning of the treatment (~week 1–3) (Kyle et al., 2014; Maurer et al., 2022), returning to baseline levels by 3 months (Kyle et al., 2014). Because of the conditioned sleep pattern, SOL and WASO remain similar in the early days of SRT implementation, provoking a decrease in TST and sleep deprivation effects as a consequence. Since patients are "prohibited" to compensate for sleep, the intervention anticipates sleep deprivation, enhancing the sleep drive. This drive works as a sleep pressure that imposes the SOL abbreviation and fills up the gap of wakefulness that exists between the fragmented sleep periods, decreasing the awakenings frequency. See the illustrations in Fig. 12.4. Nevertheless, sleep window titration will cancel the effect-sizes. As soon as the protocol adjustments provide TIB extension, soon the TST enhances, gradually reaching the adequate time of sleep, which in turn diminishes and finally cancels the sleep deprivation effects. At the beginning of SRT intervention, patients should be warned that their condition will get worse before it gets better, they will feel more sleep-deprived and tired in the beginning of the treatment and by the end of it will be feeling more restful and satisfied about their sleep.

Sleep deprivation effect-size may be worse among those with sleep misperception. Some patients with sleep misperception report a TST of less than 5 h, sometimes they affirm to sleep only 3 h every night. In such cases, it is not advisable to set the sleep window to less than 5 h to avoid subjecting the patient to severe sleep deprivation. Even so, TIB may be extremely insufficient to recover sleep needs in a way that sleep deprivation effects may be more pronounced, especially in the next days following the beginning of SRT implementation. For such cases, it is important to ask for the sleep diaries between sessions to closely follow the SRT effects and analyze if there is a need to anticipate the sleep window titration, avoiding perpetuation of severe sleep deprivation, especially if sleep perception and sleep pattern improved.

Although sleep deprivation effect-size is temporary, it used to be the main factor for resistance to adhere to SRT. As patients with insomnia usually try to compensate for the sleep deficits prolonging the time in bed, they hardly believe that the promotion of new habits and behavior in an opposite way could help them. For that, they may be uncommitted to adhere to the purpose strategies of SRT.

To help adherence, a session of sleep psychoeducation encompassing sleep–wake physiology and rhythmicity prior to SRT intervention is strongly recommended. When patients understand the principles that substantiate the technique and the conditioned pattern of behavior that maintain the vicious cycle of insomnia, they tend to collaborate with the protocol proposals.

Such cases point out that nonpharmacological insomnia intervention, which includes SRT, is not a simple application of techniques but asks for a wide and deep domain of psychological knowledge and intervention. Sleep psychologists are prepared to deal with sleep's physiological, circadian, and psychological aspects often involved among insomnia patients.

12.10 SRT Indication, Adaptation, and Careful Application

In general, SRT may be indicated for patients with initial, maintenance, or terminal insomnia (Spielman et al., 2011) that exhibit SE less than 85% (80% in seniors). Nevertheless, SRT results may be narrow or even useless in some cases of terminal insomnia or short objective sleep duration phenotype insomnia (TST <6 h), asking for other approaches to benefit the patient and sleep recovery.

Some patients that complain of insomnia, but do not report daytime impairment and/or drowsiness, may have enough TST despite a poor pattern or may be hypervigilant. In the first case, especially when patients are non-adherent to SRT strict protocol, sleep compression should be addressed by a gradual TIB reduction (Lichstein et al., 2011), respecting sleep schedules regularity in order to slowly promote a better sleep pattern (consolidated) and to avoid greater sleep deprivation effects, coping with adherence. In the second case, when the psychological aspects of hypervigilance are well treated, the patient becomes more relaxed, returning to report drowsiness as before the insomnia disorder was developed. Hypervigilance is often associated with short objective sleep duration phenotype insomnia (TST <6 h) (Vgontzas et al., 2013). Many psychological strategies and methods should be addressed for such cases, such as mindfulness and ACT. For that, see ACT-I deeply described in part 4. The same approach could help patients with terminal insomnia that usually get up as soon as they wake up.

Patients with circadian rhythm disorders, such as advanced or late phase, usually present social jet lag, complaining of insomnia symptoms. For that, SRT may regularize sleep schedules and promote TST homogeneity between work and free days, thereby restoring daytime well-being.

Patients with sleep-disordered breathing (SDB) comorbid to insomnia may also suffer from an intensified sleep deprivation. Although SRT could help to consolidate the sleep pattern, it will not be enough to promote total sleep satisfaction, since SDB harms the sleep quality. In such cases, the professional applying SRT must recognize SDB symptomatology, referring the patient to a sleep physician.

Although there is no impediment to SRT intervention in insomnia comorbid to other conditions, work or health conditions that can be strongly affected and harmful by sleep deprivation effects ask for critical analyses about SRT applicability. Air traffic controllers, airplane pilots, bus and truck drivers, machine operators in factories, and others that work within high-risk roles and under absence of surveillance may be at risk under sleep deprivation caused or potentialized by SRT. Similarly, patients that suffer from parasomnias, epilepsies, and some severe psychiatric conditions may have the worsening of the condition triggered by the sleep deprivation.

Sleep deprivation effect-size may be worse among those with sleep misperception. Some patients with sleep misperception report a TST of less than 5 h, sometimes they affirm to sleep only 3 h every night. In such cases, the sleep window is not recommended to be less than 5 h. However, some patients even adhering to a sleep window of 5 h continue to report sleep misperception, complaining of fragmentation or even extended awareness periods. In such cases, the sleep window prescribed should be maintained and relaxation strategies and psychological approaches should be addressed to decrease hypervigilance. In some rare cases, the sleep window could be briefly abbreviated. However, it is recommended to do it with supervision of a sleep psychologist very experienced in SRT management.

Finally, for seniors who live alone, sleep deprivation increases the risk of falling, asking for an SRT adaptation that offers a cadence on the steps of the process:

$$\boxed{TBR \rightarrow \text{avoidance of naps during the day} \rightarrow \text{TIBR}}$$

It is suggested to start the TIBR with a more extended sleep window and be progressively shortened.

The needs for SRT adaption reinforce the necessity for a wide and deep sleep knowledge and psychological approaches to be addressed for as long as the non-pharmacological insomnia interventions lasts.

References

American Academy of Sleep Medicine. (2014). International classification of sleep disorders. American Academy of Sleep Medicine.

Belfer, S. J., Bashaw, A. G., Perlis, M. L., & Kayser, M. S. (2021). A Drosophila model of sleep restriction therapy for insomnia. *Molecular Psychiatry, 26*(2), 492–507. https://doi.org/10.1038/s41380-019-0376-6

Borbély, A. A., & Achermann, P. (1999). Sleep homeostasis and models of sleep regulation. *Journal of Biological Rhythms, 14*(6), 557–568. https://doi.org/10.1177/074873099129000894

Borbély, A. A., Daan, S., Wirz-Justice, A., & Deboer, T. (2016). The two-process model of sleep regulation: A reappraisal. *Journal of Sleep Research, 25*(2), 131–143. https://doi.org/10.1111/jsr.12371

Buysse, D. J., Germain, A., Moul, D. E., Franzen, P. L., Brar, L. K., Fletcher, M. E., Begley, A., Houck, P. R., Mazumdar, S., Reynolds, C. F., 3rd, & Monk, T. H. (2011). Efficacy of brief behavioral treatment for chronic insomnia in older adults. *Archives of Internal Medicine, 171*(10), 887–895. https://doi.org/10.1001/archinternmed.2010.535

Edinger, J. D., & Means, M. K. (2005). Cognitive-behavioral therapy for primary insomnia. *Clinical Psychology Review, 25*(5), 539–558. https://doi.org/10.1016/j.cpr.2005.04.003

Epstein, D. R., Sidani, S., Bootzin, R. R., & Belyea, M. J. (2012). Dismantling multicomponent behavioral treatment for insomnia in older adults: A randomized controlled trial. *Sleep, 35*(6), 797–805. https://doi.org/10.5665/sleep.1878

Kalmbach, D. A., Cheng, P., Arnedt, J. T., Anderson, J. R., Roth, T., Fellman-Couture, C., Williams, R. A., & Drake, C. L. (2019). Treating insomnia improves depression, maladaptive thinking, and hyperarousal in postmenopausal women: Comparing cognitive-behavioral therapy for insomnia (CBTI), sleep restriction therapy, and sleep hygiene education. *Sleep Medicine, 55*, 124–134. https://doi.org/10.1016/j.sleep.2018.11.019

Kang, J.-H., & Chen, S.-C. (2009). Effects of an irregular bedtime schedule on sleep quality, daytime sleepiness, and fatigue among university students in Taiwan. *BMC Public Health, 9*(1), 248.

Kyle, S. D., Miller, C. B., Rogers, Z., Siriwardena, A. N., Macmahon, K. M., & Espie, C. A. (2014). Sleep restriction therapy for insomnia is associated with reduced objective total sleep time, increased daytime somnolence, and objectively impaired vigilance: Implications for the clinical management of insomnia disorder. *Sleep, 37*(2), 229–237. https://doi.org/10.5665/sleep.3386

Lichstein, K. L., Justin Thomas, T. S., & McCurry, S. M. (2011). Sleep Compression. In M. Perlis, M. Aloia, B. Kuhn (Eds.), BSM treatment protocols for insomnia, part 1: chapter 5. (Practical Resources for the Mental Health Professional, Behavioral Treatments for Sleep Disorders) (p. 55-59, ISSN 18730450, ISBN 9780123815224). Academic Press. https://doi.org/10.1016/B978-0-12-381522-4.00001-8

Manber, R., Bootzin, R. R., Acebo, C., & Carskadon, M. A. (1996). The effects of regularizing sleep- wake schedules on daytime sleepiness. *Sleep, 19*(5), 432–441.

Maurer, L. F., Espie, C. A., Omlin, X., Reid, M. J., Sharman, R., Gavriloff, D., Emsley, R., & Kyle, S. D. (2020). Isolating the role of time in bed restriction in the treatment of insomnia: A randomized, controlled, dismantling trial comparing sleep restriction therapy with time in bed regularization. *Sleep, 43*(11), zsaa096. https://doi.org/10.1093/sleep/zsaa096

Maurer, L. F., Schneider, J., Miller, C. B., Espie, C. A., & Kyle, S. D. (2021). The clinical effects of sleep restriction therapy for insomnia: A meta-analysis of randomised controlled trials. *Sleep Medicine Reviews, 58*, 101493. https://doi.org/10.1016/j.smrv.2021.101493

Maurer, L. F., Espie, C. A., Omlin, X., Emsley, R., & Kyle, S. D. (2022). The effect of sleep restriction therapy for insomnia on sleep pressure and arousal: A randomized controlled mechanistic trial. *Sleep, 45*(1), zsab223. https://doi.org/10.1093/sleep/zsab223

Miller, C. B., Espie, C. A., Epstein, D. R., Friedman, L., Morin, C. M., Pigeon, W. R., Spielman, A. J., & Kyle, S. D. (2014). The evidence base of sleep restriction therapy for treating insomnia disorder. *Sleep Medicine Reviews, 18*(5), 415–424. https://doi.org/10.1016/j.smrv.2014.01.006

Rösler, L., van der Lande, G., Leerssen, J., Cox, R., Ramautar, J. R., & van Someren, E. J. W. (2023). Actigraphy in studies on insomnia: Worth the effort? *Journal of Sleep Research, 32*(1), e13750. https://doi.org/10.1111/jsr.13750

Spielman, A. J., Saskin, P., & Thorpy, M. J. (1987a). Treatment of chronic insomnia by restriction of time in bed. *Sleep, 10*(1), 45–56.

Spielman, A. J., Yang, C. M., & Glovinsky, P. B. (2011). Sleep restriction therapy. In M. Perlis, M. Aloia, & B. Kuhn (Eds.), *BSM treatment protocols for insomnia, part I; chapter 1* (Practical resources for the mental health professional, behavioral treatments for sleep disorders) (p. 9–19, ISSN 18730450, ISBN 9780123815224). Academic Press. https://doi.org/10.1016/B978-0-12-381522-4.00001-8

Vgontzas, A. N., Fernandez-Mendoza, J., Liao, D., & Bixler, E. O. (2013). Insomnia with objective short sleep duration: The most biologically severe phenotype of the disorder. *Sleep Medicine Reviews, 17*(4), 241–254. https://doi.org/10.1016/j.smrv.2012.09.005

Part IV
ACT for Insomnia

Chapter 13
Acceptance and Commitment Therapy

Michaele Terena Saban-Bernauer and Roberta Kovac

Acceptance and Commitment Therapy (ACT) is a psychotherapeutic treatment approach that is part of contemporary contextual behavioral therapies, also called 3rd wave of Behavioral Therapies (Hayes, 2004). Its philosophical root is Functional Contextualism, which suggests observing the phenomena in their interaction with the context. In the case of behavior, the root metaphor of Functional Contextualism is the observation of action in context (Pepper, 1942), considering the impossibility of dissociating this relationship (action can only be understood in context, and context is only defined depending on the action) (Biglan & Hayes, 1996). ACT is based on a theoretical body of Contextual Behavioral Science, which presents models and theories based on evolutionary science, the principles of behavioral learning and Relational Frame Theory (RFT), a theoretical approach to language and human cognition (Hayes et al., 2001).

According to its main proponent, ACT addresses human suffering based on a transdiagnostic model of psychopathology, called psychological inflexibility (Hayes, 2019). The way language and cognition interact with direct contingencies can produce an inability to persist or change behavior in the service of long-term ends (Hayes & Smith, 2005). Thus, the authors define psychological distress as a corollary of verbal processes, both as a primary source of psychopathology and as processes that exacerbate the impact of other sources of psychopathology. ACT differentiates two types of suffering: the pain that is felt in the lived experience and the suffering derived from it, which involves thoughts about the pain, remembering,

M. T. Saban-Bernauer (✉)
School of Permanent Education, Clinics Hospital, Faculty of Medicine,
University of São Paulo, Sao Paulo, Brazil

R. Kovac
Paradigma Center of Behavioral Science and Technology, Sao Paulo, Brazil
e-mail: roberta.kovac@institutopar.org

R. El Rafihi-Ferreira (ed.), *Acceptance and Commitment Therapy for Insomnia*,
https://doi.org/10.1007/978-3-031-50710-6_13

fearing that it will happen again, relating to other experiences, deriving new rules and self-rules, and other cognitive processes that, according to the RFT, imply trained verbal relations that emerge in a given situation. Pain is lived suffering, experienced directly from immediate aversive contingencies, and psychological suffering comes from our ability to relate events.

The proposed treatment for this type of verbal distress, presented by ACT, then aims to promote psychological flexibility, defined as the "ability to contact the present moment more fully as a conscious human being, and to change or persist in behavior when it serves the purpose ends valued by the individual" (Hayes et al., 2006, p. 7). In this way, ACT does not have as its primary objective the relief of suffering, but it aims to promote a more meaningful life, even if this implies being open to challenging feelings, thoughts, sensations, and memories.

The conception of human suffering, according to ACT, is based on the assumption of "the ubiquity of human suffering" (Hooper & Larsson, 2015). Hayes et al. (1999) open ACT's landmark book with the sentence: "The most remarkable fact of human existence is how difficult it is for human beings to be happy" (p. 1). Similarly, Luoma et al. (2007) argue: "It is impossible to build a human life untouched by suffering" (p. 1).

These statements above illustrate the proposal of ACT and the model of psychopathology that it defends, that suffering is an inevitable product of the experience of human beings and that the origin of psychological suffering would be in the very behavior that seems to be exclusively human – verbal behavior (or language and cognition).

This understanding of human psychological suffering, which has an intervention and treatment proposal in ACT, is supported by experimental findings and the theoretical narrative of the Theory of Relational Frames (Hayes et al., 2001), which proposes that the central element definer in all human verbal activities is arbitrarily applicable relational responding (AARR). Relational responding constitutes responding to a relationship between events, or relating events in certain ways, based on (arbitrary) social conventions. It is understood that relational responding impacts the function of basic behavioral processes or, as stated by Hayes, Wilson, and Barnes-Holmes (2001), "relational responding is operant behavior that affects the operant learning processes themselves" (p. 45).

According to Dougher (1998), derived relational responding and the transfer of function resulting from it explain how words and other symbols can come to affect behavior. According to the author:

> (…) words participate in equivalence classes with the events to which they relate in the world and, in this way, acquire many of the functions of these events. This explains how the description of eating a sour lemon can elicit salivation or how a warning that a given substance is poisonous can cause it to be avoided (Dougher, 1998, p. 588).

Hayes et al. (2012) describe how this process of transformation of functions inherent to language processes can create an expansion of sources of control and impact on suffering for verbally competent humans:

> When nonhumans are exposed to aversive stimuli, they react in a very predictable way. They engage in avoidance behavior, emit stress-related responses, become aggressive, or

> collapse into a state of immobility. These reactions to aversive events usually have a limited time and are linked to the presence of conditioned or unconditioned stimuli. Behaviors related to these situations typically return to baseline levels once the aversive event is removed and autonomic responses subside. Humans are very different creatures, primarily because of their ability to engage in symbolic activity. Humans can carry aversive events with them, create similarities and dissimilarities between events and form relationships between historical events and current events based on constructed (arbitrary, conventional) similarities. Humans can create predictions about situations that have not yet been experienced. Humans can respond as if an aversive event were present even though that event occurred decades ago. The power of the indirect functions of language and cognition creates the potential for psychological distress in the absence of immediate environmental cues; however, these are the same cognitive skills that most aid human advancement (Hayes et al., 2012, p. 17).

Therefore, supported in this understanding of human psychological suffering, marked by attempts to control private events – feelings, thoughts, body sensations, and memories to avoid suffering (Hayes & Smith, 2005), ACT presents strategies and interventions focused on predicting and influencing the events that produce this suffering, called "Experiential Avoidance."

Experiential avoidance is initially defined as the "phenomenon that occurs when a person is unwilling to stay in touch with a particular private experience (body sensations, emotions, thoughts, memories, behavioral predispositions) and takes steps to change the form or frequency of these events and the context that caused them" (Biglan & Hayes, 1996).

In this way, it is understood that psychological suffering occurs when verbal processes interfere with behavior in a way that is harmful to the individual, in particular, in an attempt to control the frequency or presence of private events and, by doing so, produce a restriction or limitation of other aspects of life.

Numerous problems that arise in the clinical context are related to the way the person tries to control or modify their thoughts (negative, demeaning of themselves, or catastrophic about the future), their emotions (sadness, anxiety, anger), body sensations, or memories. At the same time, it is known that private experiences are made up of derived relational repertoire and that relational networks work by addition and not by subtraction, which makes it clinically impossible to eliminate aversive cognitive and emotional events (Hayes et al., 2012).

From the point of view of ACT, anxiety, depression, and insomnia, among other forms of psychological suffering, are the products of situations and are not a problem in themselves. They signal a larger problematic context and a behavioral pattern of wanting to control the discomfort generated, instead of acting in the original context of the problem. The intervention proposal on this type of suffering, presented by ACT, includes changing verbal contexts in such a way that the limitations imposed by the dominance of verbally established functions and by experiential avoidance are transformed (Hayes et al. 2012).

According to Hayes et al. (2013), the ACT-based intervention enables the creation of non-literal, non-evaluative contexts, which reduce unnecessary regulatory functions of cognitive events and increase contact with the ongoing process (thinking, feeling, evaluating, judging, remembering) as opposed to the content of what is thought, felt, remembered. Included in this intervention are strategies identified as acceptance, cognitive defusion, contact with the present moment, self as context, clarification of values and actions committed to them. These six processes are often illustrated using the image of the "Hexaflex," a hexagonal shape in which each vertex corresponds to one of the six processes that promote psychological flexibility (Fig. 13.1)

To illustrate psychological inflexibility and its six processes, consider insomnia in this prism. Many events can keep us awake at night, as well as thoughts, feelings, and memories, in the same way, can make falling asleep more difficult. Sometimes, something reminds us of a bad situation, or recurring thoughts appear and eventually generate uncomfortable sensations. Hardly a concrete experience is happening at bedtime, (a fight when you're about to fall asleep that keeps you up at night, for example). What happens is suffering arising from verbal behavior: unpleasant thoughts, feelings, sensations, and memories that we tend to try to control. An important part of the insomnia process involves thoughts like "I need to stop thinking about that," and "I have to go back to sleep." To manage distress, we engage in experiential avoidance responses that serve as distractions from discomfort. They often work, at least temporarily, but the problem that generated the unpleasant thoughts and feelings that keep us losing sleep has not been addressed.

In some situations, what we try to do is mentally "solve the problem," and find a solution. However, many of the problems that keep us awake at night and that constitute the type of psychological distress described here are "no solution" problems

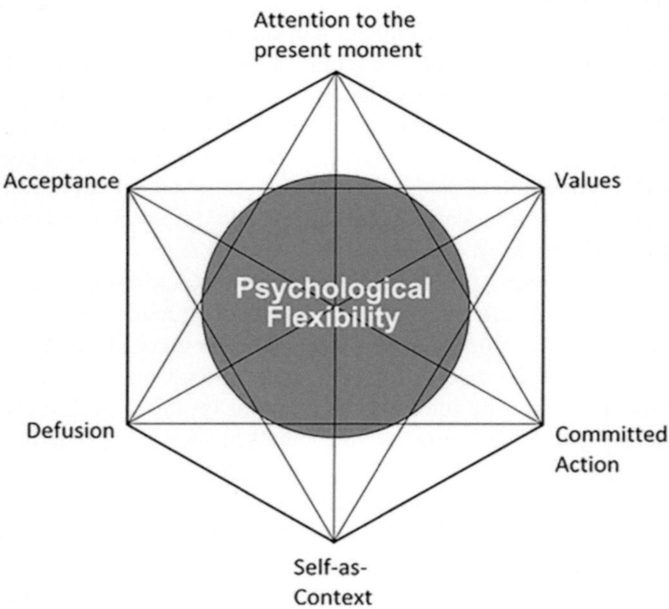

Fig. 13.1 Hexaflex. (Copyright Steven C. Hayes. Used by permission)

("I can't feel this"; "I should have said/done/thought of this sooner"/ "what will happen if I do X, Y, or Z") – problems unlikely to be solved lying in bed, at bedtime.

Thus, experiential avoidance responses are like "killing the messenger." The messenger appears to warn that the kingdom is at war, and experiential avoidance – what we do to try to control the discomfort – works like killing the messenger while the kingdom continues in flames. This is because taking action toward what is important and making life changes that make it more meaningful requires experiencing situations that in the past were challenging, learning to deal with them and including them in some (productive) way in your experience. How to get through the war. And this is difficult.

Restoring or cultivating important relationships, changing behaviors, making life changes, all this evokes many emotions and challenging thoughts. And if the focus of treatment is to avoid suffering, the patient will avoid making the changes that are important to them. So the focus of ACT-based intervention, as already mentioned, is Psychological Flexibility – being psychologically flexible to feel, think, and remember what comes along in the direction of what is important to you.

During the therapeutic process, the therapist creates alternative verbal contexts, through experiential exercises, metaphors, and questions to train skills and promote psychological flexibility (creative hopelessness, acceptance, defusion, mindfulness, self as context, values, and actions toward them).

In Creative Hopelessness, we investigate the different forms of experiential avoidance that the client presents and their effect on eliminating/controlling suffering in the short term – immediate consequences – and in the long term. Generally, experiential avoidance works in the short term, but as the original problem situation is not resolved, the feeling or thought returns and there is a need to avoid it again. This usually generates significant limitations in the person's life, mainly because it competes with larger goals. The finding of this pattern generates hopelessness in trying to control private events, as this attempt to control is not effective in the long term and generates costs. This step paves the way for the acceptance process.

Acceptance for ACT means experiencing private events openly and non-judgmentally, in a self-compassionate way. Technically, it is a type of exposure intervention carried out in a special way, because instead of exposing an anxiogenic stimulus, it exposes the person to their own anxiety, fear, sadness, or another private event that is being avoided. This change in focus of the object of exposure (from an external stimulus to a private event), enables a much broader change, because in addition to the specific situation in question, other related contingencies, in which the avoidance of feeling/thought/sensation/memory is present, they will also tend to be affected. During exposure to the private aversive event, observation and self-care responses are trained.

Another process related to the management of suffering is cognitive defusion. This process refers to the ability to observe thoughts as behaviors (and not from the content they report). Thinking is behaving, emitting sound responses, seeing images, and establishing relationships between events. Such responses abound in our species and like any other behavior, it has its learning history. We learned, in defusion interventions, to notice that thoughts are learned in our history, that is, for the discomfort of the type "why do *I* think these things," we observe how we learn to think in certain ways and not in others and to relate in different ways because we have been taught to do so. When we think, we tend to think that our thoughts are absolute truths and are reflecting reality. This experience with thinking is useful in countless situations in which what we think effectively describes the experienced contingencies. But in several other situations, especially those linked to psychological suffering, taking the content of the thought literally can be very paralyzing or insomnia-provoking (such as "I am a failure, I will never succeed, I have always been a problem"). The defusion process then involves observing language as behavior and differentiating direct functions (arising from experience) from attributed ones (evaluations, judgments, and other learned relationships).

The conception of self as context corresponds to another set of relations arising from language that generates the notion of "I." The ability to perceive oneself is typically human and constructed by language. The conception of "I" that ACT trains is not linked to specific contents of how the person is or is not, thinks or feels, but rather as the place, the locus where thoughts, feelings, sensations, memories, and actions occur. A place as a perspective from which the entire experience can be experienced. This context constitutes a hierarchical relationship in which the "I" contains private events and actions. This form of self-perception facilitates psychological flexibility and contact with difficult private content.

Just like the self as a context, the practice of mindfulness is present in all processes as a prerequisite. It is the ability to observe without judgment and in an open way. Mindfulness means the exercise of directing attention. During ACT's therapeutic processes, we train the client to pay attention to the external and internal environment, as well as their actions and their consequences in the short, medium, and long terms.

The processes of observation and self-observation, such as the change in the way of relating to private events, also make it possible to clarify values. This process is the investigation of what is important to the individual and how they want to be in the course of their life. This elucidation of values guides the therapeutic process and becomes its mission – to transform life toward individual values. From these definitions, the client establishes objectives and concrete actions to carry out this new way of living that is important to them. When carrying out these actions, all other learning and training processes of psychological flexibility are also put into practice, with an emphasis on accepting private events that appear in experiences and observing thoughts as they appear and not based on what is said.

When the client acquires fluency in these processes, the treatment ends.

References

Biglan, A., & Hayes, S. C. (1996). Should the behavioral sciences become more pragmatic? The case for functional contextualism in research on human behavior. *Applied and Preventive Psychology: Current Scientific Perspectives, 5*, 47–57.

Dougher, M. J. (1998). Stimulus equivalence and the untrained acquisition of stimulus functions. *Behavior Therapy, 29*(4), 577–591. https://doi.org/10.1016/S0005-7894(98)80018-X
Hayes, S. C., & Smith, S. (2005). *Get out of your mind get & into your life*. New Harbinger Publications, Inc..
Hayes, S., Strosahl, K., & Wilson, K. (1999/2012). *Acceptance and commitment therapy: An experiential approach to behavior change*. The Guilford Press.
Hayes, S., Barnes-Holmes, D., & Roche, B. (2001). *Relational frame theory: A post-Skinnerian account of human language and cognition*. Kluwer Academic/Plenum Publishers.
Hayes, S. C. (2004). Acceptance and Commitment Therapy, Relational Frame Theory, and the Third Wave of Behavioral and Cognitive Therapies. Behavior Therapy, *35*(4), 639–665. https://doi.org/10.1016/S0005-7894(04)80013-3
Hayes, S. C., Luoma, J. B., Bond, F. W., Masuda, A., & Lillis, J. (2006). Acceptance and commitment therapy: Model, processes and outcomes. *Behaviour Research and Therapy, 44*, 1–25. https://doi.org/10.1016/j.brat.2005.06.006
Hayes, S. C., Levin, M., Plumb-Vilardaga, J., Villatte, J., & Pistorello, J. (2013). Acceptance and Commitment Therapy and contextual behavioral science: Examining the progress of a distinctive model of behavioral and cognitive therapy. Behavior Therapy (44), 180–198.
Hayes, S. (2019). A Liberated Mind: How to Pivot Toward What Matters. New York: Avery.
Hayes, S. C, Wilson, K. G., & Barnes-Holmes, D. Derived Relational Responding as learned behavior. In: Hayes, S. C., Barnes-Holmes, D., & Roche, B. (Eds.). (2001). Relational Frame Theory: A Post-Skinnerian account of human language and cognition. New York: Plenum Press.
Hooper, N., & Larsson, A. (2015). *The research journey of acceptance and commitment therapy (ACT)*. Palgrave Macmillan. https://doi.org/10.1057/9781137440174
Luoma, J. B., Hayes, S. C., & Walser, R. D. (2007). *Learning ACT: An acceptance and commitment therapy skills-training manual for therapists*. New Harbinger Publications.
Pepper, S. (1942). *World hypotheses: A study in evidence*. University of California Press.
Hayes, S. C., Wilson, K. G., & Barnes-Holmes, D. (2001). Derived Relational Responding as learned behavior. In: Hayes, S. C., Barnes-Holmes, D., & Roche, B. (Eds.). *Relational Frame Theory: A Post-Skinnerian account of human language and cognition*. New York: Plenum Press.

Chapter 14
Evidence of Acceptance and Commitment Therapy-Based Therapies for Insomnia

Léo Paulos-Guarnieri, Ila Marques Porto Linares, and Renatha El Rafihi-Ferreira

A large number of studies are currently investigating the effects of Acceptance and Commitment Therapy (ACT) interventions on different disorders and conditions. The website of the Association for Contextual Behavioral Science (ACBS) contains a list of more than 1000 randomized clinical trials[1] and of more than 400 systematic reviews and/or meta-analyses[2] investigating ACT.

Gloster et al. (2020) recently systematized the evidence on ACT in order to evaluate the effects of ACT interventions for a variety of conditions, comparing different groups. For this purpose, the authors included 20 meta-analysis studies whose results showed that ACT has benefits for complaints such as depression, anxiety, substance use, and chronic pain. In addition to reducing these complaints, the studies have demonstrated beneficial effects for variables such as quality of life, psychological flexibility, and well-being. ACT was superior when compared with non-active control groups or with passive interventions. However, there were no significant differences between ACT and CBT.

The data analyzed by Gloster et al. (2020) can have different implications. The study suggests that ACT is a viable option for different conditions since it provided

Léo Paulos-Guarnieri receives research support from the São Paulo Research Foundation (FAPESP) [grant #2020/107486; #2023/06859-5].

[1] https://contextualscience.org/act_randomized_controlled_trials_1986_to_present

[2] https://contextualscience.org/metaanalyses_and_systematic_scoping_or_narrative_reviews_of_the_act_evidenc

L. Paulos-Guarnieri (✉) · I. M. P. Linares
Faculty of Medicine at the University of São Paulo, Sao Paulo, Brazil

R. El Rafihi-Ferreira
Department of Clinical Psychology, University of São Paulo, Sao Paulo, Brazil
e-mail: rerafihi@usp.br

R. El Rafihi-Ferreira (ed.), *Acceptance and Commitment Therapy for Insomnia*,
https://doi.org/10.1007/978-3-031-50710-6_14

favorable results in different meta-analyses involving different disorders (Gloster et al., 2020). This scenario also supports the transdiagnostic proposal of ACT (Dindo et al., 2017; Gloster et al., 2020; Ong et al., 2020), in which psychological flexibility is an important aspect of health (Kashdan et al., 2010). The proposal of promoting psychological flexibility expands the notion of mental health beyond the absence of symptoms by also considering the promotion of quality of life, well-being, functioning, and psychological flexibility (Dindo et al., 2017; Gloster et al., 2020).

The implications of the study by Gloster et al. (2020) are important; however, no systematic reviews or meta-analyses of ACT focusing on insomnia were available at the time when that study was published. At present, there are two systematic reviews on ACT for insomnia and sleep quality (Paulos-Guarnieri et al., 2022; Salari et al., 2020) and one systematic review with meta-analysis (Ruan et al., 2022). And what do these studies show?

The review by Salari et al. (2020) evaluated the effects of interventions that used ACT for insomnia with and without comorbidities, with sleep patterns and sleep quality as outcomes. Nineteen articles demonstrated a positive and significant impact of the interventions on insomnia severity, sleep quality, daytime sleepiness, dysfunctional beliefs and attitudes about sleep, acceptance of sleep problems, and parameters of sleep efficiency such as sleep latency, wakefulness after sleep onset, and total sleep time (Salari et al., 2020).

Paulos-Guarnieri et al. (2022) conducted a systematic review on interventions using ACT for insomnia as the primary outcome. The 11 articles included in the review reported significant improvements in insomnia severity and sleep parameters, as well as in secondary outcomes such as dysfunctional beliefs and attitudes about sleep, acceptance of sleep problems, daytime sleepiness, and cognitive suppression (Paulos-Guarnieri et al., 2022). Evaluation of the components of the interventions suggested that ACT can be applied as monotherapy for insomnia (Acceptance and Commitment Therapy for Insomnia, ACT-I) or combined with stimulus control and sleep restriction components (Acceptance and Commitment Therapy-Based Behavioral Intervention for Insomnia, ACT-BBI-I). Both modalities produced favorable results in terms of reducing the severity of insomnia (Paulos-Guarnieri et al., 2022)

Ruan et al. (2022) carried out a systematic review with meta-analysis of randomized clinical trials using ACT for insomnia and sleep quality, with the first meta-analysis of ACT involving these outcomes. Eighteen studies were included. Meta-analyses were performed to assess the effects of ACT on the sleep and insomnia of participants and on the sleep of participants with other diseases or conditions. The results showed that ACT provided better results in terms of reducing insomnia symptoms and dysfunctional beliefs and attitudes about sleep when compared with the waiting-list and psychoeducation control groups. When compared with CBT-I, ACT did not differ in terms of insomnia severity or sleep diary parameters. At the end, the authors highlight that, given the limitations in the methodological qualities of the included studies, caution is necessary when interpreting and generalizing the meta-analysis results (Ruan et al., 2022). Nevertheless, the authors suggest that ACT could be an effective approach to treating insomnia and improving sleep quality.

14.1 Systematization and Synthesis of Reviews on ACT for Insomnia and/or Sleep Quality

This section systematizes and synthesizes the results of the articles included in the latest reviews on the topic (Paulos-Guarnieri et al., 2022; Salari et al., 2020; Ruan et al., 2022), removing duplicate or repeated articles. Although the reviews have different objectives, as well as different inclusion and exclusion criteria, the information of the studies was arranged in tables to show the evidence found so far and which aspects future studies should explore. Two tables were built for this purpose. Table 14.1 includes randomized clinical trials and Table 14.2 studies with other designs. In both tables, the articles were organized according to year of publication, highlighting whether insomnia was the primary or secondary outcome in the studies and the general characteristics of the participants.

Table 14.1 Randomized clinical trials

Year	Authors	Primary outcome	Participants
Insomnia as primary outcome			
2015	Baik	Insomnia	Adults
2019	Lappalainen et al.	Insomnia	Adults
2021	El Rafihi-Ferreira et al.	Chronic insomnia	Adults
2021	Chapatout et al.	Chronic insomnia and hypnotic addiction	Adults
2021	Haung et al.	Insomnia	Elderly adults
2021	Zakiei et al.	Insomnia	Adults
2022	Chen et al.	Insomnia	Students
2022a, b	El Rafihi-Ferreira et al.	Chronic insomnia	Adults
Insomnia or sleep quality as secondary outcome			
2011	Westin et al.	Tinnitus	Adults
2012	Hesser et al.	Tinnitus	Adults
2013	Pelkonen and Puha	Chronic sleep problems	Adults
2015	Gao and He	Tinnitus	Adults
2017	Clarke et al.	Osteoarthritis	Elderly adults
2017	Herbert et al.	Chronic pain	Adults
2017	Lang et al.	Depression and/or anxiety	Adults
2018	Simister et al.	Fibromyalgia	Adults
2018	Mosher et al.	Breast cancer	Adults
2018	Vethe et al.	Chronic fatigue	Adults
2018	Wiklund et al.	Back, neck and/or generalized pain	Adults
2018	Zhang et al.	Gynecological cancer patients and partners	Adults
2019	Mosher et al.	Lung cancer and caregivers	Adults
2019	Wells-Di Gregorio et al.	Advanced cancer	Adults
2020	Davoudi et al.	Diabetes and neuropathic pain	Adults
2021	Rickardsson et al.	Chronic pain	Adults
2022	Monfaredi et al.	Women in menopause	Adults

Table 14.2 Other designs

Year	Authors	Primary outcome	Participants
Insomnia as primary outcome			
2010	Dalrymple et al.	Chronic insomnia	Adults
2014	Hertestein et al.	Chronic insomnia	Adults
2018	Zetteqvist et al.	Chronic insomnia and chronic pain	Adults
2019	Khazie and Zakiei	Chronic insomnia	Adults
2019	Zakiei and Khazie	Insomnia	Adults
2021	Rollinson et al.	Insomnia	Adolescents
Insomnia or sleep quality as secondary outcome			
2015	Kallestad et al.	Chronic fatigue	Adults
2017	Farhang et al.	Mental disorders	Adults
2017	Jacobsen et al.	Chronic fatigue	Adults
2020	Craner et al.	Chronic pain	Adults

As can be seen in Tables 14.1 and 14.2, 35 studies on interventions that used ACT for insomnia and sleep quality were identified among the reviews. Of these, 25 were randomized clinical trials and eight of them used insomnia as the primary outcome. Ten studies had other designs and six of them had insomnia as the primary outcome. These divisions were made in order to interpret the data of the reviews (Paulos-Guarnieri et al., 2022; Ruan et al., 2022; Salari et al., 2020). Based on the data reported in the reviews, we will discuss different aspects of ACT for insomnia: (a) the type of outcome (primary or secondary) of insomnia and/or sleep quality in the studies; (b) ACT modalities used in the interventions; (c) comparisons of ACT with CBT-I; and (d) how the ACT approach can contribute to the individualization of interventions.

14.2 Insomnia as Primary or Secondary Outcome

Insomnia was the intervention target in 14 studies; of these, eight were randomized clinical trials and six had other designs. Another 21 studies measured the effects of the intervention on insomnia and/or sleep quality, but these outcomes were not the intervention target. In the studies in which insomnia was not the target of the intervention, the most common primary outcomes were chronic pain ($n = 4$), cancer ($n = 4$), fatigue ($n = 3$), and tinnitus ($n = 3$).

To enable interpretation of the impacts of ACT on insomnia, sleep quality, or sleep parameters, the separation into primary and secondary outcomes is necessary for two reasons: first, to consider the particularities of each population and, second, to consider the differences between the protocols used. Studies whose primary outcome was insomnia involved populations in which complaints of insomnia predominated and insomnia was even diagnosed. Furthermore, these studies probably planned the interventions using the sleep topic as the main target. Unlike studies that had insomnia or sleep quality as secondary outcome, the populations had other chief complaints and the intervention protocols probably had other targets. For these reasons, caution is necessary in generalizing the data to other types of populations or to any protocol using ACT. On the other hand, ACT achieved favorable results for both patients who were diagnosed with insomnia and patients with symptoms of insomnia associated with other conditions. Thus, ACT had benefits regardless of whether or not sleep was the main target of the intervention.

The facts that ACT is aimed at developing psychological flexibility, that psychological inflexibility is transdiagnostic (Levin et al., 2014) and that studies found improvements in sleep-related outcomes suggest that psychological inflexibility and flexibility are somehow associated with insomnia and sleep quality. More studies are needed to safely affirm this statement. Nevertheless, some studies have pointed in this direction (Daly-Eichenhardt et al., 2016; McCracken et al., 2011; El Rafihi-Ferreira et al., 2022a; Zakiei et al., 2022), showing relationships of psychological flexibility or inflexibility with the severity of insomnia.

14.3 ACT Modalities for the Treatment of Insomnia

The study by Paulos-Guarnieri et al. (2022) was the only review that aimed to identify the strategies employed in each intervention using ACT for insomnia, something that could be the focus of future studies. The authors suggested two modalities in which ACT appeared to be used in the context of insomnia, namely, ACT as monotherapy for insomnia, called Acceptance and Commitment Therapy for Insomnia (ACT-I), and ACT used in combination with behavioral interventions for insomnia. (i.e., stimulus control and sleep restriction), called Acceptance and Commitment Therapy-Based Behavioral Intervention for Insomnia (ACT-BBI-I).

It is interesting to reflect on the composition of the intervention components used in the studies since different components can provide different results. Knowledge of the role of each component is also necessary in order to identify the components related to the effects of the intervention. This recommendation serves both clinicians planning individualized treatment for their patients and researchers designing protocols for intervention studies.

Understanding the roles of the components is not only important for knowing the effectiveness of ACT for insomnia and sleep quality but also for individualizing interventions. Below, when we discuss possible directions for ACT research in the context of insomnia, we will suggest research designs that can contribute to answering the questions about the individualization of interventions.

14.4 Comparison of ACT and CBT-I

It is interesting to highlight the studies that compared ACT with CBT-I (El Rafihi-Ferreira et al., 2021, 2022b). These studies revealed no significant differences when either ACT-BBI-I (El Rafihi-Ferreira et al., 2021) or ACT-I (El Rafihi-Ferreira et al., 2022b) was compared with CBT-I. The study by El Rafihi-Ferreira et al. (2022b) found higher treatment response rates in the CBT-I group within 1 week of post-treatment, while ACT-I resulted in further improvements in outcomes after 6 months. Considering that CBT-I is the recommended first-line treatment for insomnia (Edinger et al., 2021) and that not all patients adhere to this therapeutic modality, these data favor the study and implementation of ACT in the context of insomnia.

The importance of investigating which type of therapy might be more beneficial for a given patient must be highlighted. Thus, to answer the question "In which contexts may ACT be better than CBT for insomnia?" many factors, ranging from the individual characteristics of the patient to his/her context, must be investigated. For example, ACT has been shown to be beneficial for patients who are refractory to CBT-I (Dalrymple et al., 2010; Hertestein et al., 2014) and may contribute to the treatment of patients who, for different reasons, do not adhere or do not respond to CBT-I.

Outcome and process studies are important and should be complementary. While outcome studies focus on assessing whether a therapy is effective and which therapy should be applied in a given context, process studies explore the mediating and moderating factors involved in the success of treatment. Regarding outcome studies, there is currently much more research on CBT for insomnia than on ACT for insomnia. Although the effectiveness of ACT for insomnia is being explored in new studies, additional research is still needed to obtain more answers with greater potential to generalize the results.

Process studies that explore the mediating and moderating factors of interventions can increase the accuracy of the results based on characteristics of the individuals' context and of the individuals themselves. Furthermore, process studies using longitudinal measures that explore how and when changes occur are needed to understand the mechanisms involved in changing the target behavior. Such studies can provide answers to the following questions: (a) How does each intervention strategy affect sleep and what are the underlying mechanisms? (b) Which patients with certain characteristics and contexts could benefit from given interventions and strategies? (c) Which process of psychological flexibility and which behavioral strategies are related to the changes?

14.5 Contribution of ACT for the Individualization of Interventions

How do we know if ACT is the most appropriate therapy for a certain patient? When should we use ACT-I? When should we use ACT-BBI-I? How do we choose which processes of psychological inflexibility and flexibility to target? These questions are difficult to answer and highlight the complexity of a therapeutic process.

ACT is a contextual therapy whose philosophical basis is functional contextualism; hence, identification of the function of behaviors that interact with the historical and situational context is essential (Hayes et al., 1988; Hayes et al., 2012). For this purpose, functional analysis is used to identify the processes that are relevant for the intervention (Ferreira, 2021b). In addition to asking whether the therapeutic procedures are effective, one question that guides ACT is which processes are responsible for the changes (Ong et al., 2020). These approaches contribute to the individualization of cases instead of focusing on strategies for specific diagnostic disorders.

Based on these considerations, contextual therapies have been moving toward the process-based therapy (PBT) approach (Ferreira, 2021b; Ong et al., 2020). Instead of focusing on the investigation of evidence-based procedures, PBT focuses on evidence-based processes using empirical methods to evaluate pre-established procedures and outcomes (Hayes & Hoffmann, 2018; Hoffmann et al., 2021; Ong et al., 2020). Despite their differences, these therapies that make up PBT agree that clinical evidence must progress toward an understanding of the main processes of clinical change that are relevant for case formulation (Ferreira, 2021b). Functional analysis is key to PBT, privileging function over the topography of behavior (Ferreira, 2021b). The functionally described processes of change consider that it is not possible to establish a single cause since a dynamic non-linear interaction exists between many variables. These variables acquire a function within the context in which they occur. Thus, contextual interventions can confer new functions to the same events.

For clinicians, it is important to rely on functional analysis in order to identify target behaviors and the functions of these behaviors for intervention planning (Ferreira, 2021a). In the context of insomnia, target behaviors would be those that affect the homeostatic and circadian system (Borbély et al., 2016) and those related to psychological inflexibility (Hayes et al., 2012). This approach can facilitate case formulation by contributing to the identification of inflexibility processes related to elusive experiences and fusions, including insensitivity to the present moment, perspective taking, and lack of engagement (Luoma et al., 2017).

For researchers, it is important to identify future topics, for example, which processes of psychological inflexibility or flexibility may be risk or maintenance factors of insomnia. Such information will help in the field to plan prevention and treatment interventions.

In the case of clinicians, researchers, and individuals who exert both functions, it is believed that ACT can contribute to the individualization of treatments and in the quest to understand the relevant processes that affect sleep (Ong et al., 2020; Paulos-Guarnieri et al., 2022). In the context of insomnia, ACT represents a paradigm shift since it does not focus solely on reducing the symptoms and severity of insomnia but rather sees the patient as a whole in an attempt to increase quality of life and psychological flexibility (Gloster et al., 2020; Paulos-Guarnieri et al., 2022).

14.6 Directions for Future Research

There are different directions for anyone interested in studying ACT in the context of insomnia, all of them being equally encouraged and important. Different research questions will lead to different study designs (Kazdin, 2020). The following are recommended for individuals who seek to evaluate and refine the data on the effectiveness of ACT treatment for insomnia (i.e., ACT-I and ACT-BBI-I): (a) studies with high methodological quality, preferably randomized clinical trials involving large populations that evaluate both short- and long-term outcomes with long follow-ups and compare outcomes with other empirically supported therapies (e.g., CBT-I); (b) studies involving populations with not yet studied characteristics (e.g., different age groups, patients with comorbidities); (c) studies comparing different intervention formats (e.g., online versus face-to-face, self-administered versus therapist, group versus individual).

For individuals who seek to better understand how the processes of ACT interact with the disorder and insomnia symptoms, the following approaches are recommended: (a) studies that investigate the relationship between processes and the interventions used (e.g., single-subject experimental design); (b) studies that investigate the relationship of psychological inflexibility or flexibility variables with the severity of insomnia and/or sleep parameters (e.g., cross-sectional studies, longitudinal studies, moderation, mediation, and network statistical analyses); (c) studies that identify the role of each component in the intervention (e.g., dismantling studies); (d) studies that assess predictors of treatment adherence and response; (e) the use of instruments that adequately measure the ACT processes, including multidimensional instruments (e.g., MPFI; Rolffs et al., 2016, CompACT; Francis et al., 2016), unidimensional instruments (e.g., PsyFlex; Gloster et al., 2021), or specific instruments for given processes (e.g., CAQ-8; McCracken et al., 2015, CFQ; Gillanders et al., 2014, SACS; Zettle et al., 2018, VQ; Smout et al., 2014).

14.7 Final Considerations

This chapter synthesized the evidence on ACT for insomnia, focusing on the studies included in the main reviews reported in the literature (Paulos-Guarnieri et al., 2022; Salari et al., 2020; Ruan et al., 2022). This synthesis permitted to address the implications and contributions of ACT to the treatment of insomnia, highlighting insomnia as a target or not of the intervention and showing which ACT modalities are used in the interventions, their performance when compared to CBT-I, and how ACT can contribute to the individualization of interventions designed to treat insomnia and to improve sleep quality. In addition, it is expected that the possible directions for future research will encourage clinicians and researchers to refine the interventions and evidence available so far, improving the understanding of the effectiveness of interventions and focusing on the processes related to the sleep problems and sleep quality.

References[3]

*Baik, K. D. (2015). Evaluating acceptance and commitment therapy for insomnia: A randomized controlled trial (Publication No. 3726703) [Doctoral dissertation, Bowling Green State University]. ProQuest Dissertations and Theses Global.

Borbély, A. A., Daan, S., Wirz-Justice, A., & Deboer, T. (2016). The two-process model of sleep regulation: A reappraisal. *Journal of Sleep Research, 25*(2), 131–143. https://doi.org/10.1111/jsr.12371

*Chapoutot, M., Peter-Derex, L., Schoendorff, B., Faivre, T., Bastuji, H., & Putois, B. (2021). Telehealth-delivered CBT-I programme enhanced by acceptance and commitment therapy for insomnia and hypnotic dependence: A pilot randomized controlled trial. *Journal of Sleep Research, 30*(1), 6–10. https://doi.org/10.1111/jsr.13199

*Chen, Y., Hu, M. R., He, H. J., Lai, X., & Zhou, H. L. (2022). Jiena chengnuo liaofa tuanti fudao dui gaozhi nv daxuesheng shuimian zhiliang de ganyu [Intervention effect of acceptance and commitment therapy group counseling on sleep quality of female students in vocational colleges]. *China Journal of Health Psychology, 30*(4), 586–591.

*Clarke, S. P., Poulis, N., Moreton, B. J., Walsh, D. A., & Lincoln, N. B. (2017). Evaluation of a group acceptance commitment therapy intervention for people with knee or hip osteoarthritis: A pilot randomized controlled trial. *Disability and Rehabilitation, 39*(7), 663–670. https://doi.org/10.3109/09638288.2016.1160295

*Craner, J. R., Lake, E. S., Bancroft, K. A., & George, L. L. (2020). Treatment outcomes and mechanisms for an ACT-based 10-week interdisciplinary chronic pain rehabilitation program. *Pain Practice: The Official Journal of World Institute of Pain, 20*(1), 44–54. https://doi.org/10.1111/papr.12824

*Dalrymple, K. L., Fiorentino, L., Politi, M. C., & Posner, D. (2010). Incorporating principles from acceptance and commitment therapy into cognitive-behavioral therapy for insomnia: A case example. *Journal of Contemporary Psychotherapy: On the Cutting Edge of Modern Developments in Psychotherapy, 40*(4), 209–217. https://doi.org/10.1007/s10879-010-9145-1

Daly-Eichenhardt, A., Scott, W., Howard-Jones, M., Nicolaou, T., & McCracken, L. M. (2016). Changes in sleep problems and psychological flexibility following interdisciplinary acceptance and commitment therapy for chronic pain: An observational cohort study. *Frontiers in Psychology, 7*, 1326. https://doi.org/10.3389/fpsyg.2016.01326

*Davoudi, M., Taheri, A. A., Foroughi, A. A., Ahmadi, S. M., & Heshmati, K. (2020). Effectiveness of acceptance and commitment therapy (ACT) on depression and sleep quality in painful diabetic neuropathy: A randomized clinical trial. *Journal of Diabetes and Metabolic Disorders, 19*(2), 1081–1088. https://doi.org/10.1007/s40200-020-00609-x

Dindo, L., Van Liew, J. R., & Arch, J. J. (2017). Acceptance and Commitment Therapy: A transdiagnostic behavioral intervention for mental health and medical conditions. *Neurotherapeutics: The Journal of the American Society for Experimental NeuroTherapeutics, 14*(3), 546–553. https://doi.org/10.1007/s13311-017-0521-3

Edinger, J. D., Arnedt, J. T., Bertisch, S. M., Carney, C. E., Harrington, J. J., Lichstein, K. L., Sateia, M. J., Troxel, W. M., Zhou, E. S., Kazmi, U., Heald, J. L., & Martin, J. L. (2021). Behavioral and psychological treatments for chronic insomnia disorder in adults: An American Academy of Sleep Medicine systematic review, meta-analysis, and GRADE assessment. *Journal of Clinical Sleep Medicine: JCSM: Official Publication of the American Academy of Sleep Medicine, 17*(2), 263–298. https://doi.org/10.5664/jcsm.8988

*El Rafihi-Ferreira, R. E., Morin, C. M., Toscanini, A. C., Neto, F. B., Brasil, I. P., Gallinaro, J. G., Borges, D. L. G., Conway, S. G., & Hasan, R. (2021). Acceptance and commitment therapy-based behavioral intervention for insomnia: A pilot randomized controlled trial. *Revista Brasileira de Psiquiatria, 43*(5), 504–509. https://doi.org/10.1590/1516-4446-2020-0947

[3] Studies included in Tables 14.1 and 14.2 are marked with "*"

El Rafihi-Ferreira, R. E., Carmo, M. M. I. D. B. D., Bassolli, L., Hasan, R., Aizawa, I. M. N., & Toscanini, A. C. (2022a). Cognitive and psychological factors associated with severe insomnia in Brazilian women: A cross-sectional study. *Psicologia-Reflexao E Critica, 35*(1). https://doi.org/10.1186/s41155-022-00243-x

*El Rafihi-Ferreira, R. E., Morin, C. M., Hasan, R., Brasil, I. P., Ribeiro, J. L. P., & Toscanini, A. C. (2022b). A pilot randomized controlled trial (RCT) of acceptance and commitment therapy versus cognitive behavioral therapy for chronic insomnia. *Behavioral Sleep Medicine*, 1–15. https://doi.org/10.1080/15402002.2022.2071272

*Farhang, M., Ghaderi, M., Soleimani, R., & Arabshahi, F. (2017). The effectiveness of acceptance and commitment group therapy in general health, happiness, and general well-being among mental disorder patients. *Saussurea, 6*, 99–117.

Ferreira, T. A. S. (2021a). Avaliação e formulação de caso na Terapia de Aceitação e Compromisso. In C. K. M. Oshiro & T. A. S. Ferreira (Eds.), *Terapias contextuais comportamentais: análise funcional e prática clínica* (pp. 120–131). Editora Manole.

Ferreira, T. A. S. (2021b). Evidências e processos na Terapia Contextual: integração e ruptura. In C. K. M. Oshiro & T. A. S. Ferreira (Eds.), *Terapias contextuais comportamentais: análise funcional e prática clínica* (pp. 120–131). Editora Manole.

Francis, A. W., Dawson, D. L., & Golijani-Moghaddam, N. (2016). The development and validation of the comprehensive assessment of acceptance and commitment therapy processes (CompACT). *Journal of Contextual Behavioral Science, 5*(3), 134–145. https://doi.org/10.1016/j.jcbs.2016.05.003

*Gao, G. Q., & He, J. (2015). Jiena yu chengnuo liaofa dui erming zai xunlian liaofa zhiliao erming de liaoxiao guancha [Effects of acceptance and commitment therapy with tinnitus retraining therapy on patients with tinnitus]. *Chinese Journal of Modern Medicine, 25*(5), 94–99.

Gillanders, D. T., Bolderston, H., Bond, F. W., Dempster, M., Flaxman, P. E., Campbell, L., Kerr, S., Tansey, L., Noel, P., Ferenbach, C., Masley, S., Roach, L., Lloyd, J., May, L., Clarke, S., & Remington, B. (2014). The development and initial validation of the cognitive fusion questionnaire. *Behavior Therapy, 45*(1), 83–101. https://doi.org/10.1016/j.beth.2013.09.001

Gloster, A. T., Walder, N., Levin, M. E., Twohig, M. P., & Karekla, M. (2020). The empirical status of acceptance and commitment therapy: A review of meta-analyses. *Journal of Contextual Behavioral Science, 18*, 181–192. https://doi.org/10.1016/j.jcbs.2020.09.009

Gloster, A. T., Block, V. J., Klotsche, J., Villanueva, J., Rinner, M. T. B., Benoy, C., Walter, M., Karekla, M., & Bader, K. (2021). Psy-Flex: A contextually sensitive measure of psychological flexibility. *Journal of Contextual Behavioral Science, 22*, 13–23. https://doi.org/10.1016/j.jcbs.2021.09.001

Hayes, S. C., & Hofmann, S. G. (Eds.). (2018). *Process-based CBT: The science and core clinical competencies of cognitive behavioral therapy*. Context Press.

Hayes, S. C., Hayes, L. J., & Reese, H. W. (1988). Finding the philosophical core: A review of Stephen C. Pepper's World Hypotheses. *Journal of the Experimental Analysis of Behavior, 50*, 97–111.

Hayes, S. C., Strosahl, K., & Wilson, K. G. (2012). *Acceptance and commitment therapy: The process and practice of mindful change* (2nd ed.). Guilford Press.

*Herbert, M. S., Afari, N., Liu, L., Heppner, P., Rutledge, T., Williams, K., Eraly, S., VanBuskirk, K., Nguyen, C., Bondi, M., Atkinson, J. H., Golshan, S., & Wetherell, J. L. (2017). Telehealth versus in-person acceptance and commitment therapy for chronic pain: A randomized noninferiority trial. *The Journal of Pain, 18*(2), 200–211. https://doi.org/10.1016/j.jpain.2016.10.014

*Hertenstein, E., Thiel, N., Lüking, M., Külz, A. K., Schramm, E., Baglioni, C., Spiegelhalder, K., Riemann, D., & Nissen, C. (2014). Quality of life improvements after acceptance and commitment therapy in nonresponders to cognitive behavioral therapy for primary insomnia. *Psychotherapy and Psychosomatics, 83*(6), 371–373. https://doi.org/10.1159/000365173

*Hesser, H., Gustafsson, T., Lundén, C., Henrikson, O., Fattahi, K., Johnsson, E., Zetterqvist Westin, V., Carlbring, P., Mäki-Torkko, E., Kaldo, V., & Andersson, G. (2012). A randomized controlled trial of Internet-delivered cognitive behavior therapy and acceptance and com-

mitment therapy in the treatment of tinnitus. *Journal of Consulting and Clinical Psychology, 80*(4), 649–661. https://doi.org/10.1037/a0027021

Hofmann, S. G., Hayes, S. C., & Lorscheid, D. N. (2021). *Learning process-based therapy: A skills training manual for targeting the core processes of psychological change in clinical practice*. Context Press.

*Huang, L. P., Hu, M. R., Huang, Y. Y., Xia, S., Guo, T. T., Yang, Y., & Xiao, J. J. (2021). Jiena chengnuo liaofa zai laonian shuimian zhangai huanzhe jiankangjiaoyu zhong de yingyong [Application of acceptance and commitment therapy in the health education of elderly patients with sleep disorders]. *Medical Innovation of China, 18*(26), 104–107.

*Jacobsen, H. B., Kallestad, H., Landrø, N. I., Borchgrevink, P. C., & Stiles, T. C. (2017). Processes in acceptance and commitment therapy and the rehabilitation of chronic fatigue. *Scandinavian Journal of Psychology, 58*(3), 211–220. https://doi.org/10.1111/sjop.12363

*Kallestad, H., Jacobsen, H. B., Landrø, N. I., Borchgrevink, P. C., & Stiles, T. C. (2015). The role of insomnia in the treatment of chronic fatigue. *Journal of Psychosomatic Research, 78*(5), 427–432. https://doi.org/10.1016/j.jpsychores.2014.11.022

Kashdan, T. B., & Rottenberg, J. (2010). Psychological flexibility as a fundamental aspect of health. *Clinical Psychology Review, 30*(7), 865–878. https://doi.org/10.1016/j.cpr.2010.03.001

Kazdin, A. E. (2020). *Single-case research designs: Methods for clinical and applied settings* (3rd ed.). Oxford University Press.

*Khazaie, H., & Zakiei, A. (2019). Efficacy of acceptance and commitment therapy on emotional dysregulation and sleep quality in patients with chronic insomnia. *Journal of Mazandaran University of Medical Sciences, 29*(178), 52–63.

*Lang, A. J., Schnurr, P. P., Jain, S., He, F., Walser, R. D., Bolton, E., Benedek, D. M., Norman, S. B., Sylvers, P., Flashman, L., Strauss, J., Raman, R., & Chard, K. M. (2017). Randomized controlled trial of acceptance and commitment therapy for distress and impairment in OEF/OIF/OND veterans. *Psychological Trauma: Theory, Research, Practice and Policy, 9*(Suppl 1), 74–84. https://doi.org/10.1037/tra0000127

*Lappalainen, P., Langrial, S., Oinas-Kukkonen, H., Muotka, J., & Lappalainen, R. (2019). ACT for sleep – Internet-delivered self-help ACT for sub-clinical and clinical insomnia: A randomized controlled trial. *Journal of Contextual Behavioral Science, 12*, 119–127. https://doi.org/10.1016/j.jcbs.2019.04.001

Levin, M. E., MacLane, C., Daflos, S., Seeley, J., Hayes, S. C., Biglan, A., & Pistorello, J. (2014). Examining psychological inflexibility as a transdiagnostic process across psychological disorders. *Journal of Contextual Behavioral Science, 3*(3), 155–163. https://doi.org/10.1016/j.jcbs.2014.06.003

Luoma, J. B., Hayes, S. C., & Walser, R. D. (2017). Learning ACT: An Acceptance & Commitment Therapy Skills-Training Manual for Therapists. Oakland, CA: New Harbinger & Reno, NV: Context Press.

McCracken, L. M., Williams, J. L., & Tang, N. K. Y. (2011). Psychological flexibility may reduce insomnia in persons with chronic pain: A preliminary retrospective study. *Pain Medicine, 12*(6), 904–912. https://doi.org/10.1111/j.1526-4637.2011.01115.x

McCracken, L. M., Chilcot, J., & Norton, S. (2015). Further development in the assessment of psychological flexibility: A shortened committed action questionnaire (CAQ-8). *European Journal of Pain, 19*(5), 677–685. https://doi.org/10.1002/ejp.589

*Monfaredi, Z., Malakouti, J., Farvareshi, M., & Mirghafourvand, M. (2022). Effect of acceptance and commitment therapy on mood, sleep quality and quality of life in menopausal women: A randomized controlled trial. *BMC Psychiatry, 22*, 108. https://doi.org/10.1186/s12888-022-03768-8

*Mosher, C. E., Secinti, E., Li, R., Hirsh, A. T., Bricker, J., Miller, K. D., Schneider, B., Storniolo, A. M., Mina, L., Newton, E. V., Champion, V. L., & Johns, S. A. (2018). Acceptance and commitment therapy for symptom interference in metastatic breast cancer patients: A pilot randomized trial. *Supportive Care in Cancer: Official Journal of the Multinational Association of Supportive Care in Cancer, 26*(6), 1993–2004. https://doi.org/10.1007/s00520-018-4045-0

*Mosher, C. E., Secinti, E., Hirsh, A. T., Hanna, N., Einhorn, L. H., Jalal, S. I., Durm, G., Champion, V. L., & Johns, S. A. (2019). Acceptance and commitment therapy for symptom interference in advanced lung cancer and caregiver distress: A pilot randomized trial. *Journal of Pain and Symptom Management, 58*(4), 632–644. https://doi.org/10.1016/j.jpainsymman.2019.06.021

Ong, C. W., Levin, M. E., & Twohig, M. P. (2020). Beyond acceptance and commitment therapy: Process-based therapy. *The Psychological Record, 70*(4), 637–648. https://doi.org/10.1007/S40732-020-00397-Z

Paulos-Guarnieri, L., Linares, I. M. P., & Rafihi-Ferreira, R. E. (2022). Evidence and characteristics of Acceptance and Commitment Therapy (ACT)-based interventions for insomnia: A systematic review of randomized and non-randomized trials. *Journal of Contextual Behavioral Science, 23*, 1–14. https://doi.org/10.1016/j.jcbs.2021.11.001

*Pelkonen, S., & Puha, N. (2013). *Acceptance and commitment group therapy for treatment of insomnia* [Unpublished master's thesis]. University of Jyväskylä.

*Rickardsson, J., Gentili, C., Holmström, L., Zetterqvist, V., Andersson, E., Persson, J., Lekander, M., Ljótsson, B., & Wicksell, R. K. (2021). Internet-delivered acceptance and commitment therapy as microlearning for chronic pain: A randomized controlled trial with 1-year follow-up. *European Journal of Pain, 25*(5), 1012–1030. https://doi.org/10.1002/ejp.1723

Rolffs, J. L., Rogge, R. D., & Wilson, K. G. (2016). Disentangling components of flexibility via the hexaflex model: Development and validation of the multidimensional psychological flexibility inventory (MPFI). *Assessment, 25*(4), 458–482. https://doi.org/10.1177/1073191116645905

*Rollinson, R., Price, I., Gee, B., Lyons, J., Carroll, B., Wilson, J., & Clarke, T. (2021). Low-intensity sleep intervention in a youth mental health service: A case series analysis. *Behavioural and Cognitive Psychotherapy, 49*(1), 62–75. https://doi.org/10.1017/S135246582000051X

Ruan, J., Chen, S., Liang, J., Mak, Y. W., Ho, F. Y. Y., Chung, K. Y., Tong, A. K. K., Zhang, X., & Yeung, W. F. (2022). Acceptance and commitment therapy for insomnia and sleep quality: A systematic review and meta-analysis. *Journal of Contextual Behavioral Science, 26*, 139–155. https://doi.org/10.1016/j.jcbs.2022.09.002

Salari, N., Khazaie, H., Hosseinian-Far, A., Khaledi-Paveh, B., Ghasemi, H., Mohammadi, M., & Shohaimi, S. (2020). The effect of acceptance and commitment therapy on insomnia and sleep quality: A systematic review. *BMC Neurology, 20*(1), 300. https://doi.org/10.1186/s12883-020-01883-1

*Simister, H. D., Tkachuk, G. A., Shay, B. L., Vincent, N., Pear, J. J., & Skrabek, R. Q. (2018). Randomized controlled trial of online acceptance and commitment therapy for fibromyalgia. *The Journal of Pain, 19*(7), 741–753. https://doi.org/10.1016/j.jpain.2018.02.004

Smout, M., Davies, M., Burns, N., & Christie, A. (2014). Development of the valuing questionnaire (VQ). *Journal of Contextual Behavioral Science, 3*(3), 164–172. https://doi.org/10.1016/j.jcbs.2014.06.001

*Vethe, D., Kallestad, H., Jacobsen, H. B., Landrø, N. I., Borchgrevink, P. C., & Stiles, T. C. (2018). The relationship between improvement in insomnia severity and long-term outcomes in the treatment of chronic fatigue. *Frontiers in Psychology, 9*, 1764. https://doi.org/10.3389/fpsyg.2018.01764

*Wells-Di Gregorio, S. M., Marks, D. R., DeCola, J., Peng, J., Probst, D., Zaleta, A., Benson, D., Cohn, D. E., Lustberg, M., Carson, W. E., & Magalang, U. (2019). Pilot randomized controlled trial of a symptom cluster intervention in advanced cancer. *Psycho-Oncology, 28*(1), 76–84. https://doi.org/10.1002/pon.4912

*Westin, V. Z., Schulin, M., Hesser, H., Karlsson, M., Noe, R. Z., Olofsson, U., Stalby, M., Wisung, G., & Andersson, G. (2011). Acceptance and commitment therapy versus tinnitus retraining therapy in the treatment of tinnitus: A randomised controlled trial. *Behaviour Research and Therapy, 49*(11), 737–747. https://doi.org/10.1016/j.brat.2011.08.001

*Wiklund, T., Linton, S. J., Alföldi, P., & Gerdle, B. (2018). Is sleep disturbance in patients with chronic pain affected by physical exercise or ACT-based stress management? – A randomized controlled study. *BMC Musculoskeletal Disorders, 19*(1), 111. https://doi.org/10.1186/s12891-018-2020-z

*Zakiei, A., & Khazaie, H. (2019). The effectiveness of acceptance and commitment therapy on insomnia patients (A single-arm trial plan). *Journal of Turkish Sleep Medicine, 6*(3), 65–73. https://doi.org/10.4274/jtsm.galenos.2019.74745

*Zakiei, A., Khazaie, H., Rostampour, M., Lemola, S., Esmaeili, M., Dürsteler, K., Brühl, A. B., Sadeghi-Bahmani, D., & Brand, S. (2021). Acceptance and commitment therapy (ACT) improves sleep quality, experiential avoidance, and emotion regulation in individuals with insomnia – Results from a randomized interventional study. *Life (Basel, Switzerland), 11*(2), 133. https://doi.org/10.3390/life11020133

Zakiei, A., Korani, D., Sahraei, Z., Rostampour, M., & Khazaie, H. (2022). Predicting sleep quality and insomnia severity using the components of the acceptance and commitment therapy (ACT) model: A new perspective. *Journal of Contextual Behavioral Science, 26*, 227–233. https://doi.org/10.1016/j.jcbs.2022.10.006

*Zetterqvist, V., Grudin, R., Rickardsson, J., Wicksell, R. K., & Holmström, L. (2018). Acceptance-based behavioural treatment for insomnia in chronic pain: A clinical pilot study. *Journal of Contextual Behavioral Science, 9*, 72–79. https://doi.org/10.1016/j.jcbs.2018.07.003

Zettle, R., Gird, S., Webster, B., Carrasquillo-Richardson, N., Swails, J., & Burdsal, C. (2018). The self-as-context scale: Development and preliminary psychometric properties. *Journal of Contextual Behavioral Science, 10*, 64–74. https://doi.org/10.1016/j.jcbs.2018.08.010

*Zhang, H. H. (2018). *In Fuke aizheng huanzhe he peiou xinli ziyuan dui fuxing qingxu de eryuan zuoyong ji jiena chengnuo liaofa ganyu xiaoguo* [*The dyadic association between psychological resources and negative emotions among dyads of gynaecological cancer patients and spouses and the effect of the intervention based on acceptance and commitment therapy*] [Master's thesis, University of Shandong]. https://doi.org/10.27272/d.cnki.gshdu.2018.000134. China Academic Journal Network Publishing Database.

Chapter 15
A Session-by-Session Guide for Acceptance and Commitment Therapy for Insomnia

Renatha El Rafihi-Ferreira

This chapter describes an intervention protocol for insomnia complaints based on Acceptance and Commitment Therapy (ACT). Although it presents a description of the procedures to be conducted in the session, this protocol does not exclude the need for functional analysis and case formulation. The aim of functional analysis is to identify the dependency relationships between the actions of the organism and antecedent and consequent environmental events. The clinician's interest lies in investigating the determinants of the individual's behaviors.

As a clinical model, case formulation by ACT assumes the identification of processes of psychological inflexibility (experiential avoidance, cognitive fusion, dominance of the conceptualized past and future, attachment to the conceptualized self, lack of values, and inaction) and psychological flexibility (acceptance, cognitive defusion, contact with the present moment, self as context, values, and committed actions). Understanding these variables enables more effective therapeutic planning. Continuous assessment must always be present during this process. In conjunction with functional assessment, this protocol can be used flexibly, respecting the specificities of each case.

This insomnia protocol is composed of sleep psychoeducation, ACT-based interventions, and home activities. For organizational purposes, the set of therapeutic elements that make up this protocol is divided into six sessions, which can be perfectly adapted to a larger or smaller number of sessions at the therapist's discretion. The protocol can also be applied in conjunction with stimulus control and sleep restriction techniques.

The program can be applied in different formats, that is, individual, group, face-to-face, and online. It is recommended that individual sessions last approximately

R. El Rafihi-Ferreira (✉)
Department of Clinical Psychology, University of São Paulo, Sao Paulo, Brazil
e-mail: rerafihi@usp.br

R. El Rafihi-Ferreira (ed.), *Acceptance and Commitment Therapy for Insomnia*,
https://doi.org/10.1007/978-3-031-50710-6_15

50 minutes and group sessions about 120 minutes. The session-by-session protocol is described below.

15.1 First Session: Building Rapport and Introduction to Sleep

The focus of the first session is to establish a bond between the therapist and the client or group members and to provide information about the therapeutic process, sleep, and insomnia. The interventions used in session 1 are presented in Table 15.1.

1. Presentation of the therapist and client or group members

   The therapist starts with their own presentation and asks the client to answer the following questions: (1) Who am I? (2) What brought me here? (3) What do I like to do?

2. Presentation of the intervention proposal

   The therapist continues with information about the treatment, explaining that the focus will be on aspects directly related to sleep, such as habits and behaviors, and indirectly related to sleep, that is, how we deal with the discomforts of life, including sleep dissatisfaction.

3. Rules

   The therapist explains the rules of confidentiality, schedule, and absences from therapy. In the case of group intervention, the therapist emphasizes the importance of confidentiality since the participants may share very delicate and intimate content and confidentiality may be the only tool to ensure that they expose themselves and proceed with the vulnerability that ACT promotes.

Table 15.1 Interventions of session 1

Intervention	Objectives
Presentation	To introduce the therapist and client or group members To present the intervention proposal
Group/therapy rules	To clarify the confidentiality between group members or between the professional and client To explain the importance of session attendance To reinforce commitment to schedules and homework assignments
Wound metaphor	To introduce the ACT proposal To stimulate reflection based on an analogy between the metaphor and the therapeutic situation
Cartoon dynamics	To promote integration between group members or between the professional and client To encourage identification with the characters of the cartoon To discuss the experiences based on the content of the cartoons
Psychoeducation about sleep	To teach the patient or group members about sleep and its functions, effects of sleep deprivation, and insomnia
Homework assignment	To develop extra-session therapeutic activities

4. Wound metaphor
   The therapist describes the wound metaphor to the client or group.

Wound metaphor

Let's address pretty basic issues, including some you might not expect in therapy. My experience with this approach is that it can put you on a rollercoaster ride. All kinds of emotions can arise: interest, boredom, anxiety, sadness, doubt, understanding, relief, peace, anguish, discomfort, etc.

It is like treating a wound, procedures that cause even more pain will be needed so that it stops bleeding. And in the middle of the procedures, you might think that it was worse to treat it since the pain increased even more. But only by facing the discomfort of this pain will the wound stop bleeding.

Think about the following situation: Imagine that you have a wound on your body. This wound hurts and bleeds a lot. If we leave the wound and do not look at it, it will continue to bleed and hurt. Afraid of feeling even more pain, you may choose not to treat the wound. However, the wound will continue to bleed.

Whereas if we care for this wound, if we clean it, if we treat it, the wound will stop bleeding. This process is painful and you have to endure some discomfort since touching the wound causes pain. It is often necessary to clean, stitch, apply dressings, in short, to treat it. By doing this, the blood ceases.

Depending on the size of the wound, scars will remain and will remind us of the wound; however, the wound is closed and no longer bleeds.

Source: Metaphor developed by the author of this chapter.

5. Dynamics of integration

Three cartoons that portray different insomnia situations are shown (see Figs. 15.1, 15.2, and 15.3).

In the case of group intervention, different comic strips are given to each small group. In the group, each participant tells a story about the cartoon. After a few minutes, each small group shares their stories with the larger group. After all participants have told their stories, the similarities with the stories themselves are discussed.

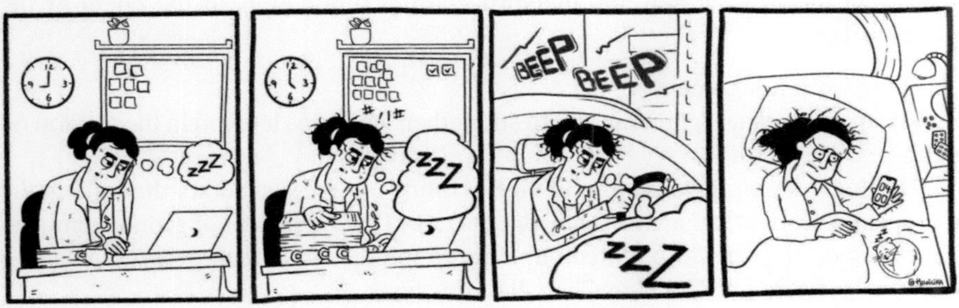

Fig. 15.1 Cartoon 1. (Source: Illustration made by the artist Helder Lira, 2023. All rights reserved ©)

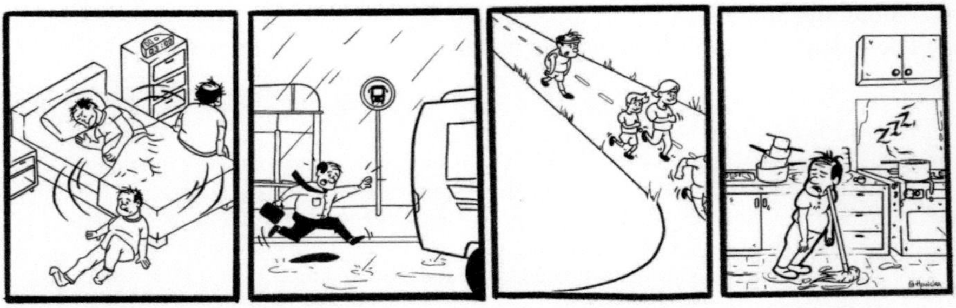

Fig. 15.2 Cartoon 2. (Source: Illustration made by the artist Helder Lira, 2023. All rights reserved ©)

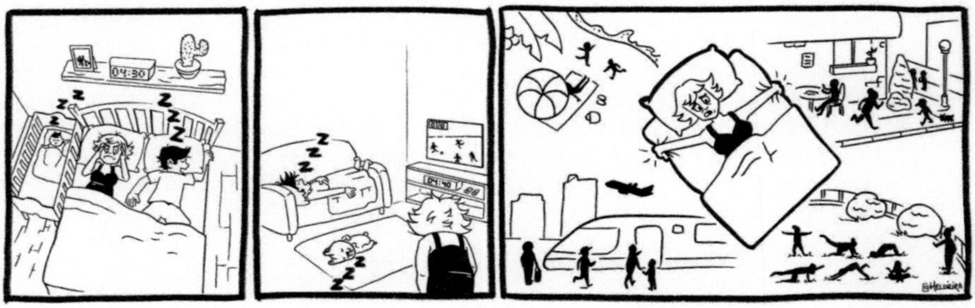

Fig. 15.3 Cartoon 3. (Source: Illustration made by the artist Helder Lira, 2023. All rights reserved ©)

In the individual intervention, the client can discuss the cartoons with the therapist, proposing their own stories.

6. Pseudoeducation about sleep

   The therapist gives a lecture about sleep to the client or group members, specifically addressing the following topics: sleep and its functions, effects of sleep deprivation, and insomnia. For the preparation of psychoeducation material, the reader can refer to the first part of this book.

   During the presentation, the therapist clarifies any doubts of the client or the group members.

7. Homework assignment

   The homework assignments aim to strengthen what was learned in the session on extra-session occasions.

   The therapist explains the importance of filling out the sleep diary throughout the therapeutic process and answers any doubts raised by the patient or group members. The sleep diaries should be filled out daily to monitor treatment progress. A sleep diary template can be found in Chap. 9 of this book.

15.2 Second Session: Sleep Hygiene and Present Moment

The second session is aimed at educating the client or group members about habits, behaviors, and activities that can promote quality sleep. In this session, mindfulness will be practiced using formal and informal exercises. The interventions used in session 2 are described in Table 15.2.

1. Review of homework

   The therapist evaluates the sleep diaries, asks the client or group members about difficulties in filling out the diary, and clarifies any doubts. Based on the sleep diary records, the client or group members report the week's feedback.

2. Psychoeducation about sleep hygiene

   The therapist gives a lecture about sleep hygiene to the client or group members, including the set of habits, behaviors, and activities that promote quality sleep. The explanation focuses on the five pillars of sleep hygiene: (1) sleep environment; (2) eating habits and substance intake; (3) routine; (4) sleep ritual; and (5) worries. The reader can refer to the Chap. 10 of this book to prepare material for psychoeducation. During the presentation, the therapist clarifies any doubts of the client or group members.

3. Delivery of supporting material (sleep hygiene booklet)

   A paper or electronic booklet with information on sleep hygiene is handed out to the client or group members. This booklet as supporting material aims to strengthen the absorption of what was learned and of the guidelines given in the psychoeducation session. Written material allows the client or group members to review the information provided in the session on extra-session occasions.

   A template of the sleep hygiene booklet can be found in the tables of the Chap. 10 of this book.

4. Mindfulness: formal versus informal practices

   The therapist explains the concept of mindfulness and mindfulness principles for insomnia and discusses formal and informal practices.

   The concept of mindfulness is defined as staying in the present moment, paying full attention. Being connected to the present moment helps the individual to assess

Table 15.2 Interventions of session 2

Intervention	Objectives
Review of homework	To review extra-session activities Feedback on established tasks
Psychoeducation about sleep – Sleep hygiene	To inform and guide the client or group members about habits and activities that promote quality sleep
Supporting material – Sleep hygiene	To hand out a paper or electronic version of a sleep hygiene booklet so that the client or group members can review the information learned in the session
Mindfulness	To explain and show formal and informal mindfulness practices
Body scan (Kabat-Zinn, 1990)	Mindfulness To establish contact with the present moment
Homework assignment	To develop extra-session therapeutic activities

what the environment offers and to react based on this perspective. Observation of the present moment focuses on assuming control of the here and now. As a practice, mindfulness aims to expand our self-awareness about how we connect with what happens within and around us (Ramos, 2015).

If we are attentive to the present moment, we are better equipped to adequately respond to what happens around us. We are often caught up in past experiences, expectations about the future, or our thoughts that distract us from what is taking place around us.

The relationship with sleep can be addressed based on the seven principles of mindfulness for insomnia proposed by Ong and Manber (2011): beginner's mind, non-striving, letting go, non-judging, acceptance, trust, and patience (see Fig. 15.4).

Mindfulness practices can be formal or informal and both types consist of training to stay in the present moment.

Formal practices consist of reserving a time of our day to an exclusive mindfulness practice such as body scan, which will be described below. On the other hand, we can practice informal exercises at any time of the day, during daily activities such as bathing, cooking, eating, walking, and driving. These activities are performed with full attention to senses (touch, smell, taste, vision, hearing), feelings, and thoughts that we are experiencing in the present moment.

5. Body scan

The therapist applies the body scan practice together with the client or group members. The practice is described below.

Body scan

Look for a comfortable place, it can be a chair, a sofa, a mattress, whatever you prefer. Position yourself comfortably. You can choose to remain seated keeping your spine straight or, if you prefer, you can lie down. If you prefer, close your eyes. Concentrate on your breathing. Observe your breathing. Feel the air moving in and out through your nostrils.

The experience of this practice is full attention to different parts of your body.

Direct your attention to your head. Explore the sensations on your scalp, on your neck until the attention reaches your forehead. Observe if there is any tension, pain, or discomfort in this region. Contemplate these sensations in a mindful, nonjudgmental way. Observe the temperature in this region. And then breathe. Go over your face, eyes, nose, lips, ears, chin. Perceive whether this region is hot, cold, or has a mild temperature.

Gradually, pay attention to your neck, working your way up to your shoulders and shoulder blades. Observe if there is any tension in this region. Breathe and return your attention to your back, observe the neck region, and go down to the lumbar region. Is there any discomfort in this region? Is the temperature in this region mild, hot, or cold?

Slowly direct your attention towards your arms, forearms, wrists, hands, and fingers. Again, observe if there is any tension in this region.

Observe the sensations in your chest, abdomen, belly. Is there any discomfort? Slowly move down to the pelvic area, thighs, knee, calf, heel, and toes. Observe if there are any points of tension or discomfort.

Explore the sensations. Pay attention whether, when you perceive pain or tension in a specific region of your body, these discomforts change naturally as you notice

(continued)

them. As you breathe with these specific parts of your body, the discomfort transforms.

Returning your attention to your breathing, say goodbye to this experience. Get in touch with the sounds of the environment where you are. Slowly move parts of your body and, when you feel comfortable, you can open your eyes.

Source: Adapted from Kabat-Zinn (1990).

TABLE 14.1 Applying Mindfulness Principles to Sleep

In the spirit of cultivating mindfulness, this program will help guide your personal inquiry into your own sleep needs and the optimal state of mind for initiation of sleep (at the beginning or middle of the night). In doing so, bring attention to changing your *relationship* to sleep rather than to the amount of sleep you get each night. As you begin to change this relationship, you might notice an improvement in the quality of your sleep. Later, you will likely see an increase in the amount of sleep you get. This approach requires discipline and consistency but follows the principles of mindfulness discussed in this program.

Beginner's Mind: Remember that each night is a new night. Be open and try Something different! What you have been doing to this point is probably not working well.

Non-striving: Sleep is a process that cannot be forced, but instead should be allowed to unfold. Putting more effort into sleeping longer or better is counterproductive.

Letting go: Attachment to sleep or your ideal sleep needs usually leads to worry about the consequences of sleeplessness. This is counterproductive and inconsistent with the natural process of letting go of the day to allow sleep to come.

Non-judging: It is easy to automatically judge the state of being awake as negative and aversive, especially if you do not sleep well for several nights. However, this negative energy can interfere with the process of sleep. One's relationship to sleep can be a fuitful subject of meditation.

Acceptance: Recognizing and accepting your current state is an important first step in choosing how to respond. If you can accept that you are not in a state of sleepiness and sleep in not likely to come soon, why not get out of bed? Many People who have trouble sleeping avoid getting out of be. Unfortunately, spending long periods of time awake in bed might condition you to being awake in bed.

Trust: Trust your sleep system and let it work for you! Trust that your mind and body can self regulate and self correct for sleep loss. Knowing that short consolidated sleep often feels more satisfying than longer fragmented sleep can help you develop trust in your sleep system. Also, sleep debt can promote good sleep as long as it is not associated with increased effort to sleep.

Patience: Be patient! it is unlikely that both the quality and quantity of your sleep will be optimal right away.

These are just some ways that the mindfulness principles are related to sleep. you might discover other connections between these principles and the process of going to sleep or falling back asleep. We encourage you to explore this for yourself and share your experience throughout this program.

Fig. 15.4 Seven principles of mindfulness for insomnia. (Source: Ong and Manber (2011). Reprinted with permission from Elsevier)

At the end of the practice, the therapist asks the client or group members for feedback on how the experience was.

6. Homework assignment

The homework assignments aim to strengthen what was learned in the session on extra-session occasions.

1. Fill out the sleep diary

The sleep diaries should be filled out weekly to monitor treatment progress. A sleep diary template can be found in Chap. 9 of this book.

2. Make changes in sleep hygiene

Knowing the habits, activities, and environments that favor sleep, it is now time to put into practice what you learned in the session on sleep hygiene and make the necessary changes. To do this, use the guidelines on sleep hygiene that can be found in the Chap. 10 of this book.

3. Write thoughts/feelings present at bedtime in the thoughts notebook

Writing about personal experiences and worries is a known tool for managing stress and ruminations, while facilitating the organization of experiences in a narrative. It may also be an extension of sleep hygiene. If you overflow with thoughts/feelings at bedtime, write them in a notebook. A template of a thoughts notebook can be found in the Chap. 10 of this book.

4. Practice the body scan mindfulness exercise daily

Practicing mindfulness daily as homework is key to developing and maintaining the ability to meditate. The body scan practice is described in this chapter.

15.3 Third Session: Creative Hopelessness and Cognitive Defusion

The third session focuses on the observation of experiential avoidance, that is, creative hopelessness. In this session, the client or group members will be guided in the assessment of attempts to control and avoid discomfort. At the same time, they are invited to observe their thoughts without judging, addressing cognitive defusion. The interventions used in session 3 are presented in Table 15.3.

1. Review of homework

The therapist evaluates the sleep diaries and asks the client or group members about changes made to sleep hygiene and about the body scan practice. The patient or group members report the week's feedback. While reviewing the homework assignment, the therapist asks the client if there have been any changes since the last session. When giving feedback to the client or group members, the therapist listens and accepts all of the client's responses. It is important to create a context of openness and welcoming regardless of the client's content. The therapist thus avoids being categorical/classifying so that the client or group members do not feel judged. Here are two phrases that usually promote welcoming: "Very interesting." and "Thank you for sharing."

Table 15.3 Interventions of session 3

Intervention	Objectives
Review of homework	To review extra-session activities Feedback on established tasks
Assessment of attempts to control and avoid discomfort	Creative hopelessness
Mindfulness practice on creative hopelessness – Insomnia	Creative hopelessness Observe the avoidance of discomfort
Tug-of-war with a monster metaphor	Creative hopelessness Acceptance
Mindfulness – Leaves on a stream	Cognitive defusion
Homework assignment	To develop extra-session therapeutic activities

2. Assessment of attempts to control and avoid discomfort

Creative hopelessness refers to the observation of contingencies that involve experiential avoidance behaviors, with relief as an immediate consequence and the subsequent reappearance of aversive stimuli that again demand the avoidance behavior (Saban, 2015).

To address creative hopelessness, the therapist proposes an activity aimed at exploring the feelings and thoughts associated with insomnia and the avoidance and control strategies used. A pen and paper are used for this activity.

The therapist asks the client or group members to recall the last time they had difficulties sleeping. Based on this memory, the patient or group members are invited to respond individually to the following questions given in the Table 15.4.

In the case of group intervention, the participants should share the answers in pairs. After sharing with the partner, the participants discuss the issues in the group. Each partner of the pair should describe what they observed in the other. This helps to synthesize and to hear yourself through the other. In that case, those who listen to the description about themselves can also complete.

When the intervention is conducted individually with the client, the therapist reserves time for the patient to complete the answers and then opens it up for discussion.

At this point, the client or group members may have difficulty identifying their emotions during insomnia. To help the participant connect with the insomnia experience, the therapist conducts the following mindfulness practice:

Mindfulness practice on creative hopelessness – Insomnia

Find a comfortable position and when you are ready, close your eyes. Focus on your breathing, feel the air come in and out through your nostrils.

Now, remember the last time you had difficulty sleeping. Where were you? As much as possible, bring to mind what the experience was like. What thoughts are appearing? Observe any emotions that arise. Name them silently. What do you feel in your body? Observe the sensations.

With the memory of this experience, connect with the environment where you are. Slowly move and, when you feel comfortable, you can open your eyes.

Source: The author.

Table 15.4 – Evaluation of control and avoidance

1. How do I feel when I cannot sleep?	Describe your feelings and sensations in face of the sleeping difficulty
2. What do I do right away?	Describe the strategies used when you have insomnia
3. Does it work as I would like? Right away and in the long term?	Describe whether the strategies are effective in the short and long terms
4. How have insomnia and the use of coping strategies transformed my life?	Describe how insomnia and strategies for coping with sleep have transformed your life
5. What will managing insomnia improve in my life?	Describe what managing insomnia may add to your life

Source: The author

After the mindfulness practice on creative hopelessness, the therapist asks whether the client or group members want to share their experience. The question remains: What if the attempt to control what we feel is in itself a problem and not the solution to sleep better?

What the client or group member generally reports is that their actions to cope with insomnia usually work at the time to get rid of the discomfort of not sleeping, yet in the long term they create bad routines that often harm them. The attempt to control sleep, thoughts, and emotions often make them even bigger and is not an effective strategy. These strategies may be effective momentarily but not in the long term, and often just distance the individual from what really matters.

3. Tug-of-war with a monster metaphor

To exemplify the cost of trying to control what you feel and think, the therapist uses the following metaphor:

Tug-of-war with a monster metaphor

This situation is like playing tug-of-war with a monster. This monster is big and very strong. It seems to be disgusting and very ugly. You can name this monster. Does it have a name? What is its name? Then imagine that between you and the monster there is a very deep well, it is so deep that it is difficult to see the end. If you lose this tug-of-war, you are going to fall into this hole that has no end. So, you struggle to pull the rope, pull, pull, but the hardest thing is that the monster pulls too, and the monster is strong and it pulls hard, it feels like you are getting closer and closer to the hole. Do you need to win this tug-of-war? The most difficult to notice here is that your work is not to win the tug-of-war. Your work is to let go of the rope.

Source: Adapted from Hayes et al. (1999).

The client or group members may often ask, "How can I do this?" The therapist responds openly, saying something like "Well, I don't know. But the first step is to realize that the tug-of-war cannot be won and that it does not have to be won." The goal is to allow the client or group members to reach their own conclusions.

4. Mindfulness – Leaves on a stream

The therapist ends the session with a mindfulness practice of observing thoughts in order to address cognitive defusion.

Leaves on a stream

Look for a comfortable place where you can sit or lie down. Focus on your breathing. Feel the air come in and out of your nostrils. And then imagine yourself in a forest. In this forest there are trees and a stream. Walk through the trees towards the stream. When you see the stream, sit down by the water and start watching the leaves detach from the trees, fly, and fall into the stream.

At this point, write your thought on a sheet of paper and observe it. Watch this thought next to the leaf detaching from the tree, flying, and falling into the serene current of a stream. A new thought, a new leaf that detaches from the tree, flies, and falls into the stream. Try to observe the thoughts that, little by little, appear in your mind like a sequence of leaves that float on the serene current of a stream.

Carefully pay attention to the leaves passing through your field of attention. Note that you are just watching your thoughts on the leaves from a distance.

When you notice that you have forgotten what you are doing, or that you have suddenly started to think about something else, or that you have become attached to a particular thought, gently return your attention to watching the leaves floating down the stream.

Slowly say goodbye to the stream, go back to walking among the trees, say goodbye to this experience, being certain that you can return to that forest to observe your thoughts at any time.

Concentrate on your breathing, on the sounds of the environment where you are and, when you feel comfortable, you can open your eyes.

Source: Adapted from Hayes et al. (2011), p. 255.

5. Homework assignment

The homework assignments aim to strengthen what was learned in the session on extra-session occasions.

1. Fill out the sleep diary

The sleep diaries should be filled out weekly to monitor treatment progress. A sleep diary template can be found in the Chap. 9 of this book.

2. Make/maintain changes in sleep hygiene

Check out the information about habits, activities, and environments that can promote sleep. Sleep hygiene guidelines can be found in the Chap. 10 of this book.

3. Write thoughts/feelings present at bedtime in a notebook. When your thoughts/feelings overflow at bedtime, write them in a notebook. A notebook template can be found in the Chap. 10 of this book.
4. Practice the mindfulness exercise daily – Leaves on a stream. Practicing mindfulness daily as homework is key to developing and maintaining the ability to meditate. The leaves on a stream practice is described in this chapter.

15.4 Fourth Session: Self as Context and Acceptance

The fourth session addresses self as context and acceptance. Self as context refers to the individual's conception of themselves. Acceptance is a process of opening to feeling and perceiving sensations without trying to avoid possible discomforts that may arise. Table 15.5 shows the interventions used in session 4 and their objectives.

1. Review of homework

The therapist evaluates the sleep diaries and asks the client or group members about maintaining the changes made in sleep hygiene and about practicing the leaves on a stream mindfulness exercise. The client or group members report the week's feedback. When reviewing the homework assignment, the therapist asks the client if there have been any changes since the last session.

2. Pain versus suffering

Pain is the feeling arising when we experience situations that cannot be avoided, such as the death of a close and loved person, unemployment, the diagnosis of a serious illness, divorce, suffering humiliation, some frustrations, or natural conditions of life. Suffering is what we do to avoid the feeling/thought/sensation or memory inherent to the situation, that is, the behaviors we develop in an attempt to avoid pain. For example: "Not going to parties to avoid feeling humiliated or isolated," "Not leaving the house to avoid having an accident," "Not enrolling in courses to avoid failure."

To avoid the pain of not sleeping and of spending a sleepless night, we often engage in avoidance behaviors (suffering). Such behaviors to avoid pain (not sleeping and/or staying up all night) include the use of medications, rituals, counting the minutes, etc. It is through avoidance behaviors that we restrict our repertoire of actions to deal with facts and difficulties. They are a defense. A situation is avoided in order not to feel, for fear of suffering. People thus restrict life. This intervention is an invitation to face the pain.

Table 15.5 Interventions of session 4

Intervention	Objectives
Review of homework	To review extra-session activities Feedback on established tasks
Pain versus suffering	Creative hopelessness Acceptance
Pudding metaphor	Creative hopelessness Suffering
Poem – The Guest House	Acceptance
Poem – The Invitation	Self as context
Front-back sheet activity	Self as context and cost of discomfort
Homework assignment	To develop extra-session therapeutic activities

3. Pudding metaphor

The therapist presents the pudding metaphor to the patient or group members to illustrate situations of suffering.

Pudding metaphor

I will tell you a story in the form of a metaphor that represents human suffering. Imagine that Carla loves puddings. Every time she eats pudding, she smears herself happily with it. She even likes to go eat pudding with her friends and appreciates the diner where they eat pudding among friends. One day, Carla ate pudding number 1 and this pudding was spoiled, which caused a lot of abdominal pain. Carla vomited and had diarrhea. It was a very uncomfortable situation. After this episode, Carla stopped eating puddings. Although pudding number 2 or number 20 was not pudding number 1, Carla did not want to taste any more pudding. Over time, in addition to no longer eating pudding, Carla stopped eating sweets resembling pudding such as blancmange and flan. Any sweet with resemblance to pudding, Carla did not try it. Carla also started to avoid the diner where she ate pudding number 1. One day, Carla's grandmother offered her a cake that looked nothing like pudding. However, the grandmother told her that the taste was very similar to that of pudding. Carla did not eat it and became suspicious of cakes. Thus, the range of sweets became more and more restricted as Carla avoided tasting them.

Source: Adapted from Saban (2015).

After presenting the metaphor, the discussion proceeds with the question: "How many puddings do we have?"

4. Acceptance and present moment – The Guest House poem

Acceptance refers to the training of feeling, of observing sensations without avoiding, noticing the emotional curve. To be in control of the world as it presents itself is to be in the present moment (Saban, 2015).

Rumi's poem "The Guest House" (Rumi, n.d.) is used to discuss how the process of accepting the uncomfortable would be. The therapist reads the poem and asks the client or group members how each of them welcomes their guests.

After discussion of the poem, the therapist proceeds with the next intervention.

5. Self as context – The Invitation poem

Self as context refers to the conception of oneself. Identifying the self as a context is addressed by reading the poem The Invitation.

The Invitation

It doesn't interest me what you do for a living. I want to know what you ache for, and if you dare to dream of meeting your heart's longing.

It doesn't interest me how old you are. I want to know if you will risk looking like a fool for love, for your dream, for the adventure of being alive.

It doesn't interest me what planets are squaring your moon. I want to know if you have touched the center of your own sorrow, if you have been opened by life's betrayals or have become shriveled and closed from fear of further pain. I want to know if you can sit with pain, mine or your own, without moving to hide it or fade it or fix it.

I want to know if you can be with joy, mine or your own, if you can dance with wildness and let the ecstasy fill you to the tips of your fingers and toes without cautioning us to be careful, to be realistic, to remember the limitations of being human.

It doesn't interest me if the story you are telling me is true. I want to know if you can disappoint another to be true to yourself; if you can bear the accusation of betrayal and not betray your own soul; if you can be faithless and therefore trustworthy.

I want to know if you can see Beauty, even when it's not pretty, everyday, and if you can source your own life from its presence.

I want to know if you can live with failure, yours and mine, and still stand on the edge of the lake and shout to the silver of the full moon, "Yes!"

It doesn't interest me to know where you live or how much money you have. I want to know if you can get up, after the night of grief and despair, weary and bruised to the bone and do what needs to be done to feed the children.

It doesn't interest me who you know or how you came to be here. I want to know if you will stand in the center of the fire with me and not shrink back.

It doesn't interest me where or what or with whom you have studied. I want to know what sustains you, from the inside, when all else falls away.

I want to know if you can be alone with yourself and if you truly like the company you keep in the empty moments.

Source: Oriah © Mountain Dreaming (Oriah, 1999).

The therapist presents the poem and asks which part the client or group members identified with and proceeds with the front-back sheet activity.

The therapist asks the client or group members to observe this sheet of paper, its front and back. The therapist then asks them to write on one side of the paper positive memories, feelings, and thoughts, and on the other side negative memories, thoughts, and feelings.

After this, the therapist asks the client or group members to read out loud what they wrote and what they would like to do with the paper. On this occasion, the therapist questions whether it would be possible to crumple or throw away the paper and points out that, even if that were possible, they would also deprive themselves of the feelings, thoughts, and memories that they identified as pleasant and positive.

Next, the client or group members are asked whether any of the elements written on the paper would represent them. At this point, the therapist highlights that the client or group members are not any of those thoughts, feelings or memories, and much less are they represented by labels.

The therapist asks the client or group members to select an action that they stop doing because of some thought, feeling or memory, and to try to perform that action. This is defined as the mission of the week.

Based on the requested activity, conditions are created for the group participants or the client to start expose themselves to contingencies, experiencing feelings, sensations, thoughts, and memories without trying to control them.

Table 15.6 Checklist – avoided and faced situations

	Situation avoided	Situation faced
Monday		
Tuesday		
Wednesday		
Thursday		
Friday		
Saturday		
Sunday		

6. Front-back sheet

A double-sided sheet of paper and a pen will be necessary for this activity. Source: Activity adapted from Costa et al. (2017).

7. Homework assignment

The homework assignments aim to strengthen what was learned in the session on extra-session occasions.

1. Fill out the sleep diary

The sleep diaries should be filled out weekly to monitor treatment progress. A sleep diary template can be found in Chap. 9 of this book.

2. Make/maintain changes in sleep hygiene

Obtain information about habits, activities, and environments that can promote sleep. For this, check out the guidelines in the Chap. 10 of this book.

3. Write thoughts/feelings present at bedtime in a notebook. A notebook template can be found in the Chap. 10 of this book.
4. Perform at least one informal mindfulness practice per day

Practicing mindfulness daily as homework is key to developing and maintaining the ability to meditate.

5. Mission of the week: Do not avoid a certain situation identified in the activity proposed in this session. Write down the situations you avoided and faced. A checklist is proposed in Table 15.6.

15.5 Fifth Session: Values and Committed Actions

Values and committed actions will be the focus of the fifth session. Values refer to the qualities of a behavior that we would like to cultivate, that is, that is important to us. The questions "How do I want my life to be?" and "How do I ideally want to behave?" help to identify these values. This stage of therapy aims to explore the individual's values, that is, to investigate how the individual wants to be and how he/she ideally wants to behave.

Table 15.7 Interventions of session 5

Intervention	Objectives
Review of homework	To review extra-session activities Feedback on established tasks
Life compass	Values clarification
Values-based committed action	Values, objectives, barriers, and actions
Metta meditation – ACT variation	Values Mindfulness
Homework assignment	To develop extra-session therapeutic activities

After these definitions, action plans targeting these values are developed. The interventions used in session 5, as well as their objectives, are presented in Table 15.7.

1. Review of homework

   The therapist evaluates the sleep diaries and asks the client or group members about maintaining the changes made in sleep hygiene, about the informal mindfulness practice, and about trying not to avoid a certain situation identified in the previous session. The client or group members report the week's feedback. When reviewing the homework assignment, the therapist asks the client if there have been any changes since the last session.

2. Values

   At this stage of treatment, it is expected that the client or group members are less involved in struggling with sleep-related thoughts and experience some improvements in sleep quality.

   Some sleep researchers believe that processes that occur during the day are just as important as those that occur at night. Consistent with this assumption, engaging in actions that target values can be important for improving psychological well-being. At this point in the intervention, the therapist helps the client or group members to assess their values.

   Values clarification helps to guide individuals toward what they really want to be and not toward what they avoid. Thus, the exercise will help the person to observe what h/she wants and what behaviors he/she needs to perform to reach their goals. At the same time, individuals will perceive how much they engage in behaviors related to the avoidance of aversive situations. Individuals often dedicate most of their time to avoidance behaviors rather than values-based behaviors. Within this context, the "life compass" activity is proposed to address values.

Life compass

The therapist explains the "life compass" activity to the client or group members and allows time so that the client or group members can complete the activity. The activity is described below.

In the main part of each large box, write a few keywords about what is important or meaningful to you in this life domain. To guide your responses, keep the following questions in mind: "What kind of person do you want to be?" "What type of personal strengths and qualities do you want to cultivate?" "How do you ideally want to behave?"

If a box seems irrelevant to you, you can leave it blank. There is no given order to fill out the boxes; thus, feel free to first fill out the boxes whose domains are most clear to you. There is no problem if the same words are repeated in different boxes; this repetition helps us to identify the core values that run through many domains of our lives.

After you have filled out all boxes, rate how important each domain is to you at this point in your life. For this, assign a score on a scale from 0 to 10 in the small top square of each box, where 0 = unimportant and 10 = extremely important.

In the small bottom square of each box, rate on a scale from 0 to 10 how much you are investing in these values at this point in your life, where 0 = not investing at all and 10 = fully investing.

Maternity/Paternity

Personal Growth

Leisure

Spirituality

Health

Work

Community and Environment

Family Relationships

Intimate Relationships

Social Relationships

____________________(any domain not mentioned)

______________________(any domain not mentioned)

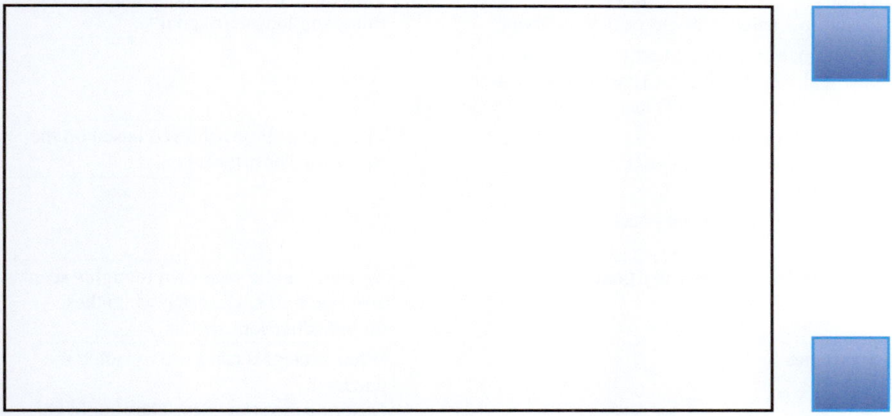

Source: Adapted from Hayes and Smith (2005).

After the activity, the client or group members share their experience.

3. Committed action

Once the values have been clarified, it is time to shift the focus to engaging in behaviors targeting these values. Commitments help boost a person's mood throughout treatment. Now the commitment should be more focused on engaging in valued activities rather than slipping back into the discomfort avoidance strategy.

Clients can experience deep emotions when they witness that they are not living up to their values. What underlies this difficulty? What quality connects us to our value? We often neglect ourselves by waiting outside and by not engaging based on this quality.

At this stage, the therapist asks the client or group members to define, based on their values, at least one goal and one action to achieve it. Short-term and long-term goals should be considered. Short-term goals are those that can be accomplished soon, while long-term goals are only achieved in the future. Having short-term goals can help you achieve your long-term goals. Within this context, the following exercise can contribute to identifying what the client or group members want and how they need to act to achieve their goals.

The client or group members can reflect on the established goals and suggest behaviors that facilitate achieving the expected results. Outlining concrete objectives whose actions can be implemented immediately is encouraged. Use the chart presented in Table 15.8 for this intervention.

By the end of this session, the client or group members will have identified some core values, as well as their goals, barriers, and target behaviors. The purpose of this exercise is to engage the client or group members in behaviors that will allow them to achieve their goals.

4. Mindfulness focused on values and committed actions

Bearing in mind the identified values, the therapist proceeds with the following mindfulness practice.

Table 15.8 Values-based committed actions

Value Describe a value that you want to cultivate	This value will be demonstrated by the following long-term goal:
To set goals, it is important that they are (1) practical, (2) attainable, (3) are in line with the current situation, and (4) take you toward your value	
Long-term goal Describe the long-term goal	This goal will be achieved based on the following short-term goals:
Short-term goals Describe the short-term goals	1. 2. 3.
Barriers to achieving my goals	Barriers can be your own thoughts seen as absolute truths. Describe when these thoughts/barriers appear
Strategies	What strategies can I use to tackle the barriers? Describe the strategies. They could be those you learned in this intervention
Values	
Goals	
Barriers to achieving my goals	
Behaviors that will allow me to achieve my goals	

Source: Adapted from Hayes and Smith (2005)

Metta meditation – ACT variation

Close your eyes and focus on your breathing. Identify a core value, for example, flexibility, compassion, love, freedom, or a value you would like to cultivate, and then imagine that value as a flash of light.

Imagine this light entering your body from the top of your head. Hence, your value is slowly filling you with a brilliant light, permeating every cell in your body.

Now visualize someone close to you with whom you have a positive relationship. Imagine that your value, represented by this light, is filling that person. Now think of other people you know, acquaintances, friends, and family, and visualize this light filling these people with your value. At this point, think of someone you have a hard time dealing with and imagine your value filling that person as well.

Imagine this light increasing and filling everyone now. Every living person is filled with this light. All people are pulsing and vibrating in this light and in this value.

Imagine yourself giving this gift to everyone and, at the same time, receiving this gift from everyone.

With the memory of this experience and connected to its value, say goodbye to this moment. Slowly move parts of your body and, when you feel comfortable, you can open your eyes.

Source: Adapted from Fletcher (2008)

5. Review of homework

The homework assignments aim to strengthen what was learned in the session on extra-session occasions.

1. Fill out the sleep diary
The sleep diaries should be filled out weekly to monitor treatment progress. A sleep diary template can be found in Chap. 9 of this book.
2. Make/maintain changes in sleep hygiene
Obtain information about habits, activities, and environments that can promote sleep. For this, check out the guidelines in the Chap. 10 of this book.
3. Write thoughts/feelings present at bedtime in a notebook. Remember, if you overflow with thoughts/feelings at bedtime, put them on paper. A notebook template can be found in the Chap. 10 of this book.
4. Observe attempts of avoidances identified in session 4.
5. Perform a behavior that meets your values established in the activity proposed in this session. Write in the checklist presented in Table 15.9 when you faced barriers to achieving the goals and when you behaved toward achieving your goals.
6. Practice Metta meditation – ACT variation daily
Practicing the mindfulness exercise daily as homework is key to developing and maintaining the ability to meditate. The Metta meditation is described in this chapter.

15.6 Sixth Session: Values and Committed Action

In session 6, values and committed actions will be reinforced based on the interventions described in Table 15.10.

Table 15.9 Barriers and pro-goal behaviors

Checklist	Facing barriers	Pro-goal behaviors
Monday		
Tuesday		
Wednesday		
Thursday		
Friday		
Saturday		
Sunday		

Table 15.10 Interventions of session 6

Intervention	Objectives
Review of homework	To review extra-session activities Feedback on established tasks
Attending your own funeral – Epitaph	Values clarification
The Unwelcomed Party Guest	Acceptance when acting toward the values
Meditation focused on values and committed actions – Tonglen meditation	Acceptance and commitment with the values
Homework assignment	To develop extra-session therapeutic activities

1. Review of homework

The therapist evaluates the sleep diaries and asks the client or group members about maintaining the changes made in sleep hygiene, about the Metta meditation practice, about the attempt of not avoiding a certain situation identified in session 4, and about behaviors that are in line with the values established in the proposed activity of session 5. The client or group members report the week's feedback. When reviewing the homework assignment, the therapist asks the client if there have been any changes since the last session.

Attending your own funeral – what message would you like to leave behind?

Have you ever noticed that, when people die, they are remembered for their virtues and their values? Try to identify someone who has died that you look up to. Think of your heroines and heroes. What was the most important inheritance of these people? My guess is that they were not material achievements or fortunes but the values reflected in their lives.

Returning now to your life. You have a certain amount of time on earth and you don't know how much. The question is "Are you going to live knowing that you are going to die?" This question is not different from the questions "Will you love knowing you will be hurt?" or "Will you commit to living the life you value knowing that, many times, it will not meet your expectations?" Or "Will you aim for success knowing that sometimes you will fail?" The potential to feel pain and the sense of vitality that arises from these experiences cannot be separated.

Being aware that we are finite can help us to take advantage of the time we have to invest in what we really believe and value. With that in mind, what message would you like to leave behind when you die? We recognize that it can be macabre to imagine the end of your life. It is not meant to be morbid but realistic.

If you could live your life the way you envisioned it, what would your values be? The question is not about what you have already done or what you expect to do. The issue is for you to observe what you expect the people closest to you to see about your life. The question is: What would be evident if you could freely choose the values of your life? How would you like to be remembered?

Source: Adapted from Hayes and Smith (2005)

2. Values

To reinforce the values addressed in the last session, the therapist proposes the following activity "Attending your own funeral – What message would you like to leave behind?" The therapist reads the activity together with the client or group members, explains the purpose, and allows time for the client or group members to complete the activity.

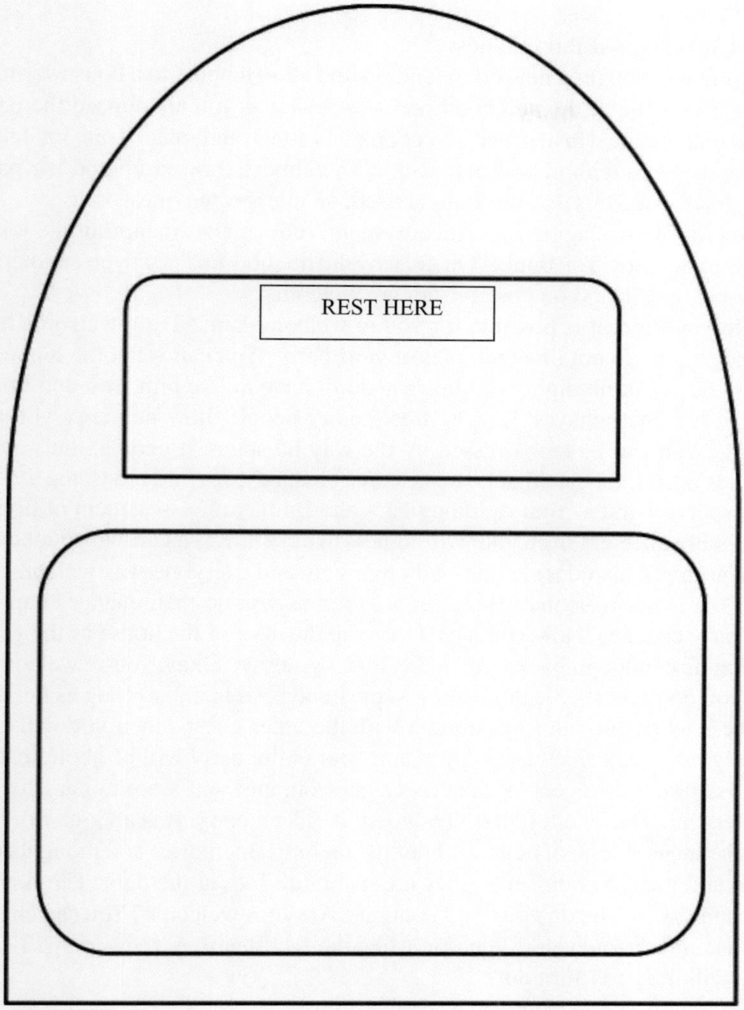

Fig. 15.5 Epitaph

With that in mind, write your epitaph in Fig. 15.5.

The therapist invites the client or group members to share their sensations and feelings during this activity.

3. Committed actions

To address acceptance during the action in pursuit of values, the therapist reads the following text together with the client or group members:

The Unwelcomed Party Guest

Imagine you bought a new house and invited all neighbors to a housewarming party. Everyone in the neighborhood was invited – you announced the party on social media (Instagram, Facebook, Twitter) and placed an invitation poster at the neighborhood mall. So, all neighbors showed up and the party was great. Suddenly Joe the Bum arrived, an unexpected guest.

Joe the Bum is aggressive, inconvenient, rude, makes inappropriate jokes, and is obnoxious. You think, "Oh no, why did he show up?" But you announced on social media and on posters: "all are welcome."

Do you think it is possible for you to welcome him? Truly welcome him, although you do not like that he is at your party? You can welcome him even if you do not think highly of him. You don't have to like him. You don't have to like how he behaves, how he treats other people, how he views you and people. You can be embarrassed by the way he stares at people, the way he offends others, the fact that he makes unnecessary jokes and brags, the way he disrespects women. Your opinion of Joe the Bum, your assessment of him, is absolutely different from your willingness to have him as a guest in your house.

You might also decide that, although you said everyone was welcome, in fact, Joe is not welcome. However, as soon as you do that, changes happen, the party changes. Now you have to stay at the door of the house as the guard so that he cannot go back to the party. Or if you say "Okay, you're welcome", but you don't really mean it, you just mean he is welcome as long as he stays in the kitchen and does not mingle with the other guests, then you will constantly have to keep an eye on him and your entire party will be about that. In the meantime, life goes on, the party goes on, and you are on guard for the unpleasant. This is not living. It is not quite like a party. It is a lot of work.

The metaphor is, of course, about the feelings, memories and thoughts that arise and that you don't like; they are just more Joes at the door. The issue is the stance you take on your own contents. Are Joes welcome? You can choose to welcome them even if you don't like the fact that they showed up? If not, how will the party turn out?

Source: Adapted from Hayes et al. (1999).

After reading the text, the therapist asks the client or group members about their impressions. The therapist guides the discussion by demonstrating that the text shows that, when we try to prevent Joe the Bum from joining the party, other undesirable reactions will manifest. Would it not be better to become "a close friend of Joe"? To understand him? To know how to deal with him? After all, he is already in your house.

Committed actions involve unpleasant events that produce discomfort because they refer to past situations with intense emotions and there is a fear of revisiting them. The idea is to realize the importance of identifying and not rejecting feelings.

Individuals commonly deny feelings, resist them, and intertwine external and internal judgments. With this attitude, individuals avoid feeling what actually manifests itself in them in terms of feeling and, therefore, they do not identify what they feel and continue to avoid it.

After reflecting on the text, the therapist proceeds with the following mindfulness practice.

Meditation focused on values and committed actions – Tonglen meditation

Find a comfortable position and settle in. Close your eyes and focus on your breathing. Breathe…

Identify a value that you consider to be fundamental. Find a word that describes this value. How do you keep this word in your mind? Observe the sensations you are experiencing in your body.

Observe if there is lightness, warmth, and a sense of openness.

Think of an image that captures what you are experiencing.

Now identify a problem that you have been struggling with.

How do you keep this problem in your mind?

Observe your bodily sensations and how you are feeling as you think about it.

Get in touch with this feeling of stress about a problem.

Think of an image that captures what you are experiencing, for example, the last time this problem occurred.

Now try some slow, long, and deep breaths.

As you inhale, think about your struggle using the image you thought of or a word to represent it. Observe any physical sensations that may arise. Breathe into this pain wherever it is located in your body.

As you exhale, remember your value using the word or image that you chose for this core value. Exhale in the sense of opening and relaxation.

Inhale again getting in touch with your pain and exhale getting in touch with your value.

Continue to touch your pain upon inhaling and your value upon exhaling.

Observe whether the pain and value start to overlap? Is it difficult to separate one from the other?

Observe this experience, this moment, and then say goodbye. Get in touch again with your breathing, focus on the sounds of your environment. Slowly move parts of your body and, when you feel comfortable, you can open your eyes.

Source: Adapted from Fletcher (2008).

4. Homework assignment

The homework assignments aim to strengthen what was learned in the session on extra-session occasions.

1. Fill out the sleep diary

The sleep diaries should be filled out weekly to monitor treatment progress. A sleep diary template can be found in Chap. 9 of this book.

2. Make/maintain changes in sleep hygiene

Obtain information about habits, activities, and environments that can promote sleep. For this, check out the guidelines in the Chap. 10 of this book.

3. Write thoughts/feelings present at bedtime in a notebook. Remember, if you overflow with thoughts/feelings at bedtime, put them on paper. A notebook template can be found in the Chap. 10 of this book.
4. Observe attempts of avoidances identified in session 4.
5. Perform a behavior that is in line with your values established in the activity proposed in the fifth session.
6. Perform Tonglen meditation with ACT variation daily.
7. Practicing the mindfulness exercise daily as homework is key to developing and maintaining the ability to meditate. The Tonglen meditation practice is described in this chapter.

5. Treatment closure and feedback

The therapist closes the treatment with the following questions:

"What did this experience change?"

The client or group members share their answers and say goodbye.

References

Costa, R. S., Soares, M. R., & Grossi, R. (2017). Estrutura das sessões de uma intervenção analítico-comportamental em grupo para pessoas diagnosticadas com transtorno bipolar. *Acta Comportamentalia, 25*(1), 57–72.

Fletcher, L. (2008). *Acceptance and commitment therapy for insomnia treatment manual*. https://contextualscience.org/act_for_sleep_problems

Hayes, S. C., & Smith, S. (2005). *Get out of your mind and into your life: The new acceptance and commitment therapy*. New Harbinger.

Hayes, S. C., Strosahl, K. D., & Wilson, K. G. (1999). *Acceptance and commitment therapy: An experiential approach to behavior change*. The Guilford Press.

Hayes, S. C., Strosahl, K. D., & Wilson, K. G. (2011). *Acceptance and commitment therapy, second edition: The process and practice of mindful change* (2nd ed.). The Guilford Press.

Kabat-Zinn, J. (1990). *Full catastrophe living: Using the wisdom of your body and mind to face stress, pain, and illness* (Reprint edition, 2013 ed.). Bantam Books.

Ong, J. C., & Manber, R. (2011). Mindfulness-based therapy for insomnia. In *Behavioral treatments for sleep disorders* (pp. 133–141). Elsevier. https://doi.org/10.1016/B978-0-12-381522-4.00014-6

Oriah "Mountain Dreamer" House from her book, THE INVITATION © 1999. Published by HarperONE, San Francisco. All rights reserved. Presented with permission of the author. www.oriah.org

Ramos, T. P. T. (2015). O Que é Mindfulness? In P. Lucena Santos, J. Pinto-Gouveia, & M. S. Oliveira (Eds.), *Terapias Comportamentais de Terceira Geração: Guia para profissionais* (pp. 59–80). Sinopsys Editora.

Rumi, J. (n.d.). The guest house. Retrieved from http://persweb.wabash.edu/facstaff/hulenp/sperit/poetry/rumi/guesthou.htmlMilton

Saban, M. T. (2015). O que é Terapia de Aceitação e Compromisso? In P. Lucena Santos, J. Pinto-Gouveia, & M. S. Oliveira (Eds.), *Terapias Comportamentais de Terceira Geração: Guia para profissionais* (pp. 179–216). Sinopsys Editora.

Chapter 16
ACT Therapeutic Processes in the ACT-I Protocol

Michaele Terena Saban-Bernauer and Roberta Kovac

This chapter describes the therapeutic processes of the Acceptance and Commitment Therapy for insomnia (ACT-I) protocol in order to better understand the strategies and execution of the exercises.

The therapeutic goal of ACT-based interventions is to promote a complex and extremely useful behavioral repertoire that will enable the effective functioning of individuals in their contexts and improve their quality of life, the so-called psychological flexibility. This repertoire consists of new approaches to deal with discomforts, symptoms, and suffering related, for example, to insomnia, which can include thoughts, feelings, physical sensations, and uncomfortable or unpleasant memories. The therapeutic process aims to create opportunities for the patient to learn to deal with these uncomfortable events in order to achieve a more meaningful life.

ACT is based on the understanding of psychological suffering that seeks, with precision, scope, and depth, to explain how inflexibility occurs and to propose interventions that will transform this suffering into its opposite – flexibility. From the point of view of ACT and supported by relational frame theory (RFT), a behavioral approach to human language and cognition (Hayes et al., 2001), typical processes of human language can induce intense psychological suffering in a person and the antidote to this suffering consists of new ways to relate to verbal and private events. According to Luoma et al. (2007), "in essence, the problem is that literal language leads to increases in pain and the tendency to overextend a problem-solving mode of thinking as a way to solve that pain. As a result, we try to escape and avoid our

M. T. Saban-Bernauer (✉)
School of Permanent Education, Clinics Hospital, Faculty of Medicine, University of São Paulo, Sao Paulo, Brazil

R. Kovac
Paradigma Center of Behavioral Science and Technology, Sao Paulo, Brazil
e-mail: roberta@paradigmaac.org

R. El Rafihi-Ferreira (ed.), *Acceptance and Commitment Therapy for Insomnia*,
https://doi.org/10.1007/978-3-031-50710-6_16

feelings, we become entangled in our thinking, we lose contact with the present, and we begin to believe and defend our own stories about ourselves" (p. 11).

Although fundamental and extremely advantageous for the human species – as they are the same cognitive abilities that contribute to human advancement and survival, this mode of functioning, enabled by symbolic behavior or by human language and cognition, causes a type of suffering that is probably exclusive to humans. From the perspective of RFT, a behavioral process is observed (arbitrary and derived relational responding) that, at the same time, (1) facilitates and favors the relationship of humans with their environment by responding to (arbitrary) relationships between events (stimuli) and thus attributing meanings (functions) to them that, in turn, affect the behavior itself. This process, which is typical of language, greatly expands the number of events and functions of the environment since it includes, in addition to present events, relationships between present and past or future events, spatially absent events, or even never known or experienced events (concepts). (2) The behavioral process forms the basis of psychological suffering. For example, reports of situations imagined in the future and memories or thoughts of situations suffered in the past themselves can produce pain in the present since both (report and situation) are bidirectionally related (Wilson et al., 2001).

In the words of Wilson and collaborators, (…) "the paradox of our species is that we have far less contact with direct sources of pain than any other species on the planet; however, through language, we are capable of suffering with a degree of intensity, constancy and pervasiveness that is literally unimaginable in the non-human world. Because of the bidirectional transformation of functions, we can judge ourselves and find ourselves 'needy'; we can imagine ideals and find our present situation unacceptable by comparison; we can reconstruct the past; we can worry about imagined futures; we can suffer with the knowledge that we will die" (Wilson et al., 2001, p. 215).

Therefore, cognitive and verbal skills, identified in their minimum unit – arbitrarily applicable relational responding, while providing an explanation of how words and other symbols can affect behavior by participating in networks of relationships between events and thus acquiring many of the functions of these events, also explain how to construct a way to relate with one's own behavior – feeling, thinking, remembering – which can amplify suffering. Favored and strengthened by recurrent cultural practices that say things like "get rid of bad feelings" or "think positive," a rigid and inflexible way of reacting to one's behavior is created – "bad" parts must be eliminated. By doing this insistently, the person ends up remaining in a vicious cycle in which, in an attempt to solve the problem, he or she engages in responses, trying to change the form, frequency, or content of their feelings, thoughts, sensations, and memories. Doing this over and over again, the individual ends up limiting their life in the long run. This mode of functioning, called experiential avoidance and psychological rigidity, represents the concept of suffering defined by ACT. Thus, the interventions proposed in ACT address suffering by targeting psychological flexibility – i.e., the abandonment of this rigid and limiting pattern of dealing with parts of one's own behavior.

The therapeutic processes described in ACT, which aim to promote psychological flexibility, are creative hopelessness, acceptance, defusion, mindfulness, self as context, values clarification, and committed action. Each of these processes will be analyzed below to illustrate the ACT protocol applied to insomnia (ACT-I). It must be noted that ACT uses experiential exercises, mindfulness practices, and metaphors to consistently and systematically address these processes in the office clinical setting. Within this context, therapy should be an opportunity to create conditions for learning this new flexible repertoire.

16.1 Creative Hopelessness

The different types of experiential avoidance commonly go unnoticed. They are not very explicit ways of trying to avoid suffering and are usually so automatic that the individual does not identify them in advance. This also occurs because noticing suffering and what we do with it are aversive processes. We start therapy by observing this pattern of experiential avoidance and its effect on:

- Avoiding short-term and long-term suffering
- How it transforms the life of the individual

This process is called creative hopelessness because the experiential avoidance pattern tends to work in the short term in an attempt to eliminate suffering momentarily; however, suffering returns in the medium and long term and the experiential avoidance itself poses restrictions because it does not solve the problem of the experienced contingencies, thus amplifying the person's suffering. Experiential avoidance only reduces the felt or imagined suffering, while the situation remains the same. For example, someone with family problems has insomnia as a consequence and takes sleeping pills. The person sleeps instantly, but the insomnia returns because the family problems are still present and their actions are focused on eliminating the insomnia and not on addressing the relationships that generate the discomfort. The process of creative hopelessness aims, in an experiential way (observing your own experience), to unravel this ineffective way of dealing with discomfort and observe its short-term (working temporarily) and medium- and long-term effects (return of the discomfort and amplification of the problem, restricting life more and more).

The insomnia protocol contains interventions that focus on this process of observing experiential avoidance and losing hope. For the exercise *Evaluating attempts to control and escape discomfort*, the client fills out a table and discusses the answers. The questions are stimuli that evoke observing responses of the experiential avoidance pattern. In Table 16.1, you will find the questions of the exercise and the description of the responses that the exercise intends to evoke.

The following exercise, *Mindfulness practice on creative hopelessness – insomnia*, dives deeper into the first question of the previous exercise about how individuals feel when they have insomnia, what they think and feel in their bodies. This

Table 16.1 Questions and responses of the evaluating attempts to control and escape discomfort exercise

How do I feel when I cannot sleep?	What do I do right away?	Does it work as I would like? Right away and in the long run?	How did this transform my life?	What will managing insomnia improve in my life?
Stimuli that evoke emotion-observing responses (covert response) at the time of insomnia. The emotions that act as aversive motivators of aversive emotion avoidance responses. Since the emotion is aversive, observing the emotion will also be aversive. The observing response is an alternative to the avoidance response and is the beginning of the acceptance process.	Stimuli that evoke an observing response of experiential avoidance. It is important that the answers here are those given at the time of insomnia, not afterwards, such as "I went to see a doctor," "I talked to people about it." The answer here refers to what the individual did at the time of insomnia, such as "I took some medication," "I thought about several things (ask to specify)," "I went to watch TV."	Experiential avoidance generally works right away to eliminate the emotion that accompanies insomnia or insomnia itself but does not change the situations that generated the emotions and insomnia in the first place. For this reason, insomnia returns and the pattern of momentarily working (if it works) and having no medium- or long-term effect is observed.	Stimuli that evoke observing responses of the limitations that experiential avoidance generates, for example, medication overuse and resulting problems, rumination, tiredness, and fatigue in the case of watching TV. It should favor the observation of the amplification of suffering in this mostly avoidance mode of functioning.	Based on a hypothetical situation, this question investigates the restrictions generated by insomnia and the attempt to control it and indicates possible positive reinforcement contingencies that are deprived because of the experiential avoidance pattern. This is the beginning of a values-related process.

mindfulness practice is both an exercise that supports creative hopelessness (conditions for observing the motivating operation of experiential avoidance) and an acceptance exercise that proposes the observation of covert responses (thoughts, feelings, sensations, and memories) without reacting to them.

The protocol proceeds with the *Tug-of-war with a monster metaphor*. The metaphor represents a strategy to describe contingencies and their functions using concrete elements. Relationships that are often abstract playfully become characters, which facilitates the observation of a specific type of functioning. According to this metaphor, insomnia or the emotions associated with insomnia correspond to the monster, the tug-of-war represents the struggle trying to control private events (thoughts, feelings, sensations, and memories), and pulling the rope corresponds to experiential avoidance and the feeling of responding in this way, i.e., struggle and war. The tension of the tug-of-war and the imminence of falling into the hole translate the fear of feeling and thinking, the fear of falling into an abyss of oneself.

Abandoning the control of private events corresponds to the therapist's proposal to let go of the rope and to relate to the monster in a new way.

Monitoring contingency elements and thus amplifying proximity, the contact with their functions, is a widely used strategy in ACT, including in metaphors, mindfulness practices, and exercises. It facilitates observation, especially when some stimuli and responses are private, and the function of the current contingency. It can also make explicit the therapeutic proposal. Metaphors in particular are a much easier elucidation to be remembered in contexts outside of the therapeutic setting, facilitating generalization. An image helps because it is easy to remember and facilitates the observation of experiential avoidances in the contexts in which it occurs in the client's life. Thus, the issues of the exercise and mindfulness practices are training and different learning opportunities, whose aim is to activate this repertoire of observing (1) one's own behavior, (2) the way the person reacts to it, and (3) the short-, medium-, and long-term effects inside and outside the therapy session.

In addition to the acceptance process, creative hopelessness or the opportunity to learn to observe emotions in the experiential avoidance contingency is especially important. The possibility of observing the emotion present during the experiential avoidance response, without reacting directly to it, potentiates the alternative of change. In contrast, engaging in typical avoidance responses – taking insomnia medication – usually produces a feeling of failure or impotence. Thinking about what could have been done or what can still be done increases worries or the feeling of being trapped in a problem with no way out. Watching TV, turning on the TV, or picking up the cell phone and viewing social media produces upset, guilt, sadness, a feeling of wasted time. The consequence of experiential avoidance is immediate relief, which is soon followed by even more uncomfortable emotions and dead-end thoughts. When people observe emotions and experiential avoidance responses in their daily lives, together with the observation of long-term losses and the resulting paralysis of life, it arises what ACT calls hopelessness in trying to control the uncontrollable, our inner world, the hopelessness regarding the strategy that has been used for so long but which, after this observation process, can prove to be clearly ineffective. A possible window is then created for a new way of relating to this inner world, acceptance.

16.2 Acceptance

Acceptance has different meanings. In ACT, acceptance is a process composed of willingness and an attitude of openness. Willingness is "the voluntary and values-based choice to enable or sustain contact with private experiences or the events that likely caused them" (Hayes et al., 1999/2012, p. 77).

Openness or psychological acceptance is "the adoption of an open, receptive, flexible, and non-judgmental posture regarding moment-to-moment experience" (Hayes et al., 1999/2012, p. 77). The posture of acceptance is also present in the mindfulness process, differing only in terms of the emphasis of acceptance on the private experience (thoughts, feelings, sensations, memories, and predispositions).

Regarding acceptance as an action (not as resignation or abandonment), being willing to get in touch with our inner world is a very important factor for behavioral change that is directly linked to values. Acting in accordance with individual values means acting in the way and in the direction that is important to the person. However, the reason why people do not do it or why they are how they are is important to them because:

1. They acted like this in the past and were punished.
2. They were taught not to act like that because it would not be accepted. This teaching can occur based on rules, differential reinforcement, vicarious learning, or modeling.
3. They were trained to relate events in a way that such an action would not be positively reinforced, would have no consequence (extinction), or would be punished.

Therefore, when people do not act coherently with what matters to them or in the direction toward what is important, it may indicate that the context in which they find themselves contains stimuli that were paired or related to aversive stimuli in their history of learning, eliciting sensations perceived as aversive and evoking covert responses such as thoughts, feelings, and memories that are also aversive. These responses possibly function as motivating operations to evoke avoidance responses, called here experiential avoidance responses since they are escape or avoidance responses to private events. Acceptance becomes a therapeutic goal when the person is faced with antecedents consisting of aversive stimuli (public or private) that do not permit escape or avoidance responses or that have even more aversive medium- to long-term consequences. The desired outcome of acceptance responses is not a change in the antecedent aversive stimulus (in terms of frequency or intensity) but rather a change in the function of this aversive event, measured by the reduction in or absence of avoidance responses and the occurrence of other (new) responses – these in the direction toward what is important to the person in the long term. To promote this action of acceptance, responses such as observation, description, tentatively dealing with extant contingencies, and approximation (desirable consequences) are trained in acceptance exercises.

Considering this proposal, learning to deal with private experiences in an open, receptive, flexible, and non-judgmental way is a key skill to be trained. Examples of experiential exercises and metaphors used for this training can be found in the *Mindfulness practice on creative hopelessness – insomnia* of the ACT-I protocol, which encourages the client to perceive feelings, sensations, and thoughts during insomnia, and in the poem *The Guest House* by Rumi (Sufi master of the nineteenth century). Using the metaphor of private events as guests of the house (and "house" here is a metaphor of the person themself, of the "I"), the poem invites to openly welcome the guests.

The poem *The Invitation* by Dreamer (2000) continues to add elements of openness to private experiences, combining committed actions, values, and self in a poetic language (see Table 16.2).

Table 16.2 ACT elements in excerpts of the poem *The Invitation*

"It doesn't interest me what you do for a living. I want to know what you ache for and if you dare to dream of meeting your heart's longing.	Values
It doesn't interest me how old you are. I want to know if you will risk looking like a fool for love, for your dream, for the adventure of being alive.	Acceptance on behalf of values-based actions
It doesn't interest me what planets are squaring your moon. I want to know if you have touched the center of your own sorrow, if you have been opened by life's betrayals or have become shriveled and closed from fear of further pain.	Values-based actions × experiential avoidance
I want to know if you can sit with pain mine or your own, without moving to hide it or fade it or fix it. I want to know if you can be with joy mine or your own, if you can dance with wildness and let the ecstasy fill you to the tips of your fingers and toes without cautioning us to be careful, to be realistic, to remember the limitations of being human.	Values-based actions and positive reinforcers
It doesn't interest me if the story you are telling me is true. I want to know if you can disappoint another to be true to yourself. If you can bear the accusation of betrayal and not betray your own soul. If you can be unfaithful and still be trustworthy.	Values-based actions in aversive and conflict situations
I want to know if you can see beauty every day even when it is not pretty. And if you can source your own life from its presence.	Values-based actions
I want to know if you can live with failure, yours and mine, and still stand at the edge of the lake and shout to the silver of the full moon: 'Yes!'	Acceptance and values-based actions
It doesn't interest me to know where you live or how much money you have. I want to know if you can get up after a night of grief and despair, weary and bruised to the bone, and do what needs to be done to feed the children.	Acceptance on behalf of values-based actions
It doesn't interest me who you know or how you came to be here. I want to know if you will stand in the center of the fire with me and not shrink back.	Acceptance on behalf of values-based actions and self as context
It doesn't interest me where or what or with whom you have studied. I want to know what sustains you from the inside when all else falls away.	Values and acceptance
I want to know if you can be alone with yourself and if you truly like the company you keep in the empty moments."	Acceptance and self-compassion

Poetry as a metaphor greatly facilitates communication of the processes proposed by the therapy, without the need to teach clients theoretical terms that may not have a function in their practical life.

The following exercise of the ACT-I protocol mixes processes of acceptance, creative hopelessness, self, and committed actions with values. The technique is designed to render feelings, thoughts and memories concrete by writing them on a paper. On one side of the paper, the participants are asked to write good memories, thoughts, and feelings, and on the other side, bad memories, thoughts and feeling. In this activity, "I" is the paper and the written words are the private events. The limitations in wanting to avoid this internal content are noted; it is observed that, by doing so, one also avoids the positive reinforcing aspects (related to what is important to the person – values). A concrete demonstration is the wish to crumple the sheet of paper, which contains good and bad memories, thoughts, and feelings. This is another way of illustrating how the process of creative hopelessness works.

When asking whether the client identifies him or herself with some written characteristic, the therapist is metaphorically investigating responses to which an individual relates by coordinating them with themselves, i.e., as an equal, as an equivalent, and, within the terms of ACT, this individual is fusing with them and considers them as inherent to themselves or to their personality. The therapeutic proposal to expand this notion of the "I" is again exemplified metaphorically and physically (concretely) by the sheet of paper, leading the person to understand that the "I" is not a written characteristic but the place that contains all aspects. This conception of the "I" is called self as context. It is produced by training multiple exemplars of the perspective of an "I" that contains all aspects of the person – thoughts, feelings, memories, sensations, actions, positive and negative, important and insignificant – therefore, an "I" that can contain all of them without defining or becoming any of these specific aspects.

At the end of the exercise, the therapist guides the client to identify with and engage in a values-guided action that was suppressed by experiential avoidance (stopped doing to avoid some thought or feeling). This action is also written on the sheet since it is part of the content and not of the "I" (the self), promoting greater flexibility, although it is a positive aspect that possibly results in positive reinforcers.

16.3 Defusion

Defusion is a term coined by the authors of ACT to describe a process using a metaphor – the opposite of fusion. Semantically, fusion designates a process in which two elements mix and transform into a third. In the case of language, fusion refers to how sound or written patterns relate to aspects of the world (so-called "referents" in language theories) that are socially agreed upon as the "meaning" of those sound or written patterns. The sound of the word "rice" fuses with a handful of white grains in such a way that it becomes "rice" – both the sound and the grains can affect us in very similar ways in certain situations. Language training is extremely extensive and, as already mentioned, represents a great differential for our species. Technically, we are trained to respond to a stimulus (sound or written word) as if it were another (object), first by pairing, then the stimuli become functional classes that interact with each other as we acquire the ability to relate events. The result of this vast training in verbal behavior is a literal world, in which we relate to events fundamentally through verbal relationships. When we eat rice without paying attention, we eat the "concept of rice"; our action of eating is conditioned to the "concept of rice" and many times we do not even feel the taste of that "rice" as a specific and unique object.

We interact with other spoken words or with sentences in the form of thoughts as if they were literal truths. This occurs because it is consistent with our history that the word "rice" is related to the actual rice. However, when we tell us things about who we are, what we like, our assessments of others and about ourselves, we act as if those words are as concrete as "rice." In therapy, when clients talk about their suffering, the word itself already generates discomfort as if it were the suffering itself. When reporting, the client is in contact with the language, i.e., indirect/attributed functions of a stimulus (experience of suffering) to another (report). The fusion between words and thoughts, emotions and memories classified as negative, bad, or uncomfortable then becomes a problem since it evokes a class of experiential avoidance responses in an attempt to get rid of these private events.

Defusion interventions consist of the observation of language as a process, separating direct (from experience) from indirect functions (attributed) and permitting the observation of behavior (verbal – thought, emotion, memory) as it actually is – a process and a product of the person's ongoing interaction with their world.

We have an idea of how we think; in practice, this behavior is much more chaotic than we imagine and is the result of learning. We believe that our thinking reflects reality, as if we were analyzing or describing the world. In practice, what we observe is what we have been trained to see in some specific way. What we do is establishing relationships between events that we have been taught to do, and we evaluate and judge those as if such comparisons were a confirmation of reality.

While acceptance is an approximation of private events, observing and feeling these events as they are, defusion is the observation of the language process, noticing it as it is and its impact on all behavior. When clients write their thoughts on a sheet of paper or look at their thought and relate it to the monster of the metaphor, the defusion process is present because they are invited to see this behavior as an ongoing process, a flowing behavior. The mindfulness practice *Leaves on a stream* is another example of a defusion exercise of the ACT-I protocol, in which the client observes the flow of thoughts.

16.4 Mindfulness

In ACT, mindfulness practices represent an extensive training of focused or expanded attention skills, either in the outer world or in the own inner world, in lived or hypothetical situations. Like most of the ACT interventions, these exercises are an alternative approach to learn to deal with the inner world, respecting it and allowing it to be as it is. As mentioned before, the training of observing responses underlies many of the practices and sometimes appears formally in the exercises. Table 16.3 shows a list of the mindfulness exercises of the ACT-I protocol, with the specification of focused and expanded attention training.

Technically, the therapist asks the client to sit down in a comfortable position in which they can stay in for a few minutes and to close the eyes if the client feels comfortable. The therapist proceeds by providing instructions and the spoken words evoke and elicit the experience that the client is invited to observe.

Table 16.3 List of the mindfulness exercises of the ACT-I protocol

Session	Mindfulness	Training
2	Body scan	Observation of the body
3	Mindfulness practice on creative hopelessness – insomnia	Observation of a situation experienced in the past in order to identify and describe context, action, thought, feeling, and sensation
3	Leaves on a stream	Observation of the flow of thoughts
5	Metta meditation (ACT variation)	Observation of thoughts, feelings, and sensations in the presence of a value
6	Meditation focused on values and committed actions – Tonglen meditation	Observation of thoughts, feelings, and sensations in the presence of a value and of the difficulty and the process of approximation of suffering followed by approximation of the value

16.5 Self as Context

Self as context is a term that designates the perception of oneself as the locus, as the perspective from which experiences unfold. The aim of this concept is to systematize the notion of "I" as the result of a continuous process of experiences, the expanded perspective of that we are "who" think and not our thoughts, we are not our feelings but "who" feel, "who" remember and even "who" act. When fusion occurs at a high frequency, we tend to describe ourselves negatively and believe that our assessment is "the truth"; however, our inner and outer experiences are constantly changing. Interventions that seek to strengthen the self as context are aimed at the person's perception of (1) what is constant and (2) what is flow, focusing the observation on the perspective from which all behaviors depart. Technically, conceptual analysis of the RFT is aimed at establishing a hierarchical relationship between the observing "I" (deictic) and thoughts, feelings, sensations, memories, and actions. In other words, they can be seen as parts of the "I." The perspective from where I can include the thoughts and feelings and observe them. Naturally or typically, our tendency is to relate such events as equivalent to the "I." Practically, it is about creating opportunities for the person to perceive, feel, and describe themselves as the "I," the place, the perspective, the origin of the action, and not the action, feeling, sensation, or thought.

The poem *The Guest House* reflects the idea that private events come and go (they are guests) and the house is the place where they transit. Likewise, the activity of writing on a sheet of paper follows the same logic of conceiving the "I" as the sheet that contains thoughts and feelings.

The process of perceiving the self/I as context promotes flexibility and greater openness to get in touch with private events since the individual is not each one of them but the *one* who notices them.

Values and Committed Action

When clients realize their experiential avoidances and the cost of them in their life (creative hopelessness); when they reach out and open up to whatever feeling (acceptance); when they observe their thoughts as flowing behaviors and not necessarily connected with each part of the experience (defusion); when they perceive themselves as the observing "I" and include all of these events in their experience (self as context), and when they observe attentively and curiously everything that presents itself (mindfulness posture), then the prerequisites for clarifying what is important to the person (values) and acting toward them (committed action) are complete.

At this stage, all trained skills are implemented for the main purpose of ACT – bringing meaning to the person's life.

The guiding questions for values clarification are:

- What is important to you?
- Who is important to you?
- How do you want to live your life?

These questions are addressed in the *Life compass* exercise, which asks the clients to describe what they consider to be important in different life domains. The clients then evaluate the priority of each domain and how much they have been dedicating themselves to them. It is interesting to note the similarities of values in the different domains of life and how they represent a pool of adjectives that reveal important characteristics of how a person is or wants to be.

In the following exercise, *Values-based committed actions*, the value is translated into concrete goals and actions and the barriers to achieving these goals are made explicit, as shown in Table 16.4.

Table 16.4 Values, goals, barriers, and behaviors in the values-based committed actions exercise

Concept	Explanation	Example
Values	What is important and how the person wants to be	Be true to the family
Goals	Concrete situation in which the value is achieved	Tell family members what bothers you (be explicit and specify what you mean)
Barriers to achieving my goals	Challenging feelings, thoughts, sensations, and memories that arise in the context (there might be external barriers such as reactions from third parties and limits; in these cases, it refers to how the person will feel in face of the reaction of third parties and alternatives regarding limits)	Anxiety, fear of the reactions of others (possible aggression from others), thoughts of ruminating about situations that the person experienced
Behaviors that allow to achieve my goals	Observable and measurable concrete actions	Schedule a conversation with the family on Tuesday, send a message to family members, get together, contextualize that you would like to clarify some things and expose how you feel, and tell the content of the discomfort

Some care is necessary at this stage of the intervention:

- Make sure that the value is a genuine value of the client and is not a way to please or feel socially accepted.
- Actions and goals need to be concrete and observable. Abstract collocations indicate experiential avoidances. In general, because it is something new, it is difficult to imagine what a concrete action would be like. In this respect, it is a creative process and a clear description facilitates the answer.
- The action must correspond to the client's skills. In the example above, if the person has never expressed themselves freely and truly, there should be time for some training such as role play.

Session 5 ends with a mindfulness practice called Metta meditation (ACT variation), which is focused on observing the sensations when acting toward values. Since the values-based actions generally addressed in therapy are often new, they may not be positively reinforced in the short term. It is therefore important that the client perceives that the reinforcement of the values-guided action lies in the action itself – being that way (intrinsic reinforcement). In the example, being truthful can and will probably generate criticism (that is why the person is not "truthful" in the first place); however, acting according to what is important to the person, being honest becomes reinforcing in the medium and long terms. Therefore, training the observation of sensations that occur in these actions increases the perception and competes with possible punishments that may result from the behavior in the natural environment.

The last session covers exercises that enhance the intrinsic positive reinforcement of the committed action and the openness to the often-inherent discomfort when acting this way.

The exercise *Attending your own funeral – What message would you like to leave behind* represents a context that strongly evokes values clarification. Remembering the finitude of life makes the time we have precious. We are going to die and what we have here, our life, the people we love, what we can do, all this will end. We do not think about death because it is aversive, but it is our human condition – finitude. How do we want to live this indeterminate time that we have? This is the answer that ACT seeks to trigger and its main purpose.

We know that this is not an easy task because it involves aversive stories that prevent individuals from acting naturally according to their values. For this reason, we address openness to suffering and all acceptance and defusion training is commonly done a priori. In the metaphor *The Unwelcome Party Guest*, Joe represents this discomfort and how experiential avoidance responses compete with values-based actions, either we are surrounding Joe or we are enjoying the party. Again, metaphorically, it is expected to produce new meanings and transform functions in such a way that the person can focus on new possibilities regarding their own behavior and new results, different from those that they have been achieving (and debating).

The protocol ends with *Meditation focused on values and committed actions – Tonglen meditation*. In this practice, breathing is used to connect with the suffering and value. The perception of these alternating sensations is analogous to the experience that the individual will go through when performing a values-guided action.

16.6 Final Considerations

The therapeutic goal of ACT – flexibility – can be divided into other more specific processes of observation and contact with the inner world in an open and compassionate way, perceiving the processes of thinking and feeling emotions. This training and the perception of self as context of these experiences enables changes in behavior from a pattern of experiential avoidance to values-guided actions that can evoke and elicit challenging experiences; the latter, however, induce, within the action itself, what is important for individuals to be and to live their life.

These processes overlap in the mindfulness exercises, metaphors, and practices that make up the ACT intervention methodology. The ACT-I protocol is an example of a studied therapeutic management applied to the population that suffers from this discomfort. The novice therapist who is venturing into ACT is advised to follow the protocol in order to try unusual exercises. The professional should first go through the protocol as a participant and then as a therapist. Since the exercises trigger emotions, the therapist must understand the proposed experience for the client from their own perspective in order to conduct the intervention properly and respectfully. The protocol can also be conducted in groups; however, individual differences in the therapeutic process cannot be fully addressed in this case.

Finally, when the therapist experiences the process and trains it, the protocol will serve as an example and suggestion of activities. The clinical management is shaped by the analysis of which observation skills and training the client requires at each point.

References

Dreamer, O. M. (2000). O Convite. Trad de Maria Helena Rangel. Editora Sextante.

Hayes, S., Strosahl, K., & Wilson, K. (1999/2012). *Acceptance and commitment therapy: An experiential approach to behavior change*. Guilford Press.

Hayes, S., Barnes-Holmes, D., & Roche, B. (2001). *Relational frame theory: A post-Skinnerian account of human language and cognition*. Kluwer Academic/Plenum Publishers.

Luoma, J. B., Hayes, S. C., & Walser, R. D. (2007). *Learning ACT: An acceptance and commitment therapy skills-training manual for therapists*. New Harbinger Publications.

Wilson, K. G., Hayes, S. C., Gregg, J., & Zettle, R. D. (2001). Psychopathology and psychotherapy. In S. C. Hayes, D. Barnes-Holmes, & B. Roche (Eds.), *Relational frame theory: A post-Skinnerian account of human language and cognition* (pp. 211–237). Kluwer Academic/Plenum Publishers.

Part V
Application of ACT-I and ACT-BBI-I

Chapter 17
Case Example: Application of ACT-I in a Group Intervention

Renatha El Rafihi-Ferreira

The present chapter describes the application of the ACT-I protocol to a group of five adults with insomnia complaints.[1] ACT-I was applied as monotherapy, i.e., stimulus control or sleep restriction techniques were not used. The chapter focuses on the description of the session-by-session protocol based on the main excerpts from the exchanges of experiences that occurred between group members that accessed some of the therapeutic elements.

The participants sought group therapy for complaints of insomnia. After being interviewed by a sleep specialist, the participants were referred to the group therapy sessions. Six sessions were held. Below is a brief description of the participants, followed by the description of the main transcribed excerpts from the six sessions.

A brief description of the participants

Raíssa (fictitious name), 22 years, single, physiotherapy student. Her main complaint was unrefreshing sleep and daytime sleepiness. She had irregular bedtime and wake-up times and fragmented sleep. As a teenager, she was diagnosed with depression and had a history of ineffective treatments. According to Raíssa, on the occasion of the group therapy, depression was not prominent and insomnia was her main complaint.

Cirley (fictitious name), 36 years, married, social worker. She had difficulty initiating sleep and reported poor bedtime control. She went through a difficult time trying repeatedly to get pregnant without success. She believes that this fact may have interfered with her ability to fall asleep.

[1] The cases reported in this book signed the free informed consent form since they are part of a research project on ACT for insomnia.

R. El Rafihi-Ferreira (✉)
Department of Clinical Psychology, University of São Paulo, Sao Paulo, Brazil
e-mail: rerafihi@usp.br

R. El Rafihi-Ferreira (ed.), *Acceptance and Commitment Therapy for Insomnia*,
https://doi.org/10.1007/978-3-031-50710-6_17

Fábio (fictitious name), 37 years, single, engineer. Extremely strict regarding sleeping habits, with difficulty in initiating and maintaining sleep and hypnotic dependence. He reported that he stopped doing several activities that he liked in order to avoid compromising his sleep. He started to reduce meetings with friends and everything that could disturb his routine and consequently compromise his hours of sleep. With insomnia, his activities were increasingly limited.

Graziela (fictitious name), 49 years, divorced, housewife. She complained mainly about initiating sleep, but also about sleep maintenance. She reported frustration with her divorce 20 years ago, feeling left out by her children, and great difficulty trusting people. She experiences a lot of tension at night and often drinks alcohol in an attempt to relax and sleep.

Ludmila (fictitious name), 59 years, married, retired. Complaint of initiating and maintaining sleep. She reported the habit of going to bed much earlier than recommended in an attempt to sleep more. She would like to be more independent, but she sees herself very closed to new activities and new friendships and very dependent on others for doing trips. As a child, she was bullied and she believes that this fact made her afraid of getting hurt when making new friends.

17.1 Session 1

1. *Presentation:* Therapist and group members introduced themselves. Each participant introduced themselves and reported the complaint, the reason for seeking the group therapy, and what they like to do. Table 17.1 shows the presentation of each participant.

1. *Group rules:* The therapist explained the rules regarding absences, schedules, and confidentiality.
1. *Wound metaphor and group dynamics:* After the description of the wound metaphor, some comic drawings of insomnia manifestations were presented. The dynamics regarding the different manifestations of insomnia present in the comic drawings brought the group members closer together. Most participants identified themselves with all the drawings and laughed a lot.
1. *Psychoeducation about sleep:* Psychoeducation was applied as Power Point slides. The group cleared questions and curiosities about sleep.
1. *Task:* At the end of the session, the therapist highlighted the importance of recording sleep patterns in the sleep diary.

Brief considerations on session 1: The group dynamics appeared to have broken the ice and promoted the integration between group members. Based on psychoeducation, the group members cleared doubts about sleep patterns, increasing their knowledge about sleep and the insomnia complaint.

Table 17.1 Presentation of the group members

Participant	Who am I? What brought me here? What do I like to do?
Raíssa	I'm Raíssa, I'm 22 years old, I'm a physiotherapy student, and I'm single. I looked for the group because I experience unrefreshing sleep, daytime sleepiness, and frequent night awakenings. I like going out with friends to dance.
Cirley	I'm Cirley, I'm 36 years old, I'm a social worker, and I'm married. My main complaint is the difficulty initiating sleep. I like to be among family and friends and in the company of children and elderly people. I love getting friends and family together to chat. I like to cook for the people in my house.
Fábio	I'm Fábio, I'm 37 years old, I'm an engineer, and I'm single. I have difficulties initiating and maintaining sleep and I am insecure about trying to sleep without medication. I love going to the cinema, theater, museum, and cultural events
Graziela	I'm Graziela, I'm 49 years old, I'm divorced, and I have two children. I have difficulties falling and staying asleep. I like to travel, discover new places and nature.
Ludmila	I'm Ludmila, I'm 59 years old, I'm retired and married, and I have two children. I have difficulty initiating and maintaining sleep. I like to watch movies and series on Netflix and to discover different places, travel.

17.2 Session 2

1. *Task revision:* For the second session, the group only completed the information in the sleep diary.
1. *Sleep hygiene:* The therapist provided explanations and guidance on sleep hygiene in Power Point. The group members asked questions during the presentation. At the end, each participant identified together with the therapist the necessary changes in sleep hygiene. Table 17.2 shows the necessary changes identified by each participant.

After the participants had identified what they needed to change in their sleep hygiene, Graziela proposed to help each other with reminders that could be sent via WhatsApp. The group was committed to making the changes during the week

1. *Mindfulness:* The therapist explained mindfulness principles for sleep and then guided the participants in a mindfulness practice, the body scan. After this practice, the members of the group explained their experience. Table 17.3 shows how each participant experienced the body scan practice.

After each participant had shared their experience, Cirley reported feeling more comfortable knowing that she was not the only one who got distracted and had difficulty concentrating and proposed to the group to charge themselves in the daily body scan task.

1. *Task:* The task established was practicing body scan daily and the changes in sleep hygiene.

Table 17.2 Changes in sleep hygiene identified by each participant

Participant	Instructions for change
Raíssa	Do not sleep with the TV on void using your cell phone before going to bed Regular bedtime and wake-up times Do not nap during the day
Cirley	Perform physical activity Do not go to bed hungry Avoid drinking too much water before going to bed
Fábio	Avoid smoking at night Do not use your cell phone before going to bed
Graziela	Avoid drinking alcohol at night Install blackout curtains on the bedroom window
Ludmila	Avoid drinking coffee during the afternoon–night period Avoid napping during the day Perform physical activity

Table 17.3 Feedback of the participants on body scan

Participant	Body scan
Raíssa	I felt so relaxed, I even wanted to sleep.
Cirley	It was very difficult for me, other thoughts invaded my mind. It was hard to concentrate.
Fábio	In the first minutes, I was able to be aware of how my body was but at the end I got distracted.
Graziela	It was a very interesting practice, I was able to surrender and concentrate on my body.
Ludmila	At first, my mind was invaded by other thoughts; however, after I persisted, I was able to concentrate and at the end I was very relaxed.
Therapist	The experience is individual and can have a different effect on each of you. The experience that each one had was interesting. Thank you for sharing.

Brief considerations on session 2: Using psychoeducation on sleep hygiene, the participants identified habits that could be modified to improve their quality of sleep. The exchange of experiences on the body scan practice facilitated identification by group members and support in performing the practice as a task assignment.

17.3 Session 3

1. *Task revision:* The third session started with exchanging experiences on the tasks established in the last session. Each participant reported the changes made during the week in sleep hygiene and body scan practice. Table 17.4 presents the report of the participants.

2. *Creative hopelessness:* After the mindfulness practice of creative hopelessness, the therapist asked some questions in order to assess attempts to control and

Table 17.4 Report on the tasks established in session 2

Participant	Tasks established in session 2
Raíssa	It was very easy for me to do the body scan practice. I really felt that it helped me relax. I even felt that I slept a little better this week. Regarding the sleep hygiene changes, I was unable to do all. For example, I did not use my cell phone at night or sleep with the TV on all week. However, keeping regular bedtime and wake-up times and not napping, I did not.
Cirley	Throughout the week I reduced my fluid intake before going to bed, I also started to eat a light snack an hour before going to bed. It felt really good to go to bed not hungry. Physical activity I'm starting little by little, I went for a walk three times this week. But I confess that the body scan practice is not easy for me. I think I get even more anxious. I only did it for 2 days and one of those days I stopped the practice in the middle.
Fábio	I did everything that was agreed upon. I did not smoke at night and stopped using my cell phone an hour before going to bed. I did the body scan practice, and when I do it, I feel very good. But it is still difficult to sleep. I wonder when my insomnia will get better?
Graziela	Well, let's go … this week I only drank twice. It is already a step forward, right? Laughter. I've also had a blackout curtain made for my bedroom. I believe that in 2 days I will already sleep with new curtains. I chose to do the body scan practice in the morning and I felt less anxious during the day.
Ludmila	Am I the only one who was lazy not doing physical activity this week? Laughter. I still have not been able to put physical activity into practice. However, I managed not to nap during the day and reduced coffee. Since the last session, I have only been drinking coffee in the morning. The body scan relaxes me a lot, this one I managed to do every day. Of course, I was not able to be mindful during the entire meditation but I was able to observe myself at least during most part of the practice.
Therapist	It is very good to see that we are making progress and that everyone, within their limits, is committed to the tasks.

avoid discomfort. Once everyone had answered the five questions, the therapist asked the group members to share their answers. These responses are presented in Table 17.5.

3. *Tug-of-war metaphor:* After the metaphor, the group members identified what "pulling the rope" means for each of them. Figure 17.1 shows their answers. After group reflection, the proposal was to find ways to let go of the rope.

After the participants had identified and expressed what "pulling the rope" means for each of them, some participants shared how the group exchange experience was.

> It was interesting for me to hear Fábio speak, it seems that seeing the situation in the other person made me see my own avoidance. (Graziela)

> I understood the metaphor but it was difficult for me to see how the attempt of control was occurring in my sleep. While listening to Ludmila, it seems that I was able to identify my attempt at controlling as well. (Raíssa)

Table 17.5 Creative hopelessness

Participant	Exchange – creative hopelessness
Cirley	Can I talk first? I get very frustrated with not being able to fall asleep. I feel incapable! So, what do I do then? I put it into my head that I need to sleep. I keep my eyes closed, speaking in a mantra "sleep, sleep, sleep." Look, it is not working neither in the short nor in the long term. Insomnia has compromised my quality of life and controlling it would make me chase more satisfying situations for myself.
Fábio	I identify myself with you Cirley because I also feel incapable and, before the fear of not sleeping takes over, I already take my medication. It works at first but then it becomes a snowball, and here I am looking for help. Today the medication is a crutch for me. Getting off the medication and sleeping naturally would bring me my life back.
Ludmila	My feelings vary, I feel angry, angry about not being able to sleep. After all, my main strategy is to go to bed earlier in an attempt to sleep more. But it has never worked. I don't know why I keep trying. If I slept better I would have a lot more energy, I have no doubt.
Graziela	Look, bedtime is not the worst, I need to relax and I use alcohol to help me. At the time I relax, it works. But not in the long term. After the psychoeducation we had in the previous session, I started to notice that, when I drink before going to bed, I wake up many times during the night. So, it is not working. I don't know how to answer what better sleep would add to my life, I'm already used to the way it is. But of course, I would like to sleep naturally, I think I would feel more independent.
Raíssa	My problem is more with sleepiness during the day. I keep thinking that I have less energy than other people. To help myself, I stay in bed longer. But I end up compromising myself by losing most of the day. If I solved this problem, I would have more time to do other things.
Therapist	Thank you for sharing. Have you ever asked yourselves if trying to control the discomfort caused by the sleep complaint is the problem rather than the solution?
Fábio	In fact, it is very tiring to have control of everything…

> It's so hard to see this so rigid side of me, the metaphor allowed me to see it without avoiding my own judgment. And apparently I am not the only controller, laughter. I confess that it makes me feel more normal. Maybe a sense of belonging, it's not just me who suffers with my sleep. (Fábio)

After group reflection, the proposal was to find ways to let go of the rope.

4. *Mindfulness:* After the guided practice of leaves on a stream, the participants shared their experiences. Some statements are cited below:

> Watching my thoughts drift away with the leaves gave me the feeling that they were indeed just thoughts. (Ludmila)

> Unlike the body scan practice that flowed, in the leaves on a stream practice I had more difficulty concentrating and imagining my thoughts. But I still felt relaxed because I imagined myself in a forest. (Raíssa)

> This practice I managed to do and I really liked it. I felt relieved and emptying my mind as I got the thoughts out of my head and onto the leaves. (Cirley)

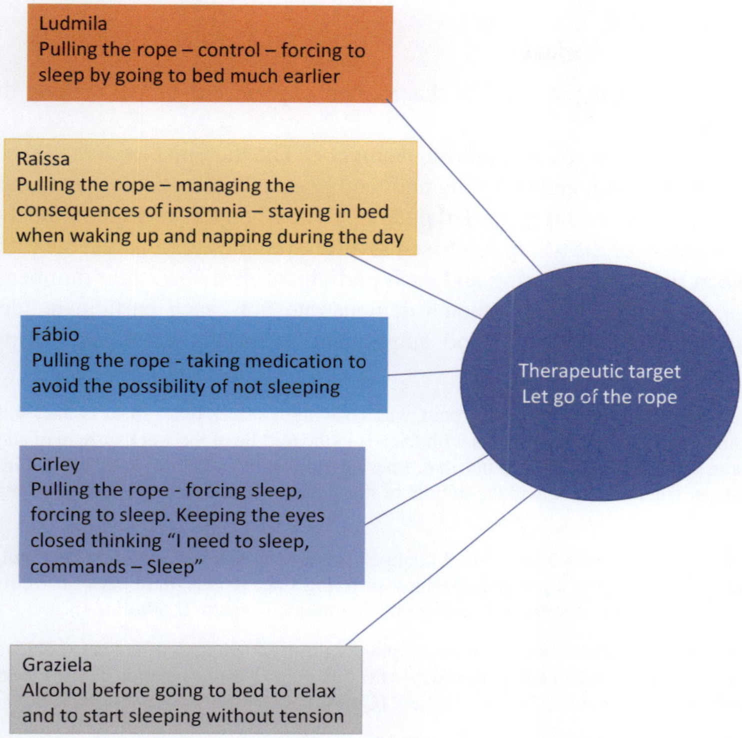

Fig. 17.1 Report of the participants on the exercise of creative hopelessness

> I was stuck in a single thought for a long time. It was difficult to let it flow down the creek but after it did, my mind went blank and I could observe my surroundings. The sound of the forest, of the birds. (Graziela)

> For me the thoughts came like a cascade, one after the other, as if it were a waterfall of thoughts. (Fábio)

4. *Tasks:* In addition to maintaining the other tasks proposed in the previous sessions, the daily use of the "leaves on a stream" practice was recommended.

Brief considerations on session 3: The use of metaphors facilitated access to control strategies. In addition, observing the behavior of others served as a model for identifying one's own behavior. The group members also showed a sense of belonging by identifying themselves with similar situations.

17.4 Session 4

1. *Task revision:* The participants shared their experiences on performing the proposed tasks.
1. *Pain* versus *suffering and pudding metaphor:* The therapist explained the difference between pain and suffering and then presented the pudding metaphor (suffering pain after eating a spoiled pudding). Based on this metaphor, the therapist and members of the group discussed several examples to illustrate the difference between pain and suffering and each participant described their number 1 puddings. The following statements demonstrate how each participant identified pain (pudding number 1) and subsequent sufferings based on the pudding metaphor.

> My number 1 pudding, my primary pain, was a bad night's sleep that I spent awake, without sleeping, after going to the movies with friends in the middle of the week instead of staying at home and sleeping early… After that, I never again went to the movies, I decline invitations from friends to events in the middle of the week, afraid of having another bad night's sleep. (Fábio)

> In childhood they bullied me when I changed schools. It was very painful. This bullying situation is my number 1 pudding. And my suffering since then is that I back off from new friendships, social relations for fear of being "humiliated" again. (Ludmila)

> It is really hard to admit, but my number 1 pudding is my frustration of not being able to get pregnant. And to avoid getting in touch with this pain, I avoid meeting friends who are mothers or going to events full of children. (Cirley)

> The divorce 20 years ago was very painful for me, it was frustrating. It hurt so much that today I close myself to new relationships for fear of further frustration. Once I almost opened up but I self-sabotaged myself, I think it was a way to avoid the possibility of pain. (Graziela)

> Oh, I don't know if I am as sure as you are about my number 1 pudding, but a few years ago I had psychiatric treatment for depression and it did not work. I was so frustrated that today I don't trust new psychiatric or psychological treatments. Maybe that is my pudding. But I am here…so I am opening myself up to the pain or not?. (Raíssa)

> Listening to our reports gives the feeling that we have much more suffering than pain. For example, I am a pain controller. In order not to have a sleepless night, I avoid many things that could leave me more relaxed and happier. (Fábio)

1. *Reading of poems:* The session continued with the reading and discussion of two poems that indirectly covered the processes of acceptance and self as context.
1. *Sheet activity:* The last activity of session 4 was to write positive memories, feelings, and thoughts on one side of the paper and negative ones on the other side. At the end of the activity, the therapist asked what each participant would like to do with the paper, as can be seen in the following statements:

> I will save it to look at the positive and negative points of life. It would be great if I could throw away just the negative ones. (Ludmila)

> I would crumple and throw away the negative points. (Cirley)

Table 17.6 Positive and negative points of the participant Ludmila

Positive	Negative
Childhood friendships	Dependence
Good family relationship	Lack of freedom
Large family	Death of loved ones
Experiences – travel, etc.	Childhood bullying
	Decision to marry just to please others (society, family)

I would burn this paper. (Raíssa)

Can I just keep the positive part?. (Graziela)

I would also keep only the positive part. (Fábio)

But not, if you crumple or burn the paper, the positive side is gone too. And if you keep it, the negative side will also be kept. (Therapist)

For life to be complete, we need the whole sheet, don't we?. (Cirley)

And that means opening yourself up to the pain. (Graziela)

Would anyone like to share their paper?. (Therapist)

I would. (Ludmila)

Table 17.6 lists the positive and negative points of Ludmila.

1. *Tasks:* After exchange, the tasks of the week were determined. In addition to the tasks already maintained in the other weeks, the task of the week would be to identify a situation that has been avoided and to face it. The participants said goodbye and the session ended.

Brief considerations on session 4: The use of the metaphor raised awareness of behaviors to avoid discomfort. The sheet activity enabled to accept what is considered "negative" and uncomfortable as part of life. The group discussion promoted openness to report the experience and learning by observing the behavior of the others.

17.5 Session 5

1. *Task revision:* The therapist asked about the tasks and the group reported their progress of the week. Cirley shared the task established in the last session, as can be seen in the following statement.

I completed the mission of the week. I called a very dear friend that I had been avoiding…her friendship does me a lot of good, but since she has recently become a mother, I am frustrated that I'm not. But even considering this discomfort, I went to visit her and I had very pleasant moments, I felt welcomed and I was happy that I faced it. (Cirley)

I was very happy to hear that, you know, I have been thinking very fondly of each one of you in the group before the sessions. I keep asking myself "How is Cirley doing this week, how has the group been committed to the tasks, do we help each other?"…. (Ludmila)

1. *Values clarification:* "Life compass" proposal. After the participants completed the life compass activity, the therapist started a dialogue with the group, expressed in the following statements:

Well, I see that everyone has completed the activity. Would anyone like to share how they felt doing this exercise?

This activity made me rethink a lot what I am neglecting and in what I am investing. I have noticed that I am neglecting important aspects of my social relations and personal growth. The values I would like to develop and cultivate in these areas are "openness" and "autonomy".

I want to open myself up to new relationships, I have been closing myself for years for fear of being rejected and humiliated. I want to have an open attitude to meet new people, new places, experience different things. This is also in line with my search for independence and, somehow, freedom. I depend a lot on my kids and husband for outings. I would like not to depend on a family member to go out and have fun, I really want to be independent. I dream of taking a trip alone and experiencing what it is like to be without family around. Knowing myself better, being only with myself. (Ludmila)

Thank you for sharing, Ludmila. What do you think prevents you from seeking autonomy, freedom and openness?. (Therapist)

I believe that on the one hand it is convenience. I am accommodated. I settled for my husband to choose all the trips and I just follow. These days I have asked myself if I like the trips he plans. I would like to plan and do whatever I choose, at least once in my life. But deep down, I am afraid I won't be able to. (Ludmila)

Ludmila, it was very good to listening to you because I feel something different. In my case, I think I am too bossy and it hurts my relationships. Because I want things my way. During the activity, I reflected on what values I would like to cultivate in my family relationships, especially with my children. I noticed that I neglect my family relationships due to a lack of tolerance. There is a value that I want to cultivate, tolerance. I find it difficult to hear the wish of the other when this wish does not include me. I feel disadvantaged and rejected. For example, on Easter my son let me know that he would have lunch with his wife's family. I was very aggressive since I expected him to have lunch with me. I realize that, by doing this, I put an even greater distance between him and me. I want to be more tolerant in my relationships. (Graziela)

Listening to Graziela's speech, I identified myself with some aspects, maybe we human beings perceive the desire of the other as rejection when it does not include us and we attack out of fear? But the children grow up and have other interests and activities…This activity made me reflect a lot; however, unlike Graziela who attacks when she feels rejected, I agree with the others, afraid of being rejected, often not revealing what I think, what I want. A need to please. It even seems silly but when I go to a restaurant with a group of friends or family and they ask what I want to eat, I always eat the same thing as the other person orders and I end up sharing the dish, I never choose what I actually want to eat. (Cirley)

I thought a lot about my health. I think I need to develop self-care. Could this be considered a value? Self-care? I thought I need to take care of my body, my food, my mental health. I haven't been doing this. (Raíssa)

Do you have any clue as to why you are not developing self-care?. (Therapist)

Physical activity often causes discomfort, pain, and I end up not persisting. Lack of persistence, determination, laziness. There are so many reasons but I think mainly because it is not comfortable to feel the initial discomforts when you start the gym. (Raíssa)

Raíssa, I understand you but I will tell you one thing, the discomfort is temporary, with time physical activity starts to give results, it improves your mood, improves your health, and then you will like it. You just have to endure the initial discomfort a little. (Fábio)

I give up many things because of this initial discomfort. (Raíssa)

I see that you are noticing the barriers to cultivating your values and are identifying what you are trying to avoid, this is a very important step. (Therapist)

In my case, do I see that I am too controlling? Is this my barrier to achieving what I want, the kind of person I want to be?. (Fábio)

And what do you want? What kind of person do you want to be?. (Therapist)

I want to be more flexible because I stop living by trying to control everything. I love art, I love going to the movies, going to events, and I am so rigid in my routine that I don't allow myself. That's it, I want to cultivate flexibility. This value, flexibility, was recurrent during the life compass activity. At my own work I compromise myself by being too rigid and methodical. (Fábio)

Fábio, I am going to use the same line of reasoning as you for me, regarding self-care. At the beginning it will be difficult to be flexible, trying to control less, but after the initial discomfort you will have advantages in cultivating flexibility. (Raíssa)

After exchanging their thoughts about values clarification, the therapist explored with the participants committed actions based on values.

1. *Committed actions:* To address committed actions, the therapist asked the participants to organize their goals in a chart, the barriers that make it difficult to achieve these goals, and which actions could be adopted to achieve the goals. At the end, the participants exchanged the following charts with the group (Table 17.7).

4. After exchange of the reasons identified by the participants that prevent them from behaving in accordance with their values, a mindfulness practice on values and committed actions was performed.
4. Committed actions were also the focus of the task of this session.

Brief considerations on session 5: After the life compass activity and further reflection on barriers to achieving values-based goals, the participants had clarity about avoidance-based versus values-based behaviors. The members of the group supported and encouraged each other to take committed actions.

17.6 Session 6

1. *Task revision:* The participants shared their experiences by performing the proposed tasks.

Table 17.7 Committed actions of the participants

Committed actions – Ludmila	
Value	Autonomy
Goal	Traveling alone
Barriers	Convenience, fear of not being able to fend for myself, facing trouble
Behaviors to achieve my goals	Step 1: Going out alone (going to the movies, going out for lunch) Step 2: Taking a day trip to a nearby town Step 3: Traveling to a nearby town and stay in a hotel alone.

Committed actions – Graziela	
Value	Tolerance
Goal	Accepting the children's decisions without yelling or blackmailing
Barriers	Fear of loneliness; feeling of being at a disadvantage
Behaviors to achieve my goals	Listening to the son's speech without attacking him Not manipulating the situation Enduring the discomfort of occasionally not being included in the children's plans

Committed actions – Fábio	
Value	Flexibility
Goal	Having a less rigid routine, allowing exceptions
Barriers	Fear of not sleeping well Fear of breaking routine and compromising sleep
Behaviors to achieve my goals	Going to the movies on Tuesday with a friend

Committed actions – Raíssa	
Value	Self-care
Goal	Performing physical activity
Barriers	Muscle soreness from adaptation to the gym
Behaviors to achieve my goals	1. Start walking 3×/week 2. Enrolling in the gym

Committed actions – Cirley	
Value	Honesty
Goal	Exposing my wishes and thoughts
Barriers	Possibility of conflict
Behaviors to achieve my goals	1. When in a group, choosing what I really want to eat at the restaurant 2. Defending my opinion in conversation with friends

1. *Attending your own funeral – epitaph:* The proposal of reflecting on what message the participants would like to leave when they die elicited emotion in some of them and reinforced their values. The cited statements denote the impact of the activity on each member of the group.

   I never stopped thinking about death. Before thinking what message I would like to leave, I thought about the message I do not want to leave. I realize that many of my actions are focused on the opinion of others – what they think about me. I do not want my epitaph to contain the message "The one who lived thinking about the opinion of others". I want to be honest about my own desires and that people like me for who I am and not what I look like. Reflecting about this honesty that I want to cultivate, my epitaph would be "The one who could be trusted and who was honest with others and especially with herself". (Cirley)

I would like to be remembered as "the one who helped others, who gave herself". But not the one who was passed over or who was the dupe. Can you tell the difference? I am afraid of being the dupe and that is why I am so distrustful and aggressive that I end up not experiencing what I value so much, which is giving, openness to others, the possibility of helping, of loving. I need to learn to balance these contradictions. (Graziela)

My epitaph would be "the one who learned to fly". That's it, I am going to learn to be independent, autonomous. I am confident I will. Even late we can learn, even after 50, right?. (Ludmila)

I always wanted to be very perfect. Make great contributions to the world. That is why I have always been very disciplined at work, in health, in everything. I built myself in cement, so inflexible and so gray that I can hardly bathe in the sun. My epitaph today would be "he who fought to be an Apollo but became a statue". But I want to change that, I want to be weightless, malleable, break this statue and become a free, weightless and untied human…laughter. (Fábio)

At my memorial people would say "The one who always made me laugh", and that's right. People think I am funny. I love making people laugh. I like my mood. I am going to start committing myself and go further, for my epitaph to be "The one who makes others smile, but mostly makes herself smile". I want to make myself smile. That's why I will take care of myself. (Raíssa)

After sharing their thoughts, there was a period of silence and reflection on the content of the work.

1. *Joe the Bum:* Reading of the "Joe the Bum" parable was aimed at addressing the acceptance of feelings, thoughts and memories, as well as the action in pursuit of values. The participants identified with the character and contributed content from their experiences, as illustrated by the following statements:

I would definitely go after Joe. That is what I do with my sleep, I watch myself to see if I am going to sleep or not. In fact, this isn't quite like a party, it is a lot of work. (Cirley)

I also see myself as a gatekeeper, a watchwoman of the consequences of a bad night. I pay attention to everything that goes on in my body. I go after the Joes. (Raíssa)

I used to be like that a lot, today I let it go. If there is any discomfort, I will let it fend for itself at the party. I am not going to worry, no. But it took me a while to stop watching the Joes. (Ludmila)

I am the type who suffers before the party. I would be desperate before Joe arrived. Sometimes he does not even show up and I suffer in anticipation. I am already suffering from imagining him being inappropriate with person X or person Y. But mindfulness helps me let Joe show up and learn to live with it. What to do…. (Fabio)

In fact, that is exactly what we do, we get so worried about the Joes in our lives that time passes, life passes and what really matters? Are we following what matters? or Are we distracting ourselves with Joes?. (Graziela)

1. *Mindfulness:* After the parable, the last mindfulness practice of the protocol was performed, which focused on values and committed actions. After the practice

and a moment of silence, the therapist asked the group "What change did this experience bring about?"

I realized that I try to control everything in order to avoid feeling discomfort. And a bad night's sleep is another one of those discomforts. My relationship with sleep has been changing with therapy. (Fábio)

The therapy made me realize that I am very much of an immediatist and I have difficulties in persisting to pursue what I really want because it is far away. I need to make a commitment to reap medium- and long-term benefits. I am in the planting phase. Regarding sleep, I noticed that I have been worrying less about the consequences of insomnia. I am less neurotic. (Raíssa)

My sleep satisfaction has improved a lot. I do not even keep counting how many hours it takes me to sleep and wake up, or how many hours I slept. Of course, I estimate it to answer the diary. But I am less worried about that. I want to live, regardless of whether I have a sleep problem or not. But that does not mean my sleep hasn't improved, I am sleeping better. Laughter. (Cirley)

I had never done group therapy, but it was interesting that seeing the situation of the other made me perceive my own avoidances. Being able to share with the group and having this welcoming space was very good. (Ludmila)

The metaphors are gentler in perceiving pains than objective speech. I had the impression that discussing the metaphors in a group and seeing the others expose themselves also encouraged me to expose myself, even in the case of things that even I did not notice about myself. After the session, I continued reflecting, the pain of the other seemed so great and I was afraid to face mine. It gave me the strength to face it too, after all it is not just me who has this complaint. I am not alone. I felt supported to share my pains and discomforts with those who could understand them, after all we had common pains. (Graziela)

At the end, all participants thanked the therapist and each member for all the moments and shared experiences and the group ended.

Brief considerations on session 6: The activities proposed in session 6, such as "Attending your own funeral" and the "Joe-the-Bum parable," made the group observe finitude and to what extent each one is or is not engaged in what really matters and what they really value. The mindfulness practice reinforced values-based committed actions. The final statements demonstrated how the relationship of the participants with their own sleep was addressed.

Figures 17.2, 17.3, 17.4, 17.5, 17.6, 17.7, 17.8, 17.9, 17.10, 17.11, 17.12, 17.13, 17.14, 17.15, 17.16, 17.17, 17.18, 17.19, 17.20, and 17.21 show the average sleep parameters of each participant over the course of the sessions.

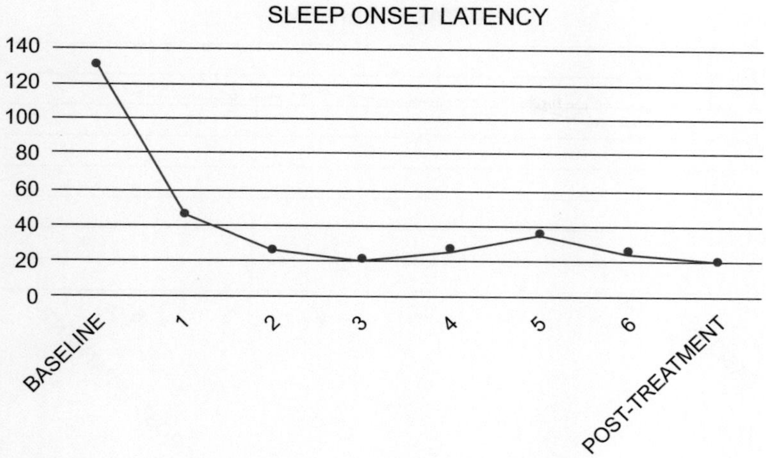

Fig. 17.2 Cirley: Sleep onset latency

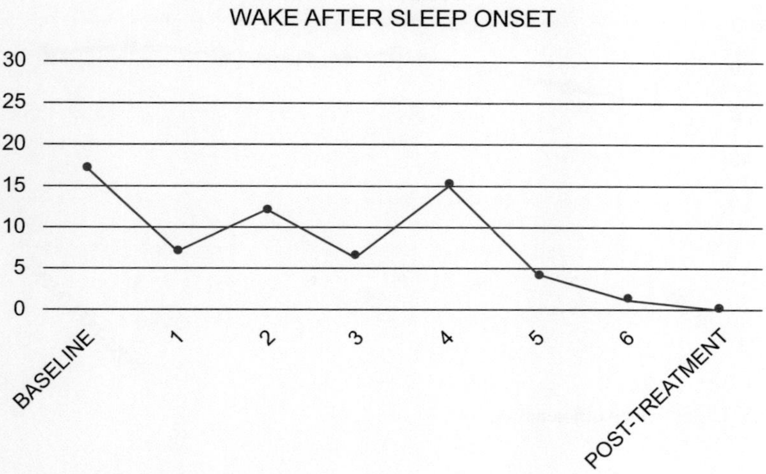

Fig. 17.3 Cirley: Wake after sleep onset

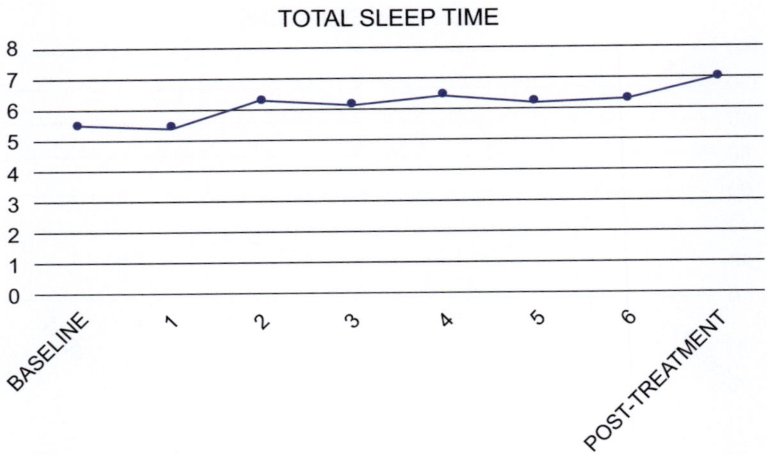

Fig. 17.4 Cirley: Total sleep time

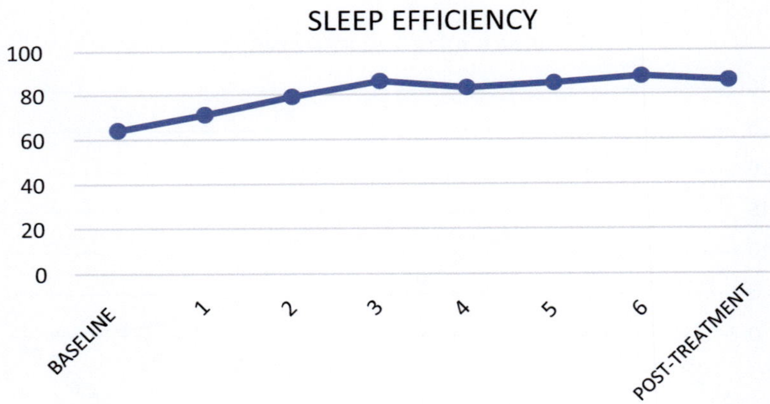

Fig. 17.5 Cirley: Sleep efficiency

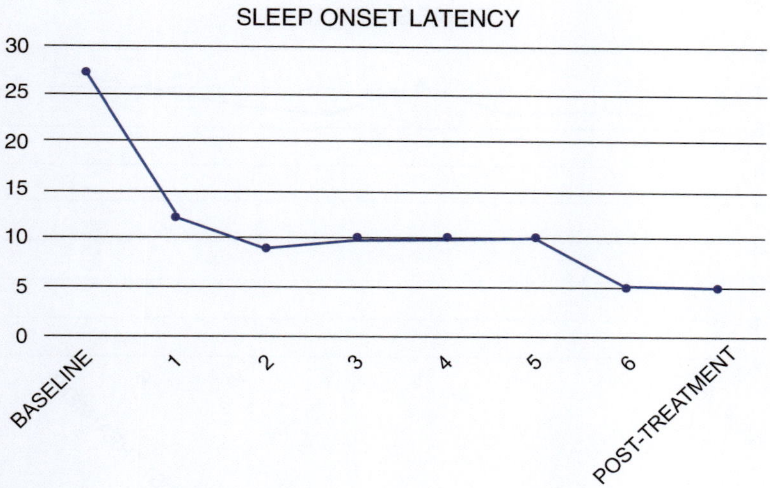

Fig. 17.6 Raíssa: Sleep onset latency

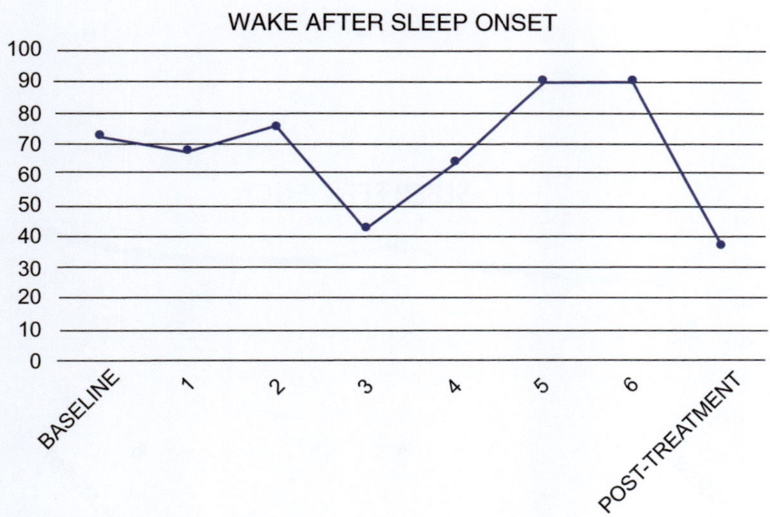

Fig. 17.7 Raíssa: Wake after sleep onset

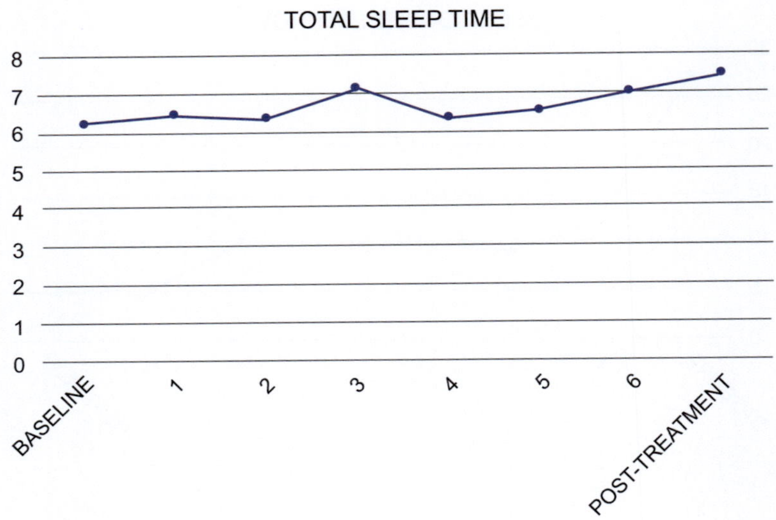

Fig. 17.8 Raíssa: Total sleep time

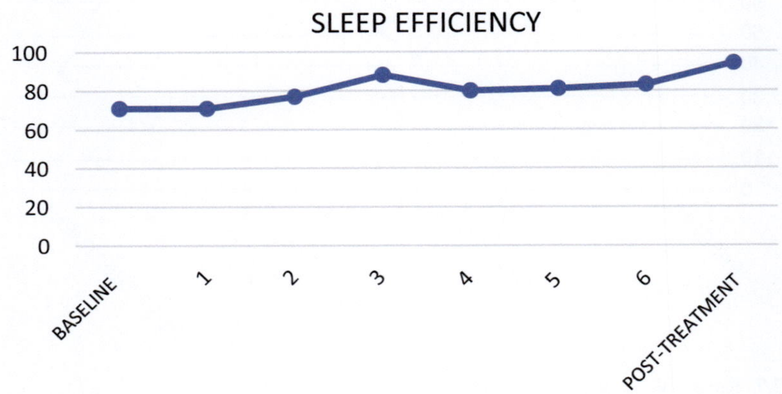

Fig. 17.9 Raíssa: Sleep efficiency

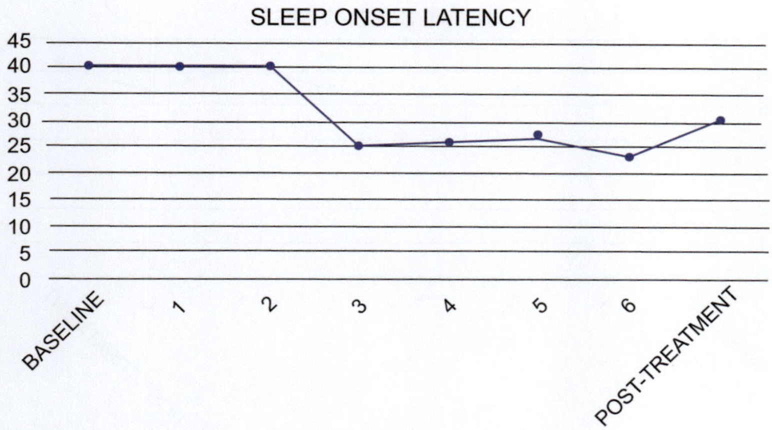

Fig. 17.10 Ludmila: Sleep onset latency

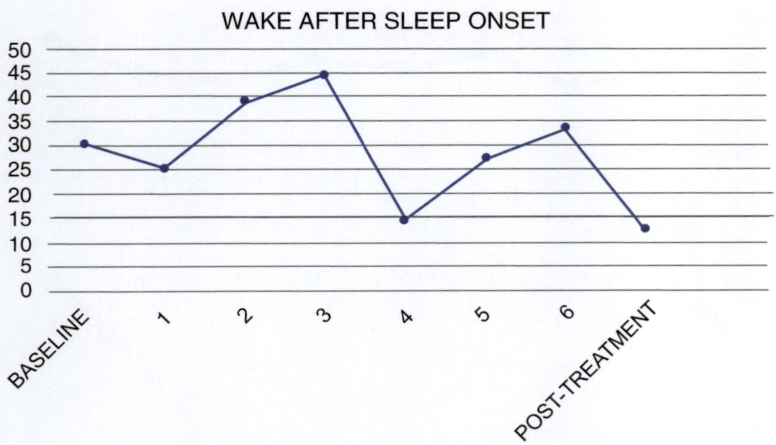

Fig. 17.11 Ludmila: Wake after sleep onset

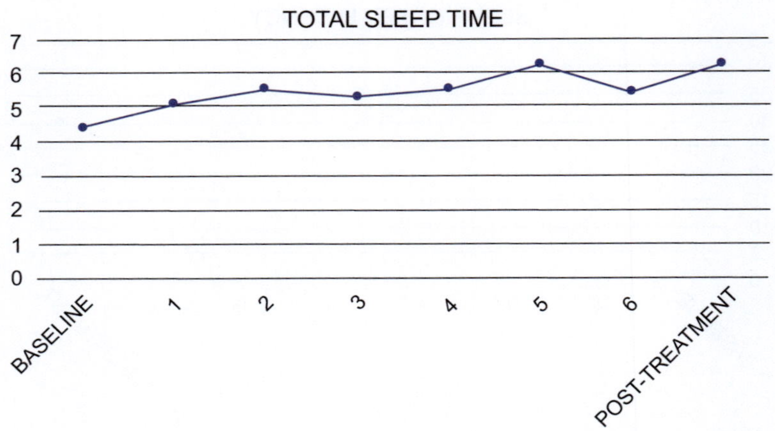

Fig. 17.12 Ludmila: Total sleep time

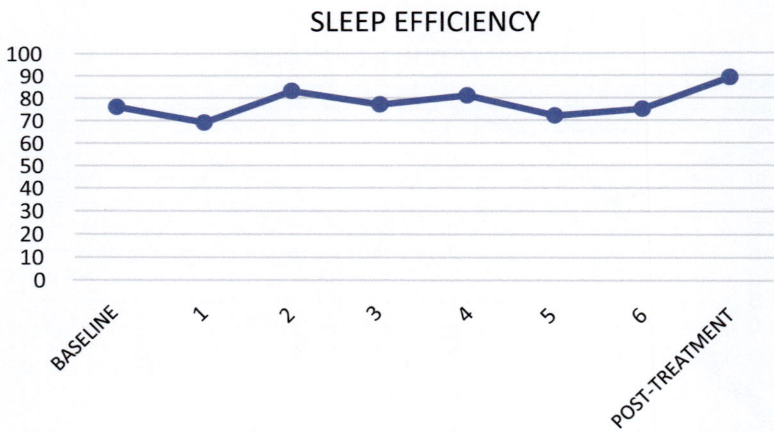

Fig. 17.13 Ludmila: Sleep efficiency

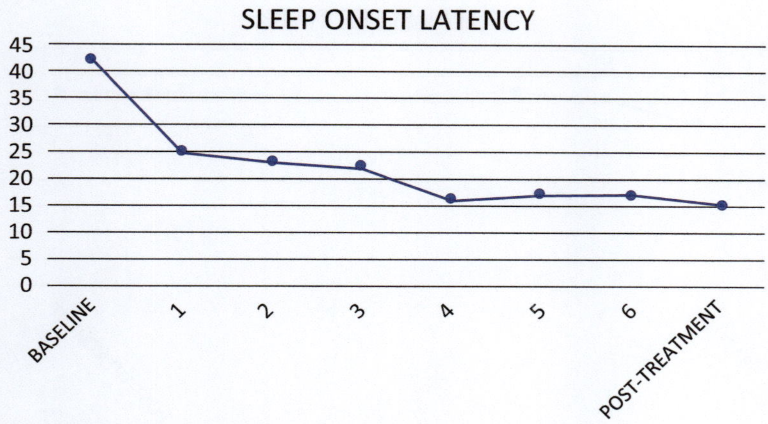

Fig. 17.14 Graziela: Sleep onset latency

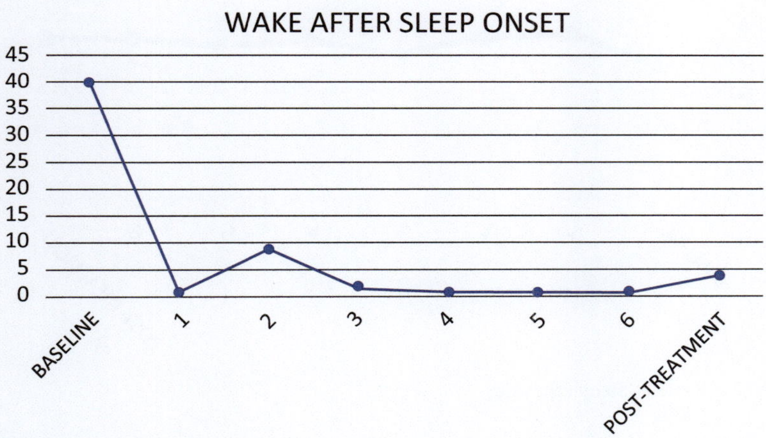

Fig. 17.15 Graziela: Wake after sleep onset

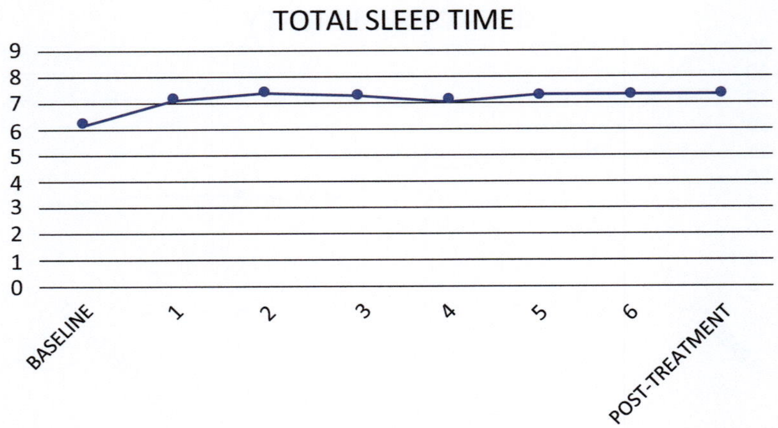

Fig. 17.16 Graziela: Total sleep time

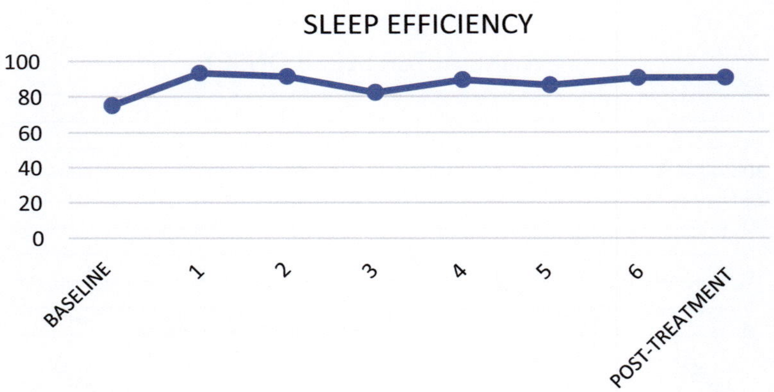

Fig. 17.17 Graziela: Sleep efficiency

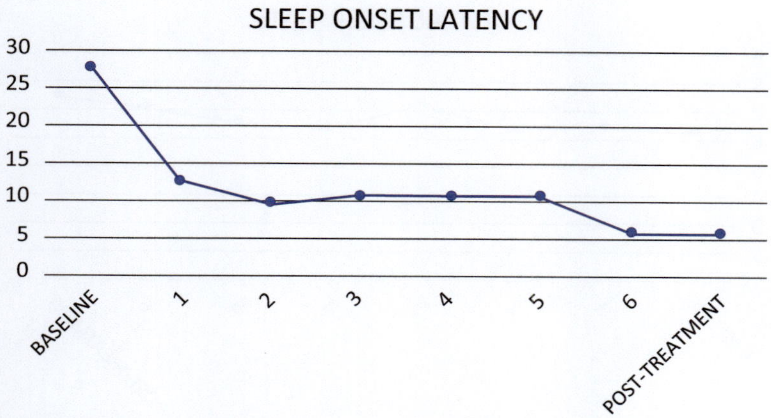

Fig. 17.18 Fabio: Sleep onset latency

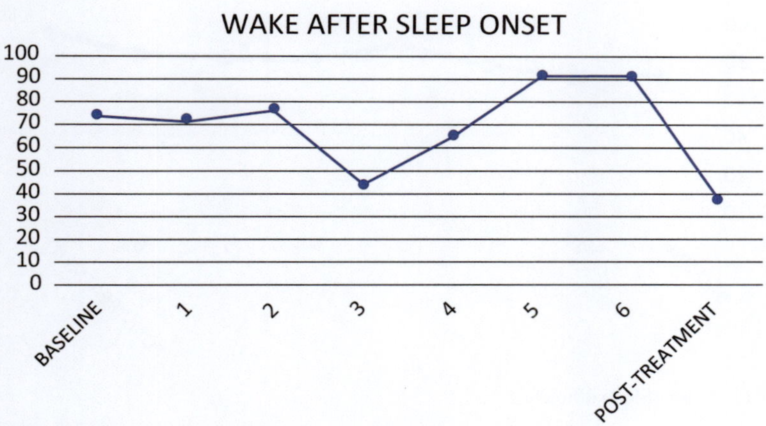

Fig. 17.19 Fabio: Wake after sleep onset

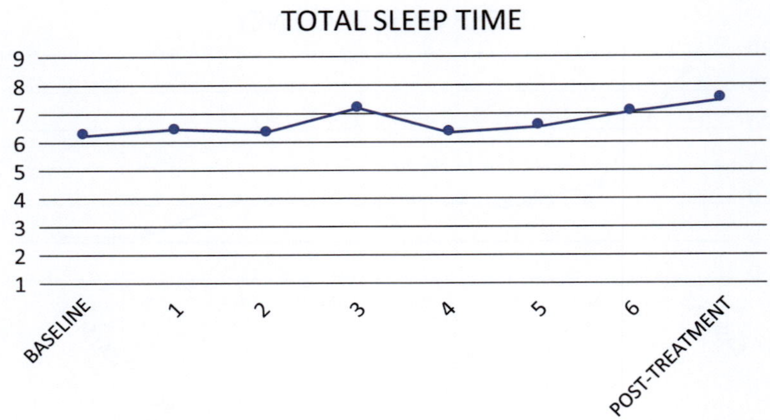

Fig. 17.20 Fabio: Total sleep time

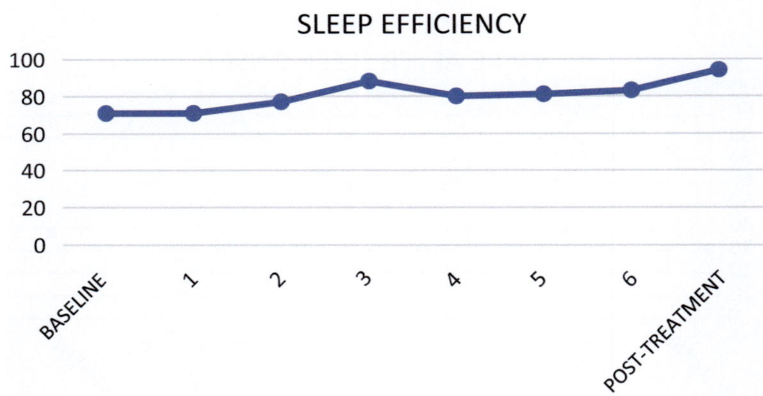

Fig. 17.21 Fabio: Sleep efficiency

17.7 Conclusion

ACT-I was found to have benefits for the sleep quality of the participants and mainly changed their relationship with their own sleep. Metaphors facilitated access to avoidance-based versus values-based behaviors. The group therapy format may have contributed to the sense of belonging and welcoming and also as a model of behavior. The present report demonstrated how group ACT-I can provide learning conditions and consequent behavior changes based on both the individual's active participation in the proposed intervention and observation of the behavior of the other group members in response to therapy.

Chapter 18
Case Example: Application of ACT-I in an Individual Intervention

Ila Marques Porto Linares

Psychotherapy for clients with insomnia complaints can be conducted in different formats, i.e., remote, face-to-face, groups, or individually. This chapter aims to describe a session-by-session outline of an ACT-based intervention for a client complaining of insomnia. The data below refer to the main points addressed in each session.[1]

18.1 First Session

Goals: Conducting anamnesis, application of scales and questionnaires, and instructions of how to fill out the sleep diary. The aim of the first session was also to start building therapeutic rapport.

Anamnesis

A. *Patient identification*: Miguel (fictious name), 52 years, a widower and accountant who lives in the city of São Paulo, Brazil.
B. *Complaint*: Difficulty in initiating and maintaining sleep.

Client: "When I realized that I was sleeping poorly, I looked online for ways to improve my sleep. It was then that I became even more concerned about the damage of sleep deprivation. I count my hours of sleep when I wake up to see if I'm sleep

[1]The cases reported in this book signed the free informed consent form since they are part of a research project on ACT for insomnia.

I. M. P. Linares (✉)
Faculty of Medicine at the University of São Paulo, Sao Paulo, Brazil

R. El Rafihi-Ferreira (ed.), *Acceptance and Commitment Therapy for Insomnia*,
https://doi.org/10.1007/978-3-031-50710-6_18

deprived and I follow all the sleep hygiene instructions I have read online, and I still do not get better."

C. *Daytime symptoms*: The client reported some symptoms that are related mainly to tiredness and concern about sleep.

Client: "I feel very tired during the day, sluggish, unproductive."
"I realize that my mood is not very good either and I spend the day thinking about how my night's sleep will be, there are days when I get very anxious."

D. *History of complaint*: When asked about his sleep history, Miguel reported that he has slept poorly since he was a child but he thought that this was normal. The client explained that he always took a long time to sleep, spending a lot of time in another activity while "sleep did not come." Fears and anxiety always seemed to be present in Miguel's life and contributed to this difficulty. He also reported that he always had at least two nocturnal awakenings. When these nocturnal awakenings occurred, Miguel usually stayed in bed waiting for sleep to return.
E. Although he always had difficulty initiating and maintaining sleep, the client reported that these symptoms intensified after his wife passed away 2 years ago.
F. *Sleep routine*: Miguel's sleep routine is very strict. Everything takes place at the same time and in the same sequence: he takes a shower at 19.00 h, he has dinner at 19.30 h, he watches the news at 20.00 h, he reads a book at 21.00 h, and he goes to bed at 22.00 h. The client usually sleeps around midnight or 01.00 in the morning. During this period, he stays in the bedroom waiting for sleep to "come." In the morning, he wakes up at 06.30 h and immediately starts his day.

Client: "It is better to stay in bed because at least I am resting my body."

G. *Personal information*: Miguel grew up in a family with many rules and coercive parenting practices. He was always pressured to perform perfectly and had few opportunities to do what he wanted to do throughout his childhood and adolescence.

At the age of 18, Miguel married his first girlfriend (Marina). The couple chose not to have children. Marriage has always been an important pillar of his life since it ensures security. His wife died unexpectedly after an acute myocardial infarction. At the time of her death, the client was very unsettled, with lowered mood, had difficulty socializing, and exhibited a hypochondriac behavior. Miguel has also slept worse every night since then, i.e., increased sleep onset latency and time to fall back to sleep after nocturnal awakenings.

The client has always been reserved and had few friends. Thus, the loss of his wife affected him even socially, given the lack of relationships in his life. Miguel prefers not to get in touch with relatives and friends from the past, as it is very unpleasant to talk about himself and he feels pressured to be the person he thinks others expect him to be. Only with Marina could he be who he really is, she understood Miguel.

Table 18.1 Objective data obtained by applying the instruments at the start of the intervention

Instrument	Score
ISI	15
PSQI	14
AAQ	26

Throughout his life, avoidance has been Miguel's main tool to deal with feelings. It therefore always seemed that everything was under his control and that nothing could unsettle him.

Client: "To avoid thinking about my worries, I spend the whole day performing some activity, even while taking a shower I read."

"Talking about how I feel makes me feel bad, so I just get on with life and do not talk about it."

"The only problem I think about is the sleep problem, the others I don't even think about."

Also from an emotional point of view, Miguel was always very rigid and had difficulty being flexible to deal with the adversities and setbacks of everyday life.

Client: "Everything has the right way of solving itself, there is no point in doing it any other way."

"I don't understand why people do not follow the rules. Everything that has rules works better."

With the death of his wife, Miguel found himself without goals in life. The couple did not have many ambitions but they have been traveling once a year to the same destination since they had gotten married. Now, the client saw no point in traveling to this destination.

Interventions: The following instruments were applied during the first session: Insomnia Severity Index (ISI), Pittsburgh Sleep Quality Index (PSQI), and Acceptance and Action Questionnaire (AAQ). In addition, the client was instructed on how to fill out the sleep diary and the therapist explained the reason for engaging in keeping this diary. The diary was filled out daily throughout the psychological intervention.

Validation of the client's complaint, welcoming, and listening are also essential in this first session in order to start building rapport. Table 18.1 shows the scores obtained with the instruments applied.

18.2 Second Session

Goals: Continuation of the process of building rapport, psychoeducation, analysis of the sleep diary, mindfulness exercise, and case formulation.

All sessions that occurred after the anamnesis session started with the therapist asking about how the client is doing, how he is perceiving himself, and what are his greatest difficulties during the process, as well as the implementation of home activities.

Client: "…it is okay but I look forward to knowing how to solve this sleep problem."

Interventions

A. Psychoeducation about sleep and its functions, as well as about the effects of sleep deprivation and the main diagnostic aspects of insomnia, was applied.

Client: "I thought all adults need eight hours per night to get enough rest. How do I know how many hours I need?"

Therapist: "This is a good question, we will need to understand this throughout the process; to obtain a reliable perception, it will be necessary to strip ourselves of the rules that we have in our head, that is, we will have to be sensitive to what we are experiencing."

B. Analysis of the sleep diary was based on understanding the following recorded sleep parameters: sleep onset latency, frequency of nighttime awakenings, time awake after sleep onset, total sleep time, total time in bed, and sleep efficiency. Table 18.2 summarizes the main parameters derived from Miguel's sleep diary.

C. *Mindfulness exercise*: To promote relaxation and attention to the present moment, a mindfulness exercise was carried out with the client. The exercise was short and was guided. In addition to in-session training, the client was instructed to perform this type of exercise not only at bedtime but throughout the subsequent days. For this purpose, the therapist made an audio recording of the exercise performed in the session.

Client: "I have a lot of difficulty with this type of exercise, I don't know if I will succeed. I will do it since it will be great if this solves the problem."

D. *Case formulation*: Case formulation is a continuous process[2] that requires the therapist to frequently revisit the approach they use to understand the case. The first time a case formulation can be performed is at the beginning of therapy.

Table 18.2 Description of the sleep parameters evaluated by the sleep diary after the first session

Parameter	Time/frequency
Sleep onset latency	120 min
Frequency of nighttime awakenings	2
Time awake after sleep onset	60 min
Total sleep time	5 h 30 min
Total time in bed	8 h 30 min
Sleep efficiency	64.7%

[2]Case formulation based on the model of Kovak and Perez.

From the perspective of ACT, the process of case formulation includes the analysis of the client's psychological flexibility and, based on that, the detailed analysis of the six processes that make up this construct. Thus, assessing how the client relates to acceptance, defusion, mindfulness, self as context, committed actions, and values is the first step necessary for structuring the intervention. Table 18.3 describes each of these processes from the perspective of Miguel's case.

Examples of experiential avoidance responses identified during the session: Miguel avoids telling details about his own sleep, only doing so when asked directly. The client reiterates that he is looking for a quick and practical solution for the sleeping difficulty. In addition, he avoids talking about any emotional issues.

Verbal responses related to the self (narrative about oneself; rules and self-rules): Miguel hardly notices the context in which the sleeping difficulty occurs, charging and judging himself most of the time (self as content). In other words, the client fuses with the rules and self-rules, which increases the difficulty in perspective taking, with consequent poor contextual self-perception.

Client: "…I will never be able to sleep satisfactorily."
"…I don't even have the capacity to sleep a whole night."
"…I don't understand, these things only happen to me. I don't sleep."
"…I slept 5 h, that means I am not in good health."

Values: The client has little clarity about his own values and seems to be quite lost.

Client: "…I don't know what is of value to me today."
"…I don't know if at some point in my life I knew what my values were."

Table 18.3 Main experiential avoidance responses

Related antecedents	What brings you to therapy? (the problem according to the client)	What have you been trying to deal with this problem (experiential avoidance)?	What happens when you try to deal with it that way (short-term consequences)?	Does this way of dealing with it help you overcome the problem (long-term consequences)?	Overall cost for life
History of psychological inflexibility and difficulty sleeping satisfactorily	Difficulty sleeping and falling back to sleep after nighttime awakenings	Sleep hygiene measures Spending the day thinking about how the night will be Staying in bed until sleep comes	Sleep hygiene measures help in not worsening the situation Increased anxiety throughout the day Bedtime aversiveness	No, he has catastrophic thoughts about sleep deprivation Spending a lot of time awake in bed exacerbates the association between bedtime and rapid sleep onset	Life "revolves around" sleep issues He avoids contact with other areas of life

"…my wife was very important to me, after she left, I lost the sense of things."
"…my life is meaningless, I lost my wife and I can't even rest."

Value-based actions: Since Miguel has little clarity about his values, it is difficult to identify values-based actions. The identification of values is therefore a prerequisite for outlining values-based actions.

In summary, analysis of each of the processes described reveals an important pattern of psychological inflexibility, which is maintained by the short-term consequences produced by the avoidance behaviors. Miguel seems quite fused with the fear of what might happen if he does not sleep, as well as with the sleep parameters such as how long he slept (cognitive fusion). In addition, he connects little to other issues of his life (inflexible attention to the now) and even has difficulty knowing what his values are.

Goals: Given the above, the therapeutic goals of the present case were (1) increasing psychological flexibility; (2) associating the bedroom with sleep; and (3) decreasing the state of physiological "alertness."

Weekly activity: Performing mindfulness exercises.

18.3 Third Session

Goals: Instructions on stimulus control, mindfulness exercise, and strategies to identify experiential avoidance and cognitive fusion.

Therapist: "Hello Miguel, how is everything?"
Client: "I am very tired, but I don't stop working because that is the right thing to do."

"I am afraid this treatment will not solve the insomnia."

Interventions

A. In an attempt to help Miguel to better associate the bedroom with sleep, he was advised to only go to bed when he was feeling sleepy and not just tired. This advice is based on stimulus control therapy, which is aimed at helping to pair stimuli, i.e., associate the bed/bedroom with falling asleep.
B. Another mindfulness exercise was conducted that Miguel should practice throughout the week.
C. In an attempt to help the client observe his experiential avoidance behaviors, activities based on metaphors were conducted so that Miguel could identify his usual attempts to control and escape the discomfort of not sleeping (experiential avoidance/acceptance).

Client: "…I understand, every time I try to control my sleep, I feel frustrated because there is no way to control it… the hard thing is to accept that I have no control."
"Every time I get into a tug-of-war with insomnia I stop doing other things in my life."
"…how am I going to accept that we can't control what we feel?"

D. In a guided experiential exercise, the therapist invited Miguel to observe his thoughts, without judgments, working on cognitive defusion.

Client: "I really get stuck in these thoughts about my sleep… as if the total number of hours I have slept is going to determine my following day."
"Thinking about insomnia all the time makes me not notice other things in my life."

Weekly activity: Performing mindfulness exercises and taking note of thoughts in the thoughts notebook before going to the bedroom.

18.4 Fourth Session

Goals: Mindfulness exercise and strategies to address self as context and acceptance.

Therapist: "Hello Miguel, how are you?"
Client: "My sleep has still not improved, but I'm doing everything you asked."

"This week I went to the park, I had not been there for a long time… it was good, I even forgot that I slept badly."

Interventions

A. Another mindfulness exercise was conducted that Miguel should practice throughout the week.
B. Using metaphors, the difference between what is real discomfort versus what we avoid in order not to take the risk of experiencing discomfort (experiential avoidance) was explained.

Client: "The real discomfort is staying awake, but what I do to avoid taking that risk is lying in bed with my eyes closed, that does not help, right? Now I understand that it only gets worse because my head does not stop while I am lying down, forcing sleep to come."
"I avoid talking to people so I don't feel judged or charged, my interactions are only with my customers, but I do everything right so I don't have any problems."
"I don't even try to meet new women since I don't want to risk losing someone again."

C. An experiential exercise was conducted so that Miguel could perceive the sensation at the same moment, training to feel something without avoiding (acceptance).

Client: "It is very difficult to accept feeling the discomfort. I have to be perfect in what I do, there can be no mistakes, that is what I have learned my whole life…"
"It is as if I needed to change my way of dealing with life. I always pretended that I did not feel anything so I would not suffer anymore, now I understand that this only makes the situation worse."

D. Finally, in an exercise in which Miguel should report positive and negative experiences of his life, an attempt was made to address the process that involves the self as context, i.e., how he perceives himself throughout all that he has lived.

Client: "hum… I understand… you cannot live only the good things, there are bad things too… I wish I could control the bad part…"
"I have many good experiences with my wife, even though I lost her. It was better to have known her, even if she is gone."
"Looking back on my life, many things have happened, it seems like there is no way I can pigeonhole myself into a single characteristic or event."

Weekly activity: Performing mindfulness exercises, trying not to avoid a certain situation identified in the activity on experiential avoidance.

18.5 Fifth Session

Goals: Mindfulness exercise and strategies to address values.

Therapist: "Hello Miguel, how is everything?"
Client: "Wow, it was hard, but I did it… I called some friends from the past, we talked a little… it was uncomfortable but it was good."

Interventions

A. Another mindfulness exercise was conducted that Miguel should practice throughout the week.
B. The issue of how we escape different situations in our lives in order to avoid discomfort and, at the same time, fail to do/be in situations that could be important was resumed.
C. Next, Miguel's values were addressed by investigating how he wants to be and how he ideally wants to behave; thus, the aim was to guide him toward what he really wants to be and not to what he avoids. For this purpose, an exercise was conducted in which the client needed to identify areas of life that are important and describe who he wants to be in each of these areas.

Client: "…wow, I had never done this kind of reflection… how hard it is to look at all of this."
"…it seems that I am discovering myself, understanding what is of value to me. I feel that I am very far from what I understand is of value to me."
"Affective relationships, health, religiosity, work, friends, leisure… all these areas are important to me. I want to be a better person in each of them… there is a lot I need to do to be closer to the direction that makes sense to me."

D. After the definition of values, the therapist explains that plans for moving toward value-based actions will be developed in the next session.

Weekly activity: Performing mindfulness exercises.

18.6 Sixth Session

Goals: Mindfulness exercise and strategies to develop values-based actions.

Therapist: "Hello Miguel, how are you?"
Client: "This week I went out with some friends, it was good…"

"I did not sleep well for a few nights, but I started thinking about the possibility of taking a trip with these friends, I think it might be good, right?"

Interventions

A. Another mindfulness exercise was conducted that Miguel should practice throughout the week.
B. Based on a story, the therapist discussed that values-based actions can involve unpleasant events, which generate discomfort. This point is clarified so that the client is aware that acting toward his own values will involve being willing to eventually feel some discomfort.

Client: "It seems like the opposite of what I have done for a long time… I avoided feeling the discomfort even if it brought my life to a standstill, but that did not matter, I had my wife, right?"

C. "Action plans" were drawn up for each of the values identified by the client in the previous session, describing (1) the values, (2) the goals that this value entails, (3) the barriers to achieving these goals, and (4) which behaviors are needed to achieve these goals despite the barriers.

Client: "Wow, I never imagined that my actions were aimless because my values were not clear to me."
"I think the main barrier to my goals is my head, I put up barriers to things so I do not risk getting hurt."

Weekly activity: Performing mindfulness exercises. The second activity is to define, based on his values, at least one goal and one short-term action to achieve it.

18.7 Seventh Session

Goals: Mindfulness exercise, resuming values and values-based actions, and termination of therapy.

Therapist: "Hello Miguel, how are you?"
Client: "I am going to travel with those friends, we are going at the end of the year."

"I am thinking about taking acting classes, I think that I need to loosen up… I realize that I have been very rigid my whole life."

Interventions

A. Reinforcing the values addressed in the last sessions through an experiential exercise regarding the legacy the client would like to leave behind when he dies.

Client: "I would like people to remember that I was a good, easygoing, cheerful person… but I think that if I died today, people would still see me differently… I am sure I want to change, get closer to my values."

B. In one more exercise, the therapist returns to the idea that we need to learn to identify feelings and not to reject them. The therapist tells a story and invites Miguel to make some reflections.

Therapist: "Would it not be better to become 'friend of our discomforts'? Understand them? Know how to deal with them?"
Client: "Now I understand that yes… now I understand that my rigidity is a way of protecting myself, but that is what I am able to do, maybe it will take time to get better."

C. A final mindfulness exercise focused on values and committed actions was conducted to terminate the session.
D. The therapist ended the session with the following question:

Therapist: "What did this experience change?"
Client: "I have been able to sleep better, I go to bed when I am sleepy… I think my life seems more fulfilled, that must have helped with sleep, right?"

"I feel that a lot of things in my head changed with this therapy, I understood how I was functioning and how this brought my life to a standstill."

Table 18.4 Objective data obtained by applying the instruments at the end of the intervention

Instrument	Score
ISI	5
PSQI	8
AAQ	12

Table 18.5 Description of the sleep parameters evaluated by the sleep diary after the therapy sessions

Parameter	Time/frequency
Sleep onset latency	15 min
Frequency of nighttime awakenings	2
Time awake after sleep onset	16 min
Total sleep time	6 h 20 min
Total time in bed	6 h 48 min
Sleep efficiency	95%

Table 18.4 shows the scores of the instruments applied in the last session. The data of the sleep diary for the week preceding the last session are presented in Table 18.5.

Weekly activity: Continuation of homework activities that were suggested along the therapy sessions.

18.8 Conclusion

As described in this chapter, Miguel exhibited a pattern of psychological inflexibility that not only contributed to the persistence of difficulties in initiating and maintaining sleep but also to the way he related to the psychological discomfort, i.e., fusing with rules and self-rules, perceiving himself in a poorly contextual way, and looking to the past or the future, without perspective of values.

Based on the case formulation, some exercises of the protocol for the treatment of insomnia described in this book were selected. The ACT-based intervention for insomnia helped Miguel relate differently to the sleeping difficulties, which resulted in lower physiological activation, greater acceptance of his difficulties, less fusion with rules and self-rules, and better understanding of his values and, therefore, of values-based actions. Despite the observed gains, the client will certainly benefit from continuation of the sessions; he was therefore referred to individualized ACT-based therapy.

Chapter 19
Case Example: Application of ACT-BBI-I in an Individual Intervention

Renatha El Rafihi-Ferreira and Ila Marques Porto Linares

Here we describe a case[1] to which the ACT protocol for insomnia was applied in combination with behavioral techniques of stimulus control and sleep restriction. This type of intervention is called Acceptance and Commitment Therapy-based Behavioral Intervention for Insomnia (ACT-BBI-I). Despite the need for further studies, ACT-BBI-I seems to meet the established criteria for an effective treatment and has been recognized as a promising therapy (Chapoutot et al., 2021; El Rafihi-Ferreira et al., 2020).

The client sought psychological treatment for complaints of insomnia and hypnotic dependence. The therapeutic process comprised an initial meeting for complaint assessment and case formulation and nine sessions of ACT-BBI-I.

19.1 First Session

The first session consisted of a thorough assessment of the main complaint, its history, daytime symptoms, and data on behaviors that interfere with sleep, including sleep routine and sleep habits. Information about the client's life history was also collected. Next, the client answered questionnaires used to assess sleep and

[1] The cases reported in this book signed the free informed consent form since they are part of a research project on ACT for insomnia.

R. El Rafihi-Ferreira (✉)
Department of Clinical Psychology, University of São Paulo, Sao Paulo, Brazil
e-mail: rerafihi@usp.br

I. M. P. Linares
Faculty of Medicine at the University of São Paulo, Sao Paulo, Brazil

R. El Rafihi-Ferreira (ed.), *Acceptance and Commitment Therapy for Insomnia*,
https://doi.org/10.1007/978-3-031-50710-6_19

psychological variables. At the end of the session, the therapist provided instructions about the use of the sleep diary. The diary was used for 14 days as baseline and throughout therapy.

Client: Marta (fictious name), female, 31 years old, single, a lawyer who studied for the exam for a career as a judge. She lived alone in an apartment in the city of São Paulo, Brazil.

Main Complaint: Difficulty falling asleep, night awakenings, hypnotic dependence.

> I am having problems falling asleep since my relationship ended 2 years ago. During this period, I started taking sleep medication (Z-drug) and since then I have not been able to sleep without the medication. The doses of the drug increased gradually, and even with the medication I wake up at night. My concern is that insomnia may affect my preparation for the exam for a career as a judge.

Daytime Symptoms: Marta reported that she feels fatigued when she wakes up and has difficulty concentrating. She was worried that fatigue will disrupt her daily study routine and afraid of failing the exam because of sleep and fatigue.

History of the Complaint

Past history: Marta did not have sleep problems in childhood. As a teenager, she had an episode of insomnia, in which she stayed up all night and performed poorly in school tests that occurred the next day.

Current history: The complaint of difficulty falling asleep started 2 years ago after the end of a relationship. Nicolas, her ex-boyfriend, ended the relationship. Marta then started complaining about difficulty falling asleep every night of the week for 3 months. She thus sought a general practitioner who prescribed zolpidem (5 mg). Marta continued to use this dosage for a while, which was then increased to 20 mg. In the first year of medication use, the only complaint was initial insomnia. After 1 year, she started to have frequent nocturnal awakenings even with the medication. Marta dreamt of becoming a judge and had been maintaining a daily study routine of 8 hours. However, due to fatigue, Marta started to increase her coffee consumption during the day in order to be able to study. She reported drinking eight cups of coffee a day. At night, she felt agitated and drank wine to relax and help her fall asleep.

Data on Behaviors That Interfere with Sleep

Sleep Environment

Marta lived in a one-bedroom apartment with a bathroom, living room, and kitchen. The bedroom comprised a bed, a study table, and a chair. The bed and pillow were comfortable and well maintained. The window had blackout curtains that kept the room dark at night. The street where Marta lived was quite noisy; even with the windows closed the environment was noisy, especially in the morning.

Eating Habits and Substance Use

Morning: When she woke up before 12.00 h, her breakfast included coffee, fruits, and eggs.

Afternoon: The lunch generally included rice, beans, and a protein source (beef, chicken, or fish). In the afternoon, Marta consumed chocolate, candies, and coffee.

Night: She generally ordered food by app. At least once a week, she had Japanese food (sushi and sashimi), pizza, hamburger, and hot dog for dinner.

Daytime Routine

Marta proposed to study for 8 hours every day; however, there were no fixed times for this activity. She usually started studying in her bed. When she studied at the table, she felt tired, took the books, and went to bed to study. It was not uncommon for her to have an afternoon nap while she studied in bed. There were also no fixed times to go to bed and to wake up. She performed physical activity twice a week, at variable times, usually in the early evening.

Sleep Routine

Most days, Marta studied until 22.00 h. However, there were days that she studied until 02.00 in the morning. After studying, she ordered food and had dinner watching TV. After dinner, she showered and opened a bottle of wine. She went to bed and drank two to three glasses of wine in order to relax while engaging in social networks using her cell phone and chatting via WhatsApp. When waking up in the morning, she usually felt sleepy and therefore extended her time in bed for at least an hour.

Worries

Marta reported frequent fear of not passing the exam for a career as a judge and that she was afraid the insomnia would affect her academic performance. She blamed herself for not studying more due to the fatigue she felt because of her insomnia.

Data on Personal Life

Marta reported having a good family relationship. She always felt cared for and wanted by the family. However, she felt that the family is very demanding regarding the performance of the children. Marta's family worked in the legal area. Her parents were judges and her younger brother recently passed the exam for a career as a judge. Marta described her mother as vain and controlling.

Marta always did well in school and had no problems with her grades, except for one situation in adolescence when she could not sleep and performed poorly on her tests. On that occasion, a friend offered her a stimulant and she subsequently performed well on the tests. She used stimulants for a few weeks as a teenager.

Marta reported having poor pain tolerance. Whenever she felt any discomfort in her body, such as headache or menstrual cramps, she immediately took dipyrone, even when the pain was mild.

From 23 to 29 years of age, Marta has dated Nicolas. She identified her dating as a positive relationship, despite criticizing her ex-boyfriend's lack of ambition. She never imagined that Nicolas would end the relationship. With the end of the relationship, Marta started to have difficulties maintaining her study routine; even so,

Table 19.1 Results of the instruments applied in the first session

Assessment instrument	Score range	Patient score
Insomnia Severity Index	0–28	22
Epworth Sleepiness Scale	0–24	5
Dysfunctional Beliefs and Attitudes About Sleep Scale	0–160	100
Sleep Problem Acceptance Questionnaire	0–60	30
Hospital Anxiety Scale	0–21	7
Hospital Depression Scale	0–21	5
Acceptance and Action Questionnaire-II	0–49	26
Daily satisfaction score	0–10	3
Sleep diary	Insomnia patterns	Patient's patterns
Sleep onset latency	30 minutes or more	35
Wake after sleep onset	30 minutes or more	40
Total sleep time	6.5	6
Sleep efficiency	Less than 85%	70
Time in bed after waking up		60–120 minutes
Total bedtime		8.15
Time going to bed		00.00 02.00
Time getting out of bed		09.00 11.15 12.15

she enrolled in two exams in the legal area and failed in both. After the end of her relationship and the failed exams, her self-charge to study intensified, as did her thoughts of worthlessness and failure. Marta reported thoughts like "I'm not good enough," "I'm a failure," "I can't rest if I don't study hard enough," "If I don't sleep, I won't pass the test." Marta mentioned that, despite the negative thoughts, she dreams of meeting a new person to build a nice relationship and of having an interesting work environment. She also wants to be able to contribute to a fairer world for women. Such thoughts were prominent before sleep.

Table 19.1 summarizes the results of the instruments applied in the first session.

19.2 Case Formulation

The process of case formulation consists of the following main steps that are interconnected and complement each other:

- Step 1: Identification of behaviors that affect the client's sleep.
- Step 2: Identification of the processes of psychological inflexibility that are contributing to the maintenance of the sleep complaint.
- Step 3: Development of intervention strategies addressing (a) behaviors focused on sleep and (b) behaviors that go beyond the sleep complaint and are aimed at psychological flexibility.

Step 1: Identification of behaviors that affect sleep (see Table 19.2).

Step 2: Identification of the processes of psychological inflexibility that are contributing to the maintenance of the sleep complaint (see Table 19.3).

At this point, it is important that the professional first determines the events reported by the client in order to subsequently identify the relationships and processes of psychological inflexibility and flexibility. Figure 19.1 illustrates how inflexibility processes may contribute to the maintenance of the insomnia complaint.

Figure 19.1 shows the processes that maintain the insomnia complaint and the use of hypnotics. The single-headed arrows indicate a single direction between events, while the double-sided arrows indicate a reciprocal relationship between events. Marta seems to be significantly fused with the fear of what might happen if she does not sleep (cognitive fusion) and is very attentive to these fears instead of paying attention to other issues (inflexible attention to the now). In an attempt to get rid of insomnia, her actions seem to perpetuate the condition. This cycle of psychological inflexibility appears to be maintained by the short-term consequences produced by Marta's avoidance behaviors.

Step 3: Development of intervention strategies

In view of the considerations in Step 2, the goals of the sleep-focused intervention were (a) regularization of schedules; (b) self-care; (c) building a routine during

Table 19.2 Systematization of behaviors that affect sleep

Routine	Stimulus control	Cognition
Irregular sleeping and waking times Lack of regular study routines Little exercise Screen exposure before bed	Spending excessive time in bed and in the bedroom Different activities in bed (studying, drinking wine, using the cell phone, sleeping)	Thoughts of worthlessness and failure

Table 19.3 Identification and examples of processes of psychological inflexibility

Psychological inflexibility process	Events identified
Inflexible attention to the now	Worry and rumination about past failures and fears of the future (not passing the exam)
Conceptualized self	"I'm not good enough" "I'm a failure"
Experiential avoidance	Taking medication for discomfort such as not sleeping, feeling pain, failing tests, etc.
Cognitive fusion	"I can't rest if I don't study hard enough" "If I don't sleep, I won't pass the test"
Lack of values	Poorly clarified values
Inaction	Poorly established routine

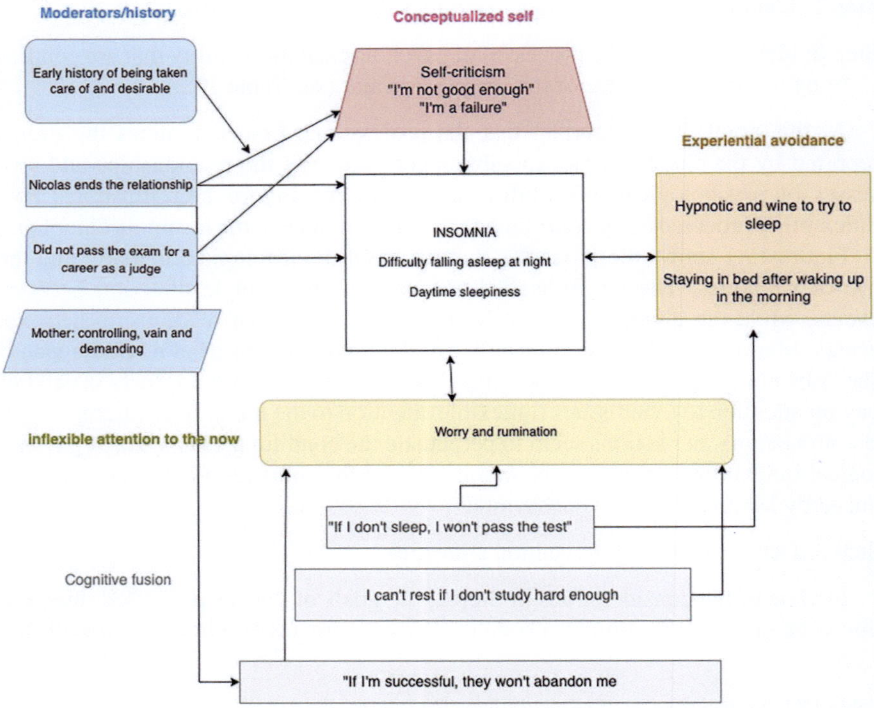

Fig. 19.1 Processes that maintain the insomnia complaint and use of hypnotics. (Source: Image from the archive of the authors)

the day; (d) using the bedroom only for sleeping and sexual activity; and (e) reduction of wake after sleep onset (WASO). The goals focusing on the development of psychological flexibility involved (1) decreasing the experiential avoidance pattern in response to the sleeping difficulties; (2) increasing contact with the present moment; and (3) taking perspective in response to events that occur and pre-sleep actions compatible with falling asleep.

The sleep-focused interventions planned for Marta are described in Table 19.4.

Figure 19.2 shows how the processes can be addressed in an attempt to develop psychological flexibility. The processes of accepting sensations and feelings of discomfort together with values-based behaviors can contribute to adhering to the behavioral components of sleep hygiene, stimulus control, and sleep restriction since some instructions of these techniques can cause discomfort. In addition, encouraging Marta to focus on the present moment could help her pay attention to what was actually happening and thus defuse her thoughts. Finally, helping the client to understand the context in which she experiences insomnia will promote an idea of self that is less content correlated and more contextual.

Table 19.4 Description of the interventions performed during each week of therapy

Weeks 1 and 2	
Regularization of schedules	Set the alarm clock at a fixed time to wake up: for example, 07.00 h
Self-care	Increase physical activity to at least four times a week, preferably in the morning
Routine	Morning: 30 minutes sunbathing Breakfast Physical activity Bath Start studying (2 hours) Afternoon: Lunch Studying (5 hours) with intervals Night: Recreational activity Dinner Relaxing activity Preparation to sleep
Stimulus control	Guidelines for using the bedroom and bed only for sleep and sex
Weeks 3–9	
Sleep restriction – week 3	01.00–07.00
Sleep restriction – week 4	00.40–07.00
Sleep restriction – week 5	00.20–07.00
Sleep restriction – week 6	00.00–07.00
Sleep restriction – week 7	23.40–07.00
Sleep restriction – week 8	23.40–07.00
Sleep restriction – week 9	23.40–07.00

19.3 Intervention Sessions

The ACT-I protocol described in this book was applied, dividing it into nine sessions. Regarding specific sleep components, psychoeducation, sleep hygiene, and stimulus control were applied in the first two sessions. Sleep restriction was started in the third week. All aspects related to psychological flexibility were addressed from sessions 3 to 9.

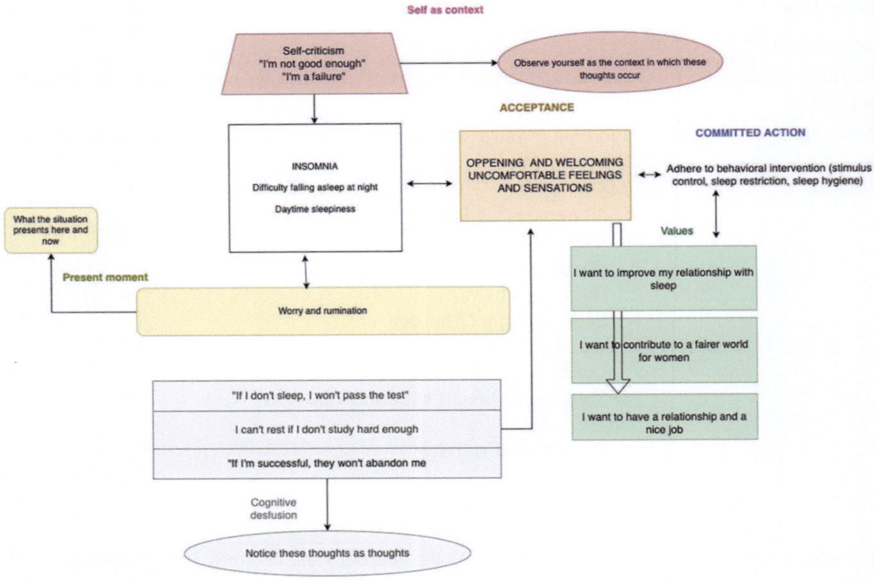

Fig. 19.2 How the psychological flexibility processes can be addressed. (Source: Image from the archive of the authors)

19.4 Assessment of Changes

Assessing the changes that occur during therapy is essential for understanding the course and outcomes of treatment. By week 7, Marta reported being satisfied and refreshed, sleeping a total of 7.20 hours. Thus, the sleep window was maintained until the end of the intervention. After application of the protocol, the questionnaires were applied again and the results are summarized in Table 19.5.

The graphs in Fig. 19.3 show Marta's sleep patterns over the course of the intervention.

After the final assessment, Marta reported being satisfied with the resolution of her sleep complaint and with the entire intervention process experienced. The case was thus closed.

Table 19.5 Results of the instruments applied after the last session

Assessment instrument	Score range	Patient score
Insomnia Severity Index	0–28	12
Epworth Sleepiness Scale	0–24	01
Dysfunctional Beliefs and Attitudes About Sleep Scale	0–160	16
Sleep Problem Acceptance Questionnaire	0–60	24
Hospital Anxiety Scale	0–21	6
Hospital Depression Scale	0–21	4
Acceptance and Action Questionnaire-II	0–49	12
Daily satisfaction score	0–10	8
Sleep diary	Insomnia patterns	Patient's patterns
Sleep onset latency	30 minutes or more	20
Wake after sleep onset	30 minutes or more	5
Total sleep time	6.5	7.20
Sleep efficiency	Less than 85%	90
Time in bed after waking up		5
Total bedtime		7.30
Time going to bed		23.40 00.40
Time getting out of bed		07.00 08.00

19.5 Conclusion

Behavioral aspects were addressed in the BBI-I interventions, while other aspects, particularly those related to psychological inflexibility, were treated using the ACT tools. Thus, ACT-BBI-I proved effective in treating the client's insomnia, reducing the so-called experiential avoidance behaviors, and promoting greater engagement in focusing on one's own values. Finally, it is worth mentioning that the establishment of a good therapeutic bond, as well as Marta's openness and engagement in the interventions, was preponderant for a good outcome.

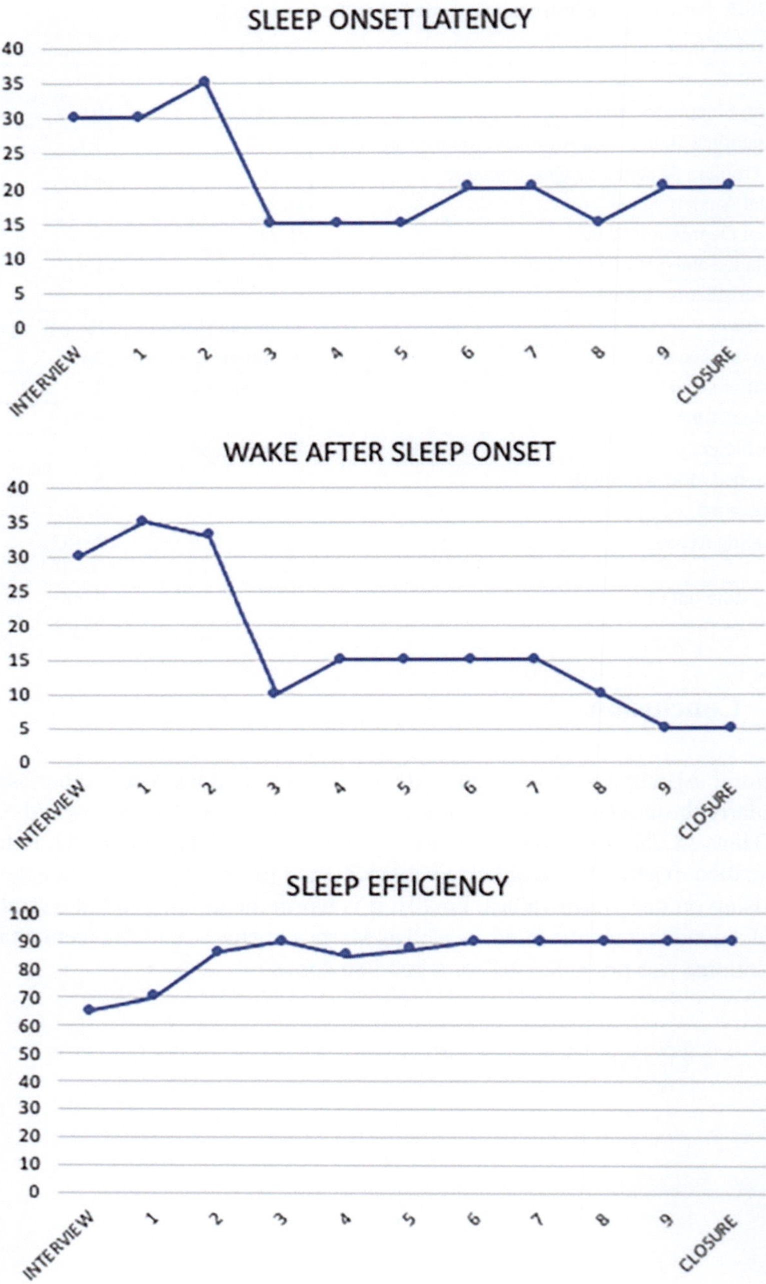

Fig. 19.3 Sleep patterns of the client before, during, and at the end of the intervention (sleep onset latency, wake after sleep onset, sleep efficiency, total sleep time, and satisfaction). (Source: Images from the archive of the authors)

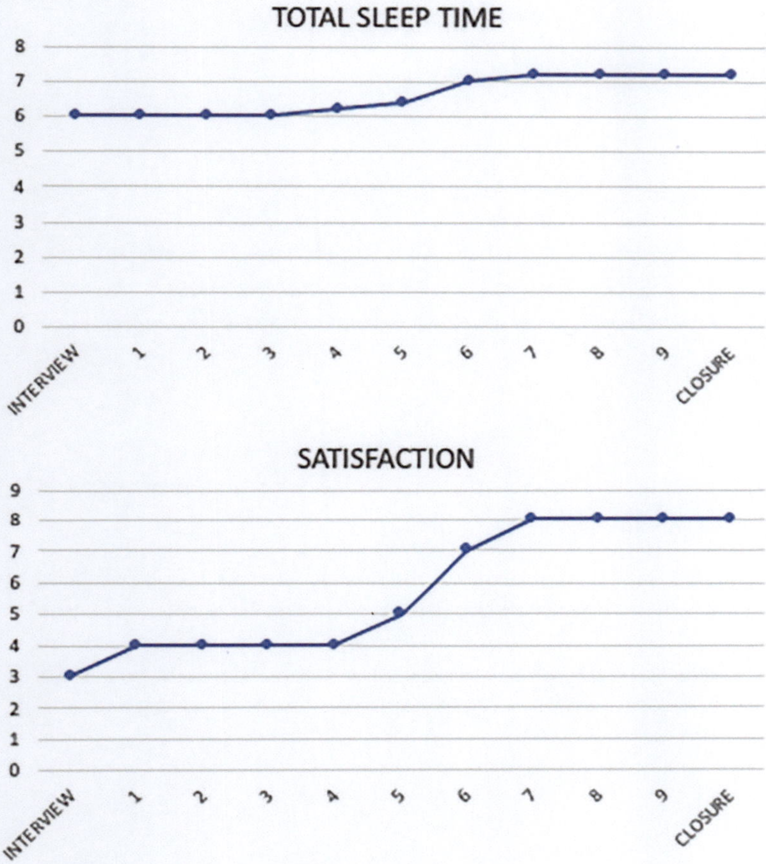

Fig. 19.3 (continued)

References

Chapoutot, M., Peter-Derex, L., Schoendorff, B., Faivre, T., Bastuji, H., & Putois, B. (2021). Telehealth-delivered CBT-I programme enhanced by acceptance and commitment therapy for insomnia and hypnotic dependence: A pilot randomized controlled trial. *Journal of Sleep Research, 30*(1), 6–10. https://doi.org/10.1111/jsr.13199

El Rafihi-Ferreira, R., Morin, C. M., Toscanini, A. C., Lotufo Neto, F., Brasil, I. S., Gallinaro, J. G., Borges, D. S., Conway, S. G., & Hasan, R. (2020). Acceptance and commitment therapy-based behavioral intervention for insomnia: A pilot randomized controlled trial. *Brazilian Journal of Psychiatry, 43*, 504–509. https://doi.org/10.1590/1516-4446-2020-0947

Index

R. El Rafihi-Ferreira (ed.), *Acceptance and Commitment Therapy for Insomnia*, https://doi.org/10.1007/978-3-031-50710-6

MIX
Papier aus verantwortungsvollen Quellen
Paper from responsible sources
FSC® C105338

If you have any concerns about our products,
you can contact us on
ProductSafety@springernature.com

In case Publisher is established outside the EU,
the EU authorized representative is:
Springer Nature Customer Service Center GmbH
Europaplatz 3, 69115 Heidelberg, Germany

Printed by Libri Plureos GmbH
in Hamburg, Germany